Blueprints

CLINICAL CASES
EMERGENCY MEDICINE

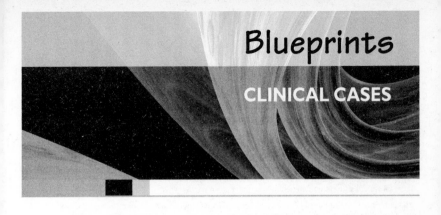

EMERGENCY MEDICINE

Christine Tsien Silvers, MD, PHD

Attending Physician, Department of Emergency Medicine
Caritas Good Samaritan Medical Center, Brockton, Massachusetts
Jordan Hospital, Plymouth, Massachusetts
Massachusetts General Hospital, Boston, Massachusetts
Research Affiliate, Children's Hospital Informatics Program,
Boston, Massachusetts

Michael R. Filbin, MD

Attending Physician, Department of Emergency Medicine
Massachusetts General Hospital, Boston, Massachusetts
Clinical Instructor, Harvard Medical School
Boston, Massachusetts

Aaron B. Caughey, MD, MPP, MPH, PHD (Series Editor)

Assistant Professor, Division of Maternal-Fetal Medicine
Department of Obstetrics & Gynecology
University of California, San Francisco
San Francisco, California

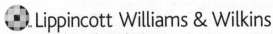 Lippincott Williams & Wilkins
a Wolters Kluwer business
Philadelphia · Baltimore · New York · London
Buenos Aires · Hong Kong · Sydney · Tokyo

Acquisitions Editor: Nancy Anastasi Duffy
Managing Editor: Stacy Sebring
Marketing Manager: Jennifer Kuklinski
Associate Production Manager: Kevin P. Johnson
Creative Director: Doug Smock
Compositor: International Typesetting and Composition
Printer: R.R. Donnelley & Sons - Crawfordsville

Printed in the United States of America

First Edition, 2002
Second Edition, 2007

Library of Congress Cataloging-in-Publication Data

Silvers, Christine Tsien.
   Clinical cases in emergency medicine / Christine Tsien Silvers,
Michael R. Filbin.—2nd ed.
      p. ; cm. — (Blueprints)
   Rev. ed. of: Blueprints clinical cases in emergency medicine / Michael R. Filbin, Christine L. Tsien.
c2002.
   Includes index.
   ISBN-13: 978-1-4051-0497-5
   ISBN-10: 1-4051-0497-X
 1. Emergency medicine.   2. Emergency medicine—Examinations, questions, etc.   I. Filbin,
Michael R.   II. Filbin, Michael R. Blueprints clinical cases in emergency medicine.   III. Title.
IV. Series.
   [DNLM: 1. Emergencies—Case Reports.   2. Emergencies—Examination Questions.
3. Emergency Medicine—Case Reports.   4. Emergency Medicine—Examination Questions.
WB 18.2 S587c 2007]

RC86.9.F554 2007
616.02'5076—dc22

                                                                            2006017089

The publishers have made every effort to trace the copyright holders for borrowed material. If they have inadvertently overlooked any, they will be pleased to make the necessary arrangements at the first opportunity.

To purchase additional copies of this book, call our customer service department at **(800) 638-3030** or fax orders to **(301) 223-2320.** International customers should call **(301) 223-2300.**

Visit Lippincott Williams & Wilkins on the Internet: http://www.LWW.com. Lippincott Williams & Wilkins customer service representatives are available from 8:30 am to 6:00 pm, EST.

                                                                07 08 09 10
                                                    2 3 4 5 6 7 8 9 10

Notice: The indications and dosages of all drugs in this book have been recommended in the medical literature and conform to the practices of the general community. The medications described and treatment prescriptions suggested do not necessarily have specific approval by the Food and Drug Administration for use in the diseases and dosages for which they are recommended. The package insert for each drug should be consulted for use and dosage as approved by the FDA. Because standards for usage change, it is advisable to keep abreast of revised recommendations, particularly those concerning new drugs.

Dedication

I am grateful to my colleagues, mentors, and friends at the Massachusetts General Hospital, Brigham and Women's Hospital, and Harvard Affiliated Emergency Medicine Residency for helping me to grow over the past four years. I would like to thank Michael Filbin, Aaron Caughey, and Selene Steneck for their vital roles in the realization of this book. I am grateful to Hsien Chyang and Bernarda Tsien, Isabelle Tsien, Marian Silvers, Nathan Silvers, Gayle Sylvia, Sola Choi, and Robert Silvers, for all of their love and support with home life to enable my academic work to progress. I am indebted to my son, Daniel, whose life has given new depth to the meaning of the word "love," and whose daily endeavors bring balance into my life.

Chris

To Dick, Jean, and Kel . . . and of course Jim, Linda, Brent, and Mandy . . . not to forget Angela, Ann, Bud, Bernard, Alice, Dennis, Marge, Leslie, Gary, and Kathy . . . oh yeah, Sammy, James, Trent, Hess, Howard, Brendan, Chris, Cindy, Joern, Jose . . . and to all the rest of my family, friends, and colleagues.

Mike

Thank you to Mike and Chris for your outstanding work on this book, as well as all of the hardworking people at both Blackwell Publishing and LWW, in particular Selene Steneck. I would also like to acknowledge the support I receive from my division, my department, and my mentors, in particular Mary Norton and Gene Washington. Finally, I thank Susan and Aidan for their inspiration.

Aaron

We would like to express our appreciation for the attendings, residents, nurses, staff members, and patients at the Harvard teaching hospitals, without whom this book would not have been possible.

November 2005

Preface

Emergency medicine is a dynamic, young specialty that has undergone a tremendous amount of growth over the past decade. As hospitals become more crowded and health care dollars further stretched, patient evaluation and diagnosis is shifting from the inpatient to outpatient and emergency settings. Emergency physicians are expected to see a large number of patients whom they have never met before in an efficient yet thorough manner, immediately stabilize those who are critically ill, develop a differential diagnosis and diagnostic plan for each patient to exclude serious illness, develop and initiate a treatment plan, and decide the most appropriate disposition.

The diagnostic tools available to the emergency physician have increased in number and sophistication over recent years. In most large hospitals and tertiary care centers, emergency diagnostics include bedside ultrasound, echocardiography, CT and MRI, vascular angiography, nuclear imaging, and cardiac stress testing. In addition to interpreting the results of these tests, emergency physicians are called upon to guide appropriate management, whether it be an immediate operation for an acute abdomen, cardiac catheterization for an acute myocardial infarction, systemic thrombolysis for an acute stroke or pulmonary embolism, emergent thoracotomy for a gunshot wound to the chest, emergent delivery for a woman whose baby is crowning, timely repair of a complex laceration, or simply close follow-up for an infant with a fever.

Many think that these decisions are within the realms of the respective specialists, but the reality of medicine today is that these decisions rest largely upon the emergency physician because the specialty services are themselves overextended and not readily available. The emergency physician needs to know how to diagnose and treat urgent as well as ambulatory conditions related to every specialty, ranging from surgical, medical, and pediatric to gynecologic and obstetric, urologic, orthopedic, neurologic, psychiatric, and dermatologic conditions. In light of these many challenges, it is not surprising that the emergency department (ED) may appear a busy, chaotic, and intimidating environment for attending physicians, residents, medical students, and patients alike. And it is precisely for the reasons just mentioned that the emergency department is a gold mine for medical education. There is no other environment in which a medical student is exposed to such a wide variety of pathology, clinical decision making, and readily available diagnostic and treatment modalities.

The greatest teaching opportunity in the emergency department, however, is the patients. As physicians, we enjoy entering a patient's room without looking at their medical records, triage notes, or any other related information. In this way, we can develop our own unbiased clinical impression, differential diagnosis, and management plan without external influences. On the inpatient wards, medical students are often assigned to interview patients who have already been evaluated by several physicians, have had their diagnostic workups completed, have been informed of their condition, and have already received treatment. This is counterproductive to the development of the thought processes required to become a competent physician. In the emergency department, students are able to evaluate patients up front, develop their own management plan, and discuss the plan with the attending emergency physician who is always present.

At the institutions in which we work, there has been a dramatic increase in the number of medical students who rotate through the emergency department. The reason for this is twofold, we think. First, emergency medicine as an academic specialty has grown over the past decade, and almost every teaching hospital ED is staffed with emergency-trained physicians who are versed in the unique aspects of the specialty and who are enthusiastic about sharing their knowledge. Second, as medical schools have changed their curriculum from one that is fact-based to one that emphasizes clinical correlation, students have realized the value of the emergency department as a clinically relevant and high-yield learning environment.

There is not enough room here to elaborate on the philosophy of patient care in the emergency department and how our approach differs from the approach on the wards, in the operating room, or in the clinic. But there are a few points that we believe are important to understand when working in the emergency department. In contrast to other clinical settings, ED patients are not scheduled for their appointments at the convenience of the physician, appointments cannot be canceled, and there is no limit to how many critically ill patients can come through the door. Considering this, emergency physicians cannot see patients one by one in order of their arrival. The patients must be seen in *parallel*, effectively in rapid sequence; and the sickest patients must be identified, given priority, and treated immediately. This may seem intuitive, but this skill is the greatest challenge for young physicians and those new to the specialty of emergency medicine.

The approach to every emergency patient involves three major steps: stabilization, diagnosis and treatment, and disposition. Stabilization refers to immediate airway management and circulatory support, popularly known as "the ABCs," for airway, breathing, and circulation. This can be as simple as walking into a patient's room and asking, "How are you?" If the patient responds appropriately, is able to string words together in an intelligent sentence, looks relatively stable, and has stable vital signs, then this first step is complete. Alternatively, stabilization can involve intubating the patient who is inadequately oxygenating or who is not protecting his or her airway, doing a cricothyrotomy for a patient in respiratory arrest from upper airway obstruction, placing a chest tube in a patient with a tension pneumothorax, defibrillating an unconscious patient in ventricular tachycardia, or placing a central line and administering fluids to a patient in hypovolemic shock.

Disposition refers to the ultimate destination of the patient when he or she leaves the emergency department; although this is the third step in the approach to the patient, it must be anticipated early in each patient's management. It is essential to determine early, often immediately after completing the history and physical, whether a patient will be able to go home or will require hospitalization. This early decision allows you to tailor your workup and to make arrangements for either discharge or admission. It is not acceptable to "sit" on patients for more than several hours, with the hope that they will improve and be able to go home. This results in poor resource utilization (e.g., space, nursing and physician staff) and suboptimal care for others in the emergency department and waiting room who may be sicker.

Finally, diagnosis and treatment is everything in between stabilization and disposition. This is the aspect of patient care that is emphasized during medical school and is what we are tested on in board exams. Likewise, diagnostics and therapeutics will be covered extensively in this book as they pertain to the emergency department.

The case-based format of this book is meant to emphasize clinical relevance and the three-pronged approach to the ED patient. Cases are presented with a history and physical similar to what would be obtained in the emergency department; in fact, nearly all of these cases present actual patients seen by the authors. The "Thought Questions" section includes several fundamental questions that a student should consider after walking out of the room in an attempt to synthesize the information obtained in the history

and physical. The "Immediate Actions" section, which is equivalent to stabilization, describes interventions that should be undertaken and tests that should be ordered immediately after obtaining
the history and physical. The "Discussion" section elaborates on
the clinical thought process and differential diagnosis that should
be formulated for each particular presentation. The "Case Continued"
section presents relevant test results and discusses the patient's
ultimate diagnosis and response to therapy. In addition, this
section discusses appropriate disposition pertaining to the patient
in question. Each chapter ends with four multiple-choice questions
in board format; these are intended to expand upon the knowledge
presented in the chapter and not simply regurgitate the information
already presented. Detailed answer explanations are provided after
each set of questions. In addition to the 60 case-based chapters in
the above-described format, we have included a separate section
for practicing questions at the end of the book, providing an additional 100 board-style, multiple-choice items. Some of these questions
are aimed at testing or expanding further upon knowledge presented
within the book, while others introduce new material in the field of
emergency medicine that could not be covered within the scope of
the 60 case-based chapters. Finally, a list of suggestions for journal
articles from the current literature is provided for the student who
wishes to pursue particular topics in greater detail. We believe the
format of this book to be ideal for understanding the nature of emergency medicine as well as for studying for the boards. We hope you
will enjoy "meeting" these patients and learning about how to take
care of them.

> Christine Tsien Silvers
> Michael Filbin
> Aaron Caughey

Acknowledgments

The authors would like to thank the reviewers, Tejal Patel (University at Buffalo), Anthony Wong MS IV (University of Arizona), and Jaime Massucci (Drexel University College of Medicine) for their useful comments and suggestions on the first edition of this book.

Contents

Preface   vii

Acknowledgments   xi

Abbreviations/Acronyms   xvii

I   Patients Presenting with Traumatic Injuries or Orthopedic Complaints   1

CASE **1**   Blow to the Head   3

CASE **2**   Abdominal Pain after Motor Vehicle Accident   11

CASE **3**   Gunshot Wound   17

CASE **4**   Pelvic Pain after Motorcycle Collision   25

CASE **5**   Stab Wound to the Neck   32

CASE **6**   Crush Injury to the Leg   39

CASE **7**   Burn   46

CASE **8**   Dog Bite   53

CASE **9**   Fall on an Outstretched Hand   58

CASE **10**   Shoulder Pain   65

CASE **11**   Knee Pain and Fever   71

CASE **12**   Hip and Sternum Pain in a Sickle-Cell Patient   77

II   Patients Presenting with Altered Mental Status and Neurologic or Psychiatric Complaints   85

CASE **13**   Acute Mental Status Change and Headache   87

CASE **14**   Acute Mental Status Change and Fever   94

CASE **15**   Weakness and Malaise   100

CASE **16**   Confusion and Hot Skin in an Elderly Man   107

CASE **17**   Homeless Alcoholic Found Unresponsive and Cold   113

CASE **18**   Fever, Confusion, and Seizure in a Prisoner   120

CASE **19**   Young Woman Found Down   126

CASE 20 Gas Bomb in the Hospital Lobby 134
CASE 21 Shaking Convulsions 141
CASE 22 Left-Sided Paralysis 148
CASE 23 Dizziness 155
CASE 24 Suicide Attempt 160

III Patients Presenting with Cardiopulmonary Complaints 167
CASE 25 Crushing Chest Pain 169
CASE 26 Tearing Chest and Back Pain 176
CASE 27 Syncope 182
CASE 28 Palpitations and Lightheadedness 188
CASE 29 Sudden Collapse in a Dialysis Patient 196
CASE 30 Shortness of Breath and Fatigue 202
CASE 31 Shortness of Breath and Chest Pain 208
CASE 32 Chest Pain and Fever 213
CASE 33 Shortness of Breath and Wheezing 219
CASE 34 Difficulty Breathing after an Insect Sting 225

IV Patients Presenting with Eye, ENT, Upper Respiratory, or Febrile Illnesses 231
CASE 35 Acute Vision Loss 233
CASE 36 Red Eye 241
CASE 37 Nosebleed 247
CASE 38 Fever and Sore Throat 252
CASE 39 Fever and Back Pain 257
CASE 40 Rapidly Spreading Skin Redness 263
CASE 41 Painful Head and Neck Rash with a Fever 269
CASE 42 Fever in an Infant 276
CASE 43 Barking Cough in a Child 282
CASE 44 Dyspnea in a Child 290

**V Patients Presenting with Abdominal
or Gastrointestinal Complaints   295**

CASE **45** Abdominal Pain Followed by Unconsciousness   297

CASE **46** Lower Abdominal Pain   302

CASE **47** Right Upper Quadrant Abdominal Pain   308

CASE **48** Left Lower Quadrant Abdominal Pain   314

CASE **49** Diffuse Abdominal Pain with Nausea and Vomiting   321

CASE **50** Weakness and Vomiting   327

CASE **51** Episodic Irritability and Vomiting in an Infant   333

CASE **52** Vomiting Blood   341

CASE **53** Buttock Pain   347

**VI Patients Presenting with Genitourinary
or Gynecologic Complaints   353**

CASE **54** Scrotal Pain   355

CASE **55** Vaginal Spotting and Pelvic Pain in Pregnancy   361

CASE **56** Sexual Assault   367

CASE **57** Acute Lower Abdominal Pain in a Young Woman   373

CASE **58** Abdominal Pain and Vaginal Odor   380

CASE **59** Heavy Vaginal Bleeding   386

CASE **60** Left Flank Pain   393

Review Q&A   399

Index   473

Abbreviations/Acronyms

AAA	abdominal aortic aneurysm
ABC	airway, breathing, and circulation
Abd	abdomen
ABG	arterial blood gas
AC	acromioclavicular; activated charcoal
ACA	anterior cerebral artery
ACE	angiotensin-converting enzyme
ACh	acetylcholine
ACLS	advanced cardiovascular life support
ACS	acute coronary syndrome
ACTH	adrenocorticotropic hormone
AF	atrial fibrillation
AKA	alcoholic ketoacidosis
ALL	allergies
ALT	alanine transaminase
AMI	acute myocardial infarction
AMS	altered mental status
Ant	anterior
AP	action potential; anteroposterior
ARDS	adult/acute respiratory distress syndrome
ARF	acute rheumatic fever
ASA	acetylsalicylic acid; aspirin
AST	aspartate transaminase
AV	atrioventricular
AVM	arteriovenous malformation
AVNRT	AV nodal reentrant tachycardia
BAL	British anti-Lewisite (dimercaprol)
βhCG	β(beta) subunit of human chorionic gonadotropin
BID	twice a day [Latin *bis in die*]
BME	bimanual examination
BP	blood pressure
BPH	benign prostatic hypertrophy
bpm	beats per minute
BPV	benign positional vertigo
BSA	body surface area
BUN	blood urea nitrogen
C	Celsius
C_N	*N*th cervical vertebra
Ca	calcium

CABG	coronary artery bypass graft
CAD	coronary artery disease
cath	catheterization
CBC	complete blood count
CBD	common bile duct
cc	cubic centimeter(s)
CC	chief complaint
CCU	cardiac care unit; coronary care unit
chem 7	chemistries, electrolytes (Na, K, Cl, CO_2, BUN, Cr, Glu)
CHF	congestive heart failure
CK	creatine kinase
CK-MB	isoenzyme of creatine kinase with muscle and brain subunits
Cl	chloride
cm	centimeter(s)
cm H_2O	centimeters water
CMT	cervical motion tenderness
CMV	cytomegalovirus
CN	cranial nerve(s)
CNS	central nervous system
CO	cardiac output; carbon monoxide
CO_2	carbon dioxide; bicarbonate
coags	coagulation panel (i.e., PT and PTT)
Code	medical emergency
COHgb	carboxyhemoglobin
COPD	chronic obstructive pulmonary disease
cort stim	cosyntropin stimulation test
CPAP	continuous positive airway pressure
CPK	creatine phosphokinase
Cr	creatinine
CRAO	central retinal artery occlusion
CRH	corticotrophin-releasing hormone
CRP	C-reactive protein
CRVO	central retinal vein occlusion
CSF	cerebrospinal fluid
c-spine	cervical spine
CT	computed tomography
CV	cardiovascular
CVA	cerebrovascular accident; costovertebral angle
CVP	central venous pressure
CXR	chest x-ray
d	day(s)
D&C	dilation and curettage
D50	50% dextrose
D50W	50% dextrose in water
D5 ½ NS	5% dextrose in one-half normal saline
D5NS	5% dextrose in normal saline
D5W	5% dextrose in water
DAI	diffuse axonal injury

DevHx	developmental history
DIC	disseminated intravascular coagulation
diff	differential
DKA	diabetic ketoacidosis
dL	deciliter(s)
DM	diabetes mellitus
DMSA	dimercaptosuccinic acid
DNA	deoxynucleic acid
DP	dorsalis pedis
DPL	diagnostic peritoneal lavage
DT	pediatric diphtheria-tetanus immunization
DTs	delirium tremens
DUB	dysfunctional uterine bleeding
DUMBELS	diarrhea, urination, miosis, bronchospasm/bronchorrhea, emesis, lacrimation, salivation
DVT	deep venous thrombosis
EA	epiploic appendagitis
EBV	Epstein-Barr virus
ED	emergency department
EDH	epidural hematoma
EDTA	ethylene diamine tetra-acetic acid
EEE	eastern equine encephalitis
EEG	electroencephalogram
EF	ejection fraction
e.g.	for example [Latin *exempli gratia*]
EGDT	early goal-directed therapy
EKG	electrocardiogram
EMS	emergency medical services
ENT	ears, nose, and throat; otolaryngology
EOM	extraocular motion(s); extraocular movement(s); extraocular muscle(s)
EOMI	extraocular muscles intact
ERCP	endoscopic retrograde cholangiopancreatography
ERP	effective refractory period
ESR	erythrocyte sedimentation rate
ETT	endotracheal tube
Extr	extremities
F	Fahrenheit
Fab	fragment antigen binding
FAST	focused assessment with sonography for trauma
FENa	fractional excretion of sodium
FES	fat emboli syndrome
FFA	free fatty acid
FHx	family history
F_iO_2	fractional inspired oxygen
fL	femtoliter
FM	face mask
FSH	follicular stimulating hormone

g	gram(s)
G-6-PD	glucose-6-phosphate dehydrogenase
G_nP_n	pregnancy *number*, live birth *number* [Latin *gravida, para*]
GABA	γ-aminobutyric acid (gamma-aminobutyric acid)
GABHS	group A β-hemolytic streptococcus
GAS	group A streptococcus (*Streptococcus pyogenes*)
GBS	group B streptococcus
GC	gonococcus (*Neisseria gonorrhoeae*)
GCS	Glasgow Coma Scale
GERD	gastroesophageal reflux disease
GFR	glomerular filtration rate
GI	gastrointestinal
Glu	glucose
GnRH	gonadotropin releasing hormone
GU	genitourinary
Gyn	gynecology, gynecological
H_2O	water
HACE	high altitude cerebral edema
HAPE	high altitude pulmonary edema
HAV	hepatitis A virus
HBIG	hepatitis B immune globulin
HBV	hepatitis B virus
hCG	human chorionic gonadotropin
Hct	hematocrit
HCTZ	hydrochlorothiazide
HCV	hepatitis C virus
HDCV	human diploid cell vaccine
HEENT	head, eyes, ears, nose, and throat
HHNC	hyperglycemic hyperosmolar nonketotic coma
HIB	*Haemophilus influenzae* type b
HIDA	hepatic iminodiacetic acid
HIV	human immunodeficiency virus
h/o	history of
hpf	high power field
HPI	history of present illness
hr	hour(s)
HR	heart rate
HRIG	human rabies immune globuliln
HSV	herpes simplex virus
HTN	hypertension
I&D	incision and drainage
IBD	inflammatory bowel disease
IC	internal capsule
ICH	intracerebral hematoma
ICP	intracranial pressure
ICU	intensive care unit
IDA	iminodiacetic acid
IDDM	insulin-dependent diabetes mellitus

i.e.	that is [Latin *id est*]
IJ	internal jugular
IL-1	interleukin-1
IL-6	interleukin-6
IM	intramuscular; intramuscularly
IMA	inferior mesenteric artery
Imm	immunizations
inh	inhaler
INH	isoniazid
INR	international normalized ratio
IOP	intraocular pressure
IU	international unit
IUD	intrauterine device
IUP	intrauterine pregnancy
IV	intravenous; intravenous line; intravenously
IVC	inferior vena cava
IVP	intravenous pyelogram
J	Joule(s)
JRA	juvenile rheumatoid arthritis
JVD	jugular venous distention
JVP	jugular venous pressure
K	potassium
k	thousand
KCl	potassium chloride
kg	kilogram(s)
KUB	kidneys/ureters/bladder radiograph
L	left; liter
L_N	Nth lumbar vertebra
LAD	left anterior descending (coronary artery)
LBBB	left bundle branch block
LBO	large-bowel obstruction
LDH	lactate dehydrogenase
LF	luteinizing hormone
LFTs	liver function tests
LLQ	left lower quadrant
LMP	last menstrual period
LP	lumbar puncture
LUQ	left upper quadrant
Lymph	lymphatic; lymphatics
lymphs	lymphocytes
MAP	mean arterial pressure
MAT	multifocal atrial tachycardia
MCA	middle cerebral artery
MCP	metacarpophalangeal; metacarpal-phalangeal
MDI	metered-dose inhaler
Meds	medications
MEOS	microsomal ethanol-oxidizing system
mEq	milliequivalent(s)

Mg	magnesium
mg	milligram(s)
mg%	milligram percent
MI	myocardial infarction
MICU	medical intensive care unit
min	minute(s)
mIU	milli-international unit(s)
mL	milliliter(s)
mm	millimeter(s)
mm³	cubic millimeter(s)
mm Hg	millimeters mercury
mo	month(s)
mOsm	milliosmol(s)
MR	magnetic resonance
MRA	magnetic resonance angiography
MRI	magnetic resonance imaging
MRSA	methicillin-resistent *S. aureus*
ms	millisecond(s)
MSSA	methicillin-sensitive *S. aureus*
MUDPILES	methanol, uremia, diabetic ketoacidosis, paraldehyde, infection/intoxication (alcohol, iron, isoniazid), lactic acidosis, ethylene glycol, salicylates
μ	mu (Greek)
μg	microgram(s)
μL	microliter(s)
μm	micrometer(s)
MVA	motor vehicle accident
MVC	motor vehicle collision
MVI	multivitamin
Na	sodium
NAC	*N*-Acetylcysteine
NC	nasal cannula
NCT	narrow complex tachycardia
NEC	necrotizing enterocolitis
neg	negative
Neuro	neurologic exam
NG	nasogastric
NGT	nasogastric tube
NICU	neurosurgical intensive care unit; neonatal intensive care unit
NIDDM	non-insulin-dependent diabetes mellitus
NKDA	no known drug allergies
NPH	neutral protamine Hagedorn (insulin)
NPO	nothing by mouth [Latin *nil per os*]
NPPV	noninvasive positive pressure ventilation
NS	normal saline
NSAID	nonsteroidal anti-inflammatory drug
O+	O-positive (blood type)
O–	O-negative (blood type)

O_2	oxygen
OB	obstetrics
OB/GynHx	obstetrical and gynecological history
OCP	oral contraceptive pill
OD	right eye [Latin *oculus dexter*]
OG	orogastric
OR	operating room
ORIF	open reduction with internal fixation
OS	left eye [Latin *oculus sinister*]
OTC	over-the-counter
OU	both eyes [Latin *oculus unitas*]
PA	posteroanterior
PAC	premature atrial contraction(s)
$Paco_2$	partial pressure of carbon dioxide in arterial blood
Pao_2	partial pressure of oxygen in arterial blood
PCA	patient-controlled analgesia; posterior cerebral artery
PCI	percutaneous intervention
PCP	phencyclidine; *Pneumocystis carinii* pneumonia; primary care provider
PCr	plasma creatinine
PE	physical examination; pulmonary embolism
PEFR	peak expiratory flow rate
PERRL	pupils equal, round, and reactive to light
PERRLA	pupils equal, round, and reactive to light and accommodation
Phos	phosphate
PID	pelvic inflammatory disease
plt	platelet(s)
PMHx	past medical history
PMN	polymorphonuclear leukocyte(s)
PNa	plasma sodium
PO	by mouth [Latin *per os*]
PO_4	phosphate
POC	product(s) of conception
polys	polymorphonuclear leukocytes
PPA	parapharyngeal abscess
ppd	packs per day
PPD	purified protein derivative (tuberculin skin test)
PRBC	packed red blood cells
PRN	as needed [Latin *pro re nata*]
PSHx	past surgical history
PSVT	paroxysmal supraventricular tachycardia
PT	posterior tibial; prothrombin time
PTA	peritonsillar abscess
PTSD	post-traumatic stress disorder
PTT	partial thromboplastin time
PTU	propylthiouracil
PUD	peptic ulcer disease
P_vCO_2	partial pressure of carbon dioxide in venous blood

P_vO_2	partial pressure of oxygen in venous blood
QN hr	once every N hour(s)
Q1–2 hr	once every one to two hours
Q15–30 min	once every 15 to 30 minutes
Q4–6 hr	once every four to six hours
QAM	once each morning [Latin *quaque ante meridiem*]
QD	once a day [Latin *quaque die*]
QHS	once a day at bedtime [Latin *quaque hora somni*]
QID	four times a day [Latin *quater in die*]
QOD	once every other day [Latin *quaque altera die*]
QPM	once each night [Latin *quaque post meridiem*]
QTc	corrected QT interval
R	right
RA	room air
RBBB	right bundle branch block
RBC	red blood cell(s)
RCA	right coronary artery
RLQ	right lower quadrant
RMSF	Rocky Mountain spotted fever
r/o	rule out
ROM	range of motion
RPA	retropharyngeal abscess
RPR	rapid plasma reagin
RR	respiratory rate
RRR	regular rate and rhythm
RSI	rapid sequence intubation; rapid sequence induction
RSV	respiratory syncytial virus
RUQ	right upper quadrant
RV	right ventricle; right ventricular
RVR	rapid ventricular rate
S_1	first heart sound
S_2	second heart sound
S_3	third heart sound
S_4	fourth heart sound
S_N	Nth sacral vertebra
SAB	spontaneous abortion
SAH	subarachnoid hemorrhage
Sao_2	oxygen saturation, arterial
SBI	serious bacterial infection
SBO	small-bowel obstruction
SBP	systolic blood pressure
SC	subcutaneous; subcutaneously
SCA	sickle cell anemia
SCFE	slipped capital femoral epiphysis
SDH	subdural hematoma
SEM	systolic ejection murmur
SGOT	serum glutamic-oxaloacetic transaminase (AST)
SHx	social history

SLE	systemic lupus erythematosus
SLUDGE	salivation, lacrimation, urination, diarrhea, GI cramping, emesis
SMA	superior mesenteric artery
SOB	short of breath, shortness of breath
s/p	event in past [Latin *status post*]
STAT	at once [Latin *statim*]
STD	sexually transmitted disease
STI	sexually transmitted infection
STEMI	ST-elevation myocardial infarction
strep	streptococcus (*Streptococcus pneumoniae*)
SV	stroke volume
SVG	saphenous vein graft
S_vO_2	oxygen saturation, central venous
SVT	supraventricular tachycardia
T_N	*N*th thoracic vertebra
tab	tablet(s)
TAB	therapeutic abortion
TCA	tricyclic antidepressant(s)
Td	adult tetanus-diphtheria immunization
TEE	transesophageal echocardiogram
temp	temperature
TIA	transient ischemic attack
TID	three times a day [Latin *ter in die*]
TM	tympanic membrane(s)
TNF	tissue necrosis factor
TnI	troponin I
TOA	tubo-ovarian abscess
TOC	tubo-ovarian complex
tox	toxic; toxicology; toxicologic
tPA	tissue plasminogen activator (alteplase)
TSH	thyroid-stimulating hormone
TSS	toxic shock syndrome
TURP	transurethral resection of prostate
TVS	transvaginal sonography; transvaginal sonogram
u, U	unit(s)
UA	urinalysis
UCr	urine creatinine
UNa	urine sodium
UPJ	ureteropelvic junction
URI	upper respiratory tract infection
US	ultrasound
UTI	urinary tract infection
UV	ultraviolet
UVJ	ureterovesicle junction
Vasc	vascular
VEE	Venezuelan equine encephalitis
VF	ventricular fibrillation
V/Q	ventilation-perfusion

VS	vital signs
VT	ventricular tachycardia
VZV	varicella-zoster virus
WASH	warm water, analgesic agents, stool softeners, high-fiber diet
WBC	white blood cell(s)
WCT	wide complex tachycardia
WEE	western equine encephalitis
WPW	Wolff-Parkinsom-White syndrome
yr	year(s)
2-PAM	pralidoxime chloride
3-D	three-dimensional
4-MP	4-methylpyrazole; fomepizole

I

Patients Presenting with Traumatic Injuries or Orthopedic Complaints

CASE **1**

Blow to the Head

CC: 33-year-old man with head trauma

HPI: H.T. is a 33-year-old man who was drinking heavily and got into a barroom fight, sustaining several blows to his head with a stool. He was knocked out for a couple of minutes but then woke up. He was taken to his sister's house, where he walked with assistance from the car into the house. Once inside, he developed nausea, vomited, and then fell face down onto the floor. Paramedics found him groggy, with equal and reactive pupils and an intact gag reflex; he was placed in a c-spine collar and secured to a backboard. The patient became totally unresponsive as he was wheeled into the ED.

PMHx: Unknown

Meds: Unknown

ALL: Unknown

SHx: Unknown

VS: Temp 38.1°C (100.6°F), HR 56, BP 188/98, RR 8, Sao$_2$ 98% on 15 liters O$_2$ by face mask

PE: *General:* No open head wounds or severe facial contusions. *Airway:* Oropharynx patent; trachea midline. *Breathing:* Lungs clear bilaterally; deep sonorous breathing. *Circulation:* Heart sounds regular; good radial pulses. *Rapid neuro assessment:* Unresponsive to voice; R pupil 3 mm reactive, L pupil 5 mm fixed; corneal reflexes decreased; decreased gag response; extension posturing to pain; GCS 4.

THOUGHT QUESTIONS

- What are the immediate actions for this patient?
- What are the different types of intracranial injuries?

■ Which noninvasive interventions can be done to lower intracranial pressure?

■ Which patients with head injury need to be taken to the OR immediately?

Immediate Actions:
Place on 15 liters O_2 by nonrebreather mask; place on cardiac monitor; establish large-bore IVs; administer lidocaine 100 mg IV, etomidate 20 mg IV, and succinylcholine 120 mg IV; intubate using laryngoscope and 7.5 ETT; establish mechanical ventilation; perform secondary survey; place Foley; prop head of bed to 30 degrees; order CBC, chem 7, tox screen, PT/PTT, type and hold, urinalysis; administer mannitol 70 g over first 30 minutes; obtain STAT head and c-spine CT; notify neurosurgery.

Discussion:
Head injury severity is assessed based on the mechanism of injury and the initial neurologic exam. A GCS of 8 or less, or any evidence of intracranial hemorrhage, is considered severe head injury. Types of intracranial hemorrhage include parenchymal contusions (small areas of peripheral gray matter bruising), intracerebral hematomas (ICH, larger hemorrhage deep within brain tissue caused by sheared arterioles), subarachnoid hemorrhage (SAH, blood within the CSF space—see Figure 1-1), subdural hematomas (SDH, bleeding between the dura and the subarachnoid space creating a crescent-shaped hematoma—see Figure 1-2), and epidural hematomas (EDH, bleeding between the cranium and dura creating a lenticular-shaped hematoma—see Figure 1-3).

(*Continued*)

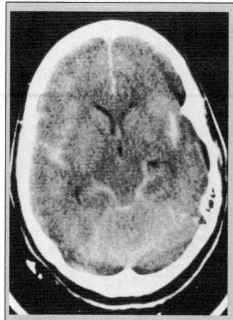

FIGURE 1-1
Noncontrast head CT shows diffuse subarachnoid hemorrhage. (*Image reprinted with permission from Harwood-Nuss A, Wolfson AB, et al. The Clinical Practice of Emergency Medicine, 3rd Ed. Philadelphia: Lippincott Williams & Wilkins, 2001.*)

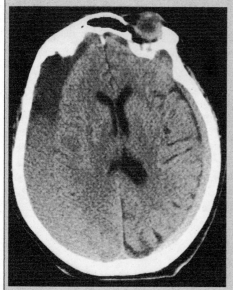

FIGURE 1-2
Noncontrast head CT shows bilateral, subacute subdural (crescent-shaped) hematomas, with varying densities and layering. (*Image reprinted with permission from Harwood-Nuss A, Wolfson AB, et al. The Clinical Practice of Emergency Medicine, 3rd Edition, Philadelphia: Lippincott Williams & Wilkins, 2001.*)

(Continued)

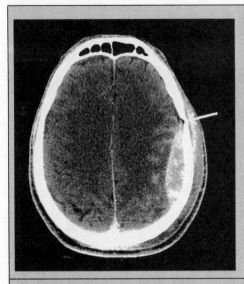

FIGURE 1-3
Noncontrast head CT shows a large epidural hematoma (lenticular-shaped hyperdensity) at the site of a temporoparietal bone fracture (arrow). (*Image courtesy of Massachusetts General Hospital, Boston.*)

The cranium is a closed space that does not allow expansion of injured, edematous brain tissue or enlarging hematomas. Rising ICP decreases cerebral perfusion and results in neuronal ischemia and death. Conservative measures for decreasing ICP include raising the head of the bed, inducing temporary hyperventilation (hypocarbia will promote cerebral vasoconstriction and thus decrease ICP), and administering mannitol (an osmotic agent that draws intracerebral edema into the vascular space).

Whether the patient needs an immediate operation depends on the CT findings and the neurologic exam. Large collections of extra-axial blood (e.g., epidural or subdural hemorrhages) should be evacuated in the OR regardless of the neurologic exam. There is controversy regarding management for a patient with a GCS of 8 or less and no large collection of extra-axial blood. There is no evidence that a craniotomy simply to relieve increased ICP results in a better outcome for these patients.

CASE CONTINUED

The secondary survey is unremarkable aside from a large scalp hematoma on the left side. The head CT reveals a left temporoparietal epidural hematoma (EDH) with an overlying temporal bone fracture (Fig. 1-3). The patient is taken directly from CT scan to the OR for a craniotomy, evacuation of the EDH, and placement of an ICP monitor. Intraoperatively, the ruptured left middle meningeal artery is identified and ligated. The patient is transferred to the ICU, where he recovers neurologic function but with permanent cognitive deficits.

QUESTIONS

1-1. A 19-year-old man is involved in a rollover motor vehicle collision. He had not been wearing a seatbelt, and is found 10 feet from his car, responsive to voice but confused. After transport from the scene to the ED, he undergoes a primary survey followed by a rapid head-to-toe assessment. He remains confused, although he answers some questions. His pupils are equal, round, and reactive. He is hemodynamically stable and goes to the CT scanner. What is the most likely finding this patient will have on his head CT?

    A. Epidural hematoma
    B. Intracerebral hematoma
    C. Subarachnoid hemorrhage
    D. Subdural hematoma
    E. Diffuse axonal injury

1-2. A male patient gets assaulted with a bat and is knocked unconscious. Within a few minutes, he wakes up and seems appropriate. Twenty minutes later, however, he seems more and more confused, and then becomes unresponsive again. Clinically, he appears to have a temporoparietal skull fracture. All other factors being equal, which age group is most likely to develop this type of head injury?

    A. Infants
    B. Children
    C. Adults, excluding elderly persons
    D. Elderly persons
    E. Prevalence is the same throughout age groups

1-3. Paramedics arrive at an alley where a 25-year-old man is unconscious with an obvious right-sided scalp wound. During transport to the ED, he opens his eyes and asks what happened. Head CT in the ED shows a small amount of extra-axial blood on the right side. While awaiting a neurosurgery consult, the patient complains of severe headache, vomits several times, and becomes unarousable. What is the most appropriate next step?

A. Obtain repeat head CT
B. Re-page the neurosurgeon
C. Obtain abdominal CT
D. Administer IV antiemetic and place NG tube to empty the stomach
E. Intubate

1-4. An 88-year-old woman with mild dementia slips on ice and hits her head on the ground. Her head CT scan shows a small crescent-shaped hyperdensity on the left side. What is the most likely source of this CT finding?

A. Left middle meningeal artery
B. Subarachnoid vessels
C. Veins bridging from dura to brain surface
D. Chronic age-related small vessel disease
E. Shearing of white matter neurons

ANSWERS

1-1. C. In the setting of severe head trauma, subarachnoid hemorrhage is the most common CT finding, present in approximately 44% of patients. SAHs are due to bleeding from subarachnoid vessels into the CSF space. On noncontrast CT scan, blood (increased density) may be seen in the interhemispheric fissures, sulci, and basilar cisterns in SAH. Subdural hematomas occur in as many as 30% of severe head injury patients. SDHs are due to bridging veins bleeding into the potential space between the dura and arachnoid layers of the meninges; SDHs appear as high-density crescent shapes adjacent to the cranium on CT scan. Intracerebral hematomas occur in approximately 12% of patients with severe head injury, seen within the deep brain parenchyma as increased-density regions on CT scan. Epidural hematomas are the least common intracranial injury, present in only about 0.5% of patients with severe head trauma. EDHs appear as high-density lenticular or biconvex collections adjacent to the cranium on CT scan. Diffuse axonal injury is very commonly associated with severe head injury. Forces imparted during the injury result in shearing of the white matter neurons, resulting in edema, increased ICP, and coma. This condition, however, has no specific associated CT findings.

1-2. C. The patient described sustains a blow to the head, causing unconsciousness followed by a "lucid interval," and then becomes unconscious again, as is classically seen in epidural hematomas. Nonelderly adults are most likely to have epidural hematomas following severe head trauma. Elderly persons as well as children are less likely to get EDHs because in both groups, the dura is adhered firmly to the skull. Children's skulls also have more elasticity, allowing the skull to tolerate a severe blow to the head with less likelihood of breaking. The majority of EDHs are associated with temporoparietal skull fractures that rupture the middle meningeal artery, in turn leading to dissection of high-pressure arterial blood between the dura and skull.

1-3. E. Sleepiness, nausea, and severe headache are common symptoms of EDHs. Other symptoms include vomiting and dizziness. Classically, patients with EDHs are described as having a decreased level of consciousness following their initial head trauma, then a "lucid interval," during which full consciousness is recovered. An EDH typically gets bigger because of its arterial source, and eventually the patient will deteriorate. The initial CT scan may be normal or show a small amount of extra-axial blood, indistinguishable from a subdural hematoma. However, as the patient's mental status deteriorates, a repeat STAT head CT will show the accumulation of epidural blood. These patients require immediate operative evacuation. **The immediate next step when a patient is vomiting and becomes unarousable, though, is to protect the airway.**

1-4. C. This patient has a CT finding consistent with a subdural hematoma (SDH). SDHs occur most frequently in elderly persons as well as alcoholics, both groups associated with brain atrophy. An atrophic brain causes stretching of the bridging vessels that traverse from the dura, which is attached to the cranium, across the subdural space to the surface of the brain. Lower mechanisms of injury, such as falls, may tear these bridging vessels and result in a subdural hematoma. Choice A is for an epidural hematoma. Choice B is for a subarachnoid hemorrhage. Choice E is for diffuse axonal injury.

SUGGESTED ADDITIONAL READINGS

Jagoda AS, Cantrill SV, Wears RL, et al. Clinical policy: neuroimaging and decision-making in adult mild traumatic brain injury in the acute setting. Ann Emerg Med 2002;40:231–249.

Nolan S. Traumatic brain injury: a review. Crit Care Nurs Q 2005;28:188–194.

Nortje J, Menon DK. Traumatic brain injury: physiology, mechanisms, and outcome. Curr Opin Neurol 2004;17:711–718.

Vincent JL, Berre J. Primer on medical management of severe brain injury. Crit Care Med 2005;33:1392–1399.

CASE 2

Abdominal Pain after Motor Vehicle Accident

 CC: 17-year-old woman in high-speed MVA

HPI: B.T. is a 17-year-old woman who was the shoulder-belt-restrained driver in an MVA at 70 mph. Her car was apparently cut off by another driver; she lost control of the car, which then rolled down an embankment and struck a tree. There was a large amount of front-end damage to the car, but no driver's door intrusion or steering wheel deformity. She did not lose consciousness. EMS finds her alert and oriented in the front seat. She is extricated, and then placed on a backboard in a cervical collar. Her vitals at the scene are HR 122 and BP 108/50. She complains of abdominal pain and left arm pain.

PMHx: None

Meds: None

ALL: NKDA

FHx: Noncontributory

SHx: Denies tobacco, alcohol, and drugs

VS: Temp 36.5°C (97.7°F), HR 107, BP 101/44, RR 28, Sao$_2$ 99% on 15 liters O$_2$ by face mask

PE: *Airway:* Patient alert; oropharynx patent; trachea midline. *Breathing:* Lungs clear bilaterally; no crepitus. *Circulation:* Well-perfused with 2+ radial and femoral pulses.

THOUGHT QUESTIONS

- What are the immediate actions for this patient?
- What is the differential diagnosis for abdominal pain in blunt trauma?

- Which studies are used to evaluate the abdomen after blunt trauma?
- What are the absolute indications for laparotomy after blunt trauma?

Immediate Actions:
Start with 15 liters O_2 by face mask, two large-bore IVs, and cardiac monitor; hang 1 liter NS; perform secondary survey; send blood for hematocrit, basic chemistries (including amylase), PT/PTT, and a blood-bank sample; place a Foley catheter and send a urinalysis and hCG; order trauma series (lateral c-spine, supine chest, and pelvis); perform bedside ultrasound; notify trauma consultants.

Discussion:
Blunt trauma to the abdomen causes injury most commonly to solid visceral organs (e.g., liver, spleen), although hollow visceral injuries (e.g., stomach, small bowel, colon, or bladder) must also be considered. Retroperitoneal injuries (e.g., kidney, duodenum, and pancreas) and diaphragmatic injuries also occur. Even though an abdominal injury may be suspected, a thorough evaluation of every major system (head, spine, thorax, abdomen, extremities) is necessary. The trauma series is used to quickly identify major injuries that require intervention (e.g., unstable c-spine, pneumothorax, or unstable pelvis). The focused assessment with sonography for trauma (FAST) exam is done with a portable ultrasound and looks specifically for blood in Morison's pouch (hepatorenal space, most dependent portion of the abdomen), in the splenorenal space, and in the pelvis. It is also used to detect hemopericardium. A diagnostic peritoneal lavage (DPL) can also be done in an unstable patient to detect intraperitoneal free blood. In a high-speed MVA in which the potential for injury is great, evaluation by CT scan is the imaging modality of choice for stable patients. Typically, head, c-spine, and abdomen CT scans are obtained. Chest CT is obtained if there is evidence of thoracic trauma or any abnormality on the portable CXR. Indications for laparotomy in blunt trauma include abdominal injury with hypotension or clinical peritonitis, hemoperitoneum by FAST or DPL, and free abdominal air by CXR or CT scan.

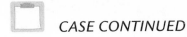

CASE CONTINUED

Secondary survey reveals an oriented patient with multiple facial abrasions and lacerations and a large contusion in her LUQ with tenderness and guarding. She has deformity of her left arm, with intact distal motor and sensory function and 2+ radial pulse. There is no overlying laceration. She receives a tetanus shot. Her labs are significant for an Hct of 33.5% and trace microscopic hematuria. The trauma series is normal. A FAST exam reveals blood in Morison's pouch (Fig. 2-1). She remains hemodynamically stable and goes for CT scans (head, neck, and abdomen), which reveal a splenic laceration with intraperitoneal free fluid. X-ray shows a supracondylar humerus fracture with 50% medial displacement. The patient is taken to the OR for exploratory laparotomy and splenectomy. Orthopedics performs an ORIF of the humerus fracture. The patient's postoperative course is uneventful and she is discharged several days later after receiving vaccines for pneumococcus, meningococcus, and *Haemophilus influenzae* (due to known increased risk of infection with encapsulated bacteria in postsplenectomy patients).

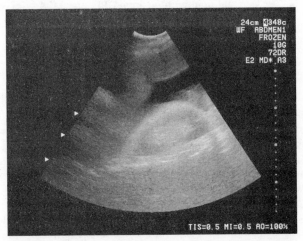

FIGURE 2-1 Abdominal ultrasound shows blood (black region) in Morison's pouch, located between the kidney and liver. (*Image courtesy of Massachusetts General Hospital, Boston, Massachusetts.*)

QUESTIONS

2-1. A 22-year-old man presents to the ED after a 15-foot fall onto concrete. He is minimally responsive and is intubated for airway control. His abdomen is mildly distended without obvious tenderness or guarding. His pelvis is unstable to palpation and is wrapped with a sheet. A FAST exam shows no intraperitoneal fluid. His blood pressure is 146/98. In the CT scanner, the head CT shows an epidural hematoma with midline shift. Neurosurgery wants to take the patient immediately to the OR for craniotomy and evacuation of hemorrhage. What is the best way to evaluate the abdomen?

A. Continue with planned CT scan before going to OR.
B. Perform DPL in OR during neurosurgical procedure.
C. If he remains stable, obtain CT abdomen after surgical procedure.
D. Perform exploratory laparotomy in OR after neurosurgical procedure.
E. Admit to ICU after neurosurgical procedure for serial abdominal exams.

2-2. Which of the following patients has an *absolute* indication for laparotomy?

A. 27-year-old man with positive DPL after MVA who is hemodynamically stable
B. 19-year-old man with splenic laceration
C. 24-year-old man with liver laceration
D. 30-year-old man with small hemoperitoneum on CT without source after MVA
E. 60-year-old woman with gunshot wound to the abdomen

2-3. A 42-year-old man is involved in a high speed MVC. He is intubated in the field for altered mental status, and two large-bore IVs are established. In the ED, his HR is 134, BP is 88/44, and oxygen saturation is 98% while being bagged through the ETT. After NG tube placement, his abdomen appears distended. Which of the following is accurate regarding his abdominal workup?

A. DPL cannot identify the presence of hemoperitoneum.
B. DPL cannot determine the etiology of hemoperitoneum.
C. Ultrasound can determine the etiology of hemoperitoneum.
D. Ultrasound can reliably image the retroperitoneum.
E. Ultrasound is the test of choice for diagnosing solid organ injury.

2-4. A 24-year-old man is involved in a high-speed MVC. Upon presentation to the ED, he is alert and complains of low abdominal pain. His HR is 124, BP 136/88, RR 18, and oxygen saturation 98% on high-flow oxygen. He complains of low abdominal pain and has pelvic tenderness to palpation. He has no blood at the urethral meatus and his prostate exam is normal. A Foley catheter is placed with return of gross blood. Which of the following tests is indicated?

    A. CT abdomen/pelvis with IV contrast alone
    B. Ultrasound of the bladder
    C. CT abdomen/pelvis with IV and transurethral contrast
    D. CT abdomen/pelvis without contrast
    E. Ultrasound of the kidneys

ANSWERS

2-1. C. This patient requires immediate surgical decompression of his epidural hematoma; therefore, no time can be spared to continue with the planned CT scan. A DPL would then be performed in the OR if the patient showed any signs of instability in order to rule out intraperitoneal bleeding as a source of instability. If positive, an exploratory laparotomy would be performed. **If the patient remains stable hemodynamically, he can wait until the neurosurgical procedure is finished and then go back to CT for completion of scans.** A patient who is unconscious cannot be evaluated with serial abdominal exams.

2-2. E. The decision to take a patient with abdominal injuries to the OR for laparotomy is clinically based, and no absolute criteria exist. It is generally understood that the following patients require immediate laparotomy: hypotensive patient with evidence of hemoperitoneum by ultrasound or DPL; clear signs of peritonitis; radiologic signs of pneumoperitoneum consistent with ruptured viscous; or significant GI bleeding by nasogastric or rectal source. In general, gunshot wounds to the abdomen require laparotomy to evaluate for perforated bowel. Patients who are hemodynamically stable may undergo CT scan to better define intra-abdominal injuries. Conservative management can be undertaken with some intra-abdominal injuries, including low-grade liver and spleen lacerations, provided that the patient has a clear sensorium and serial abdominal exams can be performed. Patients with small hemoperitoneum without an obvious source can also be managed expectantly;

however, there must be a high suspicion for hollow viscous or diaphragmatic injury that is not readily detected by abdominal CT scan.

2-3. B. Both DPL and ultrasound can determine the *presence* of hemoperitoneum, but neither can determine the *etiology* of hemoperitoneum. Bedside ultrasound cannot reliably provide information about retroperitoneal structures or solid organ injury. Ultrasound cannot detect intraperitoneal free blood until at least 500 mL has accumulated. DPL is more sensitive than ultrasound in detecting the presence of free intraperitoneal blood when the peritoneal washing is sent to the lab for red blood cell count (RBC >100,000 cells/mm^3 is positive). CT is the preferred imaging modality in hemodynamically stable patients when evaluating the abdomen and retroperitoneum.

2-4. C. Patients with gross hematuria have injuries to the kidneys, ureters, bladder, or urethra. A CT scan of the abdomen/pelvis with IV contrast will identify kidney injuries. **Retrograde injection of dye into the bladder via the urethra will identify bladder injuries, referred to as CT cystogram.** Ureteral injuries are more difficult to identify. If suspected, a CT scan with IV contrast and delayed images can be performed in order to allow time for the IV contrast to enter the ureters. It is important in trauma patients to perform a rectal exam to ensure that the prostate, and thus the urethra, is intact before placing a urinary catheter.

 SUGGESTED ADDITIONAL READINGS

American College of Emergency Physicians: Clinical policy for the initial approach to patients presenting with acute blunt trauma. Ann Emerg Med 1998;31:422–454.

Fakhry SM, Watts DD, Luchette FA. Current diagnostic approaches lack sensitivity in the diagnosis of perforated blunt small bowel injury: analysis from 275,557 trauma admissions from the EAST multi-institutional HVI trial. J Trauma 2003;54:295–306.

Lindstaedt M, Germing A, Lawo T, et al. Acute and long-term clinical significance of myocardial contusion following blunt thoracic trauma: results of a prospective study. J Trauma 2002;52:479–485.

Schiff MA, Holt VL, Daling JR. Maternal and infant outcomes after injury during pregnancy in Washington state from 1989 to 1997. J Trauma 2002;53:939–945.

Gunshot Wound

 CC: 22-year-old man with a gunshot wound to the chest

HPI: G.S. is a 22-year-old man who is shot in the left anterior chest at close range with a 38-caliber handgun. He is found by EMS to be on the ground moaning but conscious. En route to the hospital, two 16-gauge IVs are established and he is placed on oxygen. His vitals include HR 120, BP 110/60. His lung sounds are reported as decreased on the left side. Upon arrival to the ED, the patient is screaming and thrashing on the gurney.

PMHx: None

Meds: None

ALL: NKDA

VS: HR 128, SBP 90 by palpation, RR 36, Sao_2 unable to obtain

PE: *Airway:* Patient awake; oropharynx patent; trachea midline. *Breathing:* Decreased breath sounds over the left chest with crepitus upon palpation; gunshot wound 2 cm above the left nipple. *Circulation:* Thready radial pulses bilaterally with cool extremities.

THOUGHT QUESTIONS

- What immediate actions should be taken?
- What major organ systems must be considered with a gunshot wound to the chest?
- What are the indications for immediate operative intervention in penetrating chest wounds?

Immediate Actions:
Place on 15 liters O_2 by face mask; confirm two large-bore IVs already in place; place on cardiac monitor; hang 2 liters of warmed NS wide open; prepare left chest for tube thoracostomy (i.e., chest tube); perform rapid sequence intubation with etomidate 20 mg and succinylcholine 120 mg IV followed by placement of an 8.0 endotracheal tube under direct laryngoscopy; place left chest tube; call for 4 units of O+ blood (O−blood for women); perform bedside FAST exam and portable chest x-ray; notify trauma surgery and OR staff.

Discussion:
A gunshot wound to the chest requires team members to perform multiple resuscitative tasks simultaneously. The lead physician performs the primary survey and directs other team members. In any unstable patient, definitive airway control is always first priority. Once IV access is established, the patient should be intubated. Breathing is the second priority; therefore, simultaneous to the intubation, a second physician should prepare the chest, and a chest tube should be placed once the patient has been sedated and paralyzed. Circulation is the third priority, which is assessed by peripheral pulses, blood pressure, and mental status. A gunshot wound to the chest is likely to produce a large volume of blood loss; therefore, the patient should have at least two 14- or 16-gauge antecubital IVs in addition to an 8-French femoral venous line. The following organ systems are at risk with penetrating chest trauma: heart, great vessels, lungs, diaphragm, and abdomen. If the patient remains hypotensive after initial fluid resuscitation with 2 liters NS and commencement of O+ blood, he should be taken to the OR for an open thoracotomy. Other indications for OR thoracotomy include initial hemothorax with 1500 mL or more of blood, continuous drainage of greater than or equal to 300 mL/hr, or bedside ultrasound that shows pericardial fluid. A widened mediastinum on CXR should raise the suspicion for aortic injury, and the patient should receive a chest CT if stable or go directly to the OR if unstable. Lower chest wounds (e.g., below the level of the nipples) should raise the suspicion for potential intra-abdominal injury, which can be diagnosed by bedside ultrasound (i.e., by

(Continued)

detecting intraperitoneal blood), CT scan if the patient is stable, or a bedside DPL if the patient is unstable. Wounds closer to the midline should raise the suspicion for esophageal or tracheal injuries. Once injury to the heart and great vessels has been excluded, these patients should undergo bronchoscopy and esophagoscopy.

CASE CONTINUED

Upon secondary survey, an exit wound is noted in the left back about 3 cm lateral to T3. A chest tube is inserted and about 900 mL of blood is obtained. The chest tube is hooked to wall suction, with resultant continuous blood return. A portable CXR shows a narrow mediastinum, a chest tube in the left thorax, and a large hemothorax on the left (Fig. 3-1). Two units of O+ blood are infused rapidly after 2 liters of NS, but the patient remains tachycardic to the 120s and hypotensive in the 90s systolic. The patient is taken to the OR, where an open thoracotomy is performed. Bleeding is noted at the pulmonary hilum, and several pulmonary vessels are ligated. There is no evidence of mediastinal violation or aortic injury. The chest tube is left in place and the patient is admitted to the ICU, where he recovers uneventfully.

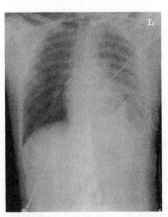

FIGURE 3-1 Upright chest x-ray with left-sided chest tube and large hemothorax. (*Image courtesy of Massachusetts General Hospital, Boston.*)

QUESTIONS

3-1. In which of the following patients is emergency department thoracotomy indicated?

A. Unbelted driver in a high-speed MVA who initially has a pulse but subsequently loses it during extrication and transport

B. Patient with a gunshot wound to the chest who is found apneic, cyanotic, cold, and pulseless in the field with a 10-minute transport time

C. Pedestrian struck by car with massive pelvic fractures who loses pulses and blood pressure 20 minutes before helipad touchdown by air transport

D. Patient with stab wound to the anterior chest who is initially stable but suddenly becomes unresponsive and pulseless

E. Unhelmeted motorcyclist who hits a highway median divider at high speed and is dragged 200 feet, who has a thready pulse

3-2. An 18-year-old male presents to the ED after sustaining a stab wound to the left anterior chest with a 4-inch blade. He is awake and cooperative, complaining of left chest pain. His pulse is 80, blood pressure 118/78, and oxygen saturation 99% on room air. He has clear breath sounds bilaterally. You see a 4-cm wound just below the nipple on the left side. What is the most appropriate management?

A. Immediate tube thoracostomy (i.e., chest tube) because the likelihood of a pneumothorax is high despite his normal physical exam

B. Gentle inspection of the wound, bedside ultrasound exam, portable chest x-ray, admission to the hospital for observation, repeat chest x-ray the following day and discharge home if normal

C. Deep probing of the wound with a cotton swab to ensure no pleural violation, portable chest x-ray, and discharge home if normal

D. Chest CT, then discharge home if no evidence of pneumothorax

E. Transthoracic echocardiography, followed if normal by transesophageal echocardiography; discharge home if both studies are normal

3-3. A 32-year-old female is shot at close range in the right anterior chest with a 38-caliber pistol. She presents to the ED intoxicated and yelling; her vitals include a pulse of 92, blood pressure of 134/84, and oxygen saturation of 97% on room air. She has clear breath sounds bilaterally. The entrance wound is just above the right breast, and an exit wound is noted in the right axilla. What is the most appropriate management of this patient?

A. IV access, portable chest x-ray, tube thoracostomy, and exploratory thoracotomy in the OR to search for cardiac or pulmonary vascular injury

B. IV access, endotracheal intubation and simultaneous placement of a right chest tube, bedside ultrasound, portable chest x-ray, and admission to the ICU if stable

C. IV access, portable chest x-ray, right chest tube placement if x-ray shows a pneumothorax or hemothorax, admission to the ICU for observation

D. IV access, endotracheal intubation, CT scan of chest to look for pneumothorax or hemothorax or injuries to the heart or great vessels

E. IV access, endotracheal intubation, ED thoracotomy to search for cardiac or pulmonary vascular injury

3-4. A 42-year-old man is stabbed in the left side with an unknown weapon during a bar fight. He presents to the ED with dyspnea, pulse of 108, blood pressure of 138/92, and oxygen saturation of 94% on room air. He has absent breath sounds on the left side; you note a small puncture wound in the midaxillary line at the level of the tenth rib. His abdominal exam is normal. Two large-bore IVs are established. What is the appropriate management of this patient?

A. Endotracheal intubation, left-sided chest tube, portable chest x-ray, and admission

B. Left-sided chest tube, portable chest x-ray, and admission

C. Left-sided chest tube, portable chest x-ray, diagnostic peritoneal lavage, and admission

D. Left-sided chest tube, portable chest x-ray, bedside abdominal ultrasound or CT scan of the abdomen, and admission

E. Endotracheal intubation, portable chest x-ray, exploratory laparotomy in the OR, and admission

ANSWERS

3-1. D. A resuscitative thoracotomy, or opening of a patient's chest in the ED, is a procedure that is not often performed but is essential in several specific circumstances. **Open thoracotomy is primarily reserved for patients who have sustained penetrating trauma to the chest and who decompensate rapidly in the trauma bay. Several specific goals of resuscitative thoracotomy include relieving pericardial tamponade, repairing a hole in the heart or a disruption of pulmonary vessels, and clamping the descending aorta.** Survival for patients who arrive in the ED pulseless following blunt trauma (e.g., motor vehicle collision, fall, crush) is negligible; therefore, thoracotomy in these patients is considered futile. There may be an indication for thoracotomy in blunt trauma if the patient acutely decompensates in the ED. For example, if massive bleeding into the pelvis or abdomen is suspected and the patient suddenly becomes pulseless, then an open thoracotomy with cross-clamping of the aorta may reduce bleeding and increase perfusion to the brain. This is, of course, a temporizing measure until the patient can be taken to the OR. Of the choices given, only answer choice D, a patient with penetrating stab wound to the chest, who is initially stable but becomes pulseless (whether on scene or in the bay), has a clear indication for ED thoracotomy. Answers A, C, and E are patients of blunt trauma who lose their pulses before reaching the ED. Answer B represents a patient who is essentially dead on arrival of EMS to the scene.

3-2. B. Stab wounds to the chest are worrisome despite an initially stable appearance of the patient. Pericardial tamponade, tension pneumothorax, or massive hemothorax can be delayed and cause acute decompensation in a young, healthy patient. The initial management includes ensuring an adequate airway, securing two large-bore IVs, checking vital signs, auscultating the lungs, and palpating for subcutaneous air. If the patient is dyspneic, has decreased breath sounds, or has abnormal vital signs, a chest tube should be placed immediately before a chest x-ray is obtained. **If the patient is stable, gentle inspection of the wound can be done; however, deep probing is discouraged because a lacerated**

artery may be inadvertently opened. It is often difficult to identify the base of a stab wound, and there is little utility in doing so. Observation and a repeat chest x-ray are usually warranted even if the initial chest x-ray is normal.

3-3. B. Pneumothorax or hemothorax is assumed present with any gunshot wound to the chest, and tube thoracostomy (i.e., chest tube) should be performed immediately after or concordant with IV access and airway management. Most gunshot wounds to the chest will require endotracheal intubation due to the high likelihood of serious injury and to facilitate further management (e.g., chest tube placement, CT scan if necessary). This is especially true if the patient is combative. A chest x-ray should be obtained only after intubation and thoracostomy have been performed. A bedside ultrasound should be done to look for pericardial blood. The mediastinum should be evaluated on the chest x-ray. A wide mediastinum is evidence for great vessel injury. An abnormal chest x-ray can be followed by a CT scan in the ED if the patient is stable. If the patient becomes unstable, an open thoracotomy is indicated.

3-4. D. Injury to the diaphragm or abdominal organs must be considered with penetrating trauma below the level of the nipples. In addition to treating the patient's pulmonary injuries, diagnostic tests must be done to exclude abdominal injury. In selected cases in which the suspicion for abdominal injury is low or in which the resources are not available, a bedside ultrasound can be done to exclude intraperitoneal blood and the patient can be admitted for serial abdominal exams and hematocrits. If the patient is stable in the ED, the optimal test is a CT scan to exclude splenic laceration or intraperitoneal blood. In an unstable patient, a diagnostic peritoneal lavage can be performed at the bedside. This involves inserting a catheter into the peritoneum and infusing 1000 mL of sterile saline. The saline is then allowed to drain back out of the peritoneum into the bag. Return of gross blood indicates intra-abdominal injury and necessitates immediate exploratory laparotomy in the OR. A clear return is sent to the lab for cell count. A red blood cell count of greater than 100,000 cells per mm^3 is very specific for intra-abdominal injury and is an indication for immediate exploratory laparotomy in the OR.

SUGGESTED ADDITIONAL READINGS

Aihara R, Millham FH, Blansfield J, et al. Emergency room
    thoracotomy for penetrating chest injury: effect of an
    institutional protocol. J Trauma 2001;50:1027–1030.
Asensio JA, Chahwan S, Forno W, et al. Penetrating esophageal
    injuries: multicenter study of the American Association for the
    Surgery of Trauma. J Trauma 2001;50:289–296.
Demetriades D, Velmahos GC. Penetrating injuries of the chest:
    indications for operation. Scand J Surg 2002;91:41–45.
Ullman EA, Donley LP, Brady WJ. Pulmonary trauma emergency
    department evaluation and management. Emerg Med Clin
    North Am 2003;21:291–313.

CASE **4**

Pelvic Pain after Motorcycle Collision

CC: 30-year-old man with pelvic pain after a motorcycle collision

HPI: M.C. is a 30-year-old man who was involved in a high-speed motorcycle accident after which he was found approximately 30 to 40 feet from his motorcycle, with his helmet still in place. He had lost consciousness initially, but is awake and alert upon EMS arrival to the scene. Vital signs prior to transport include a HR of 130 and BP of 95/palp. He does not remember what happened, and denies any alcohol or illicit drug use. He arrives in the ED on a backboard with a cervical collar in place, complaining of pain all over and especially in the pelvic area.

PMHx: Unrestrained, rear-ended motor vehicle collision one month earlier, in which he had back and neck pain

Meds: None

ALL: NKDA

SHx: Lives with his wife and two children; no tobacco or drugs, occasional alcohol

VS: Temp 37.3°C (99.1°F), HR 126, BP 88/46, RR 24, SaO$_2$ 99% on 15 liters O$_2$ by face mask

PE: *Airway:* Patient alert; oropharynx patent; trachea midline. *Breathing:* Lungs clear on the right, mildly diminished with a few crackles on the left. *Circulation:* Well-perfused with 2+ radial and femoral pulses.

THOUGHT QUESTIONS

- What are the immediate actions for this patient?
- What are some of the possible sources of hemorrhage in high-force blunt trauma?
- What associated injuries are common in patients who sustain pelvic fractures?
- How should unstable pelvic fractures be managed initially?

Immediate Actions:

Give high-flow oxygen by face mask; establish two large-bore IVs; place on cardiac monitor; bolus 2 L normal saline; perform secondary survey; send blood for hematocrit, basic chemistries (including amylase), PT/PTT, and a blood-bank sample; order trauma series (lateral c-spine, supine chest, and pelvis); perform bedside ultrasound; notify trauma consultants; place Foley catheter if prostate exam is normal and no blood is at the meatus; administer uncrossmatched type O+ blood if persistent hypotension after fluid bolus; tie sheet tightly around pelvis if x-ray shows displaced fracture.

Discussion:

The goal in hypotensive blunt trauma patients is to resuscitate and to "find the blood." The sources of hemorrhage are thoracic injuries (massive hemothorax, aortic rupture), abdominal injuries (hemoperitoneum), pelvic fractures (noncompressible arterial or venous injury), femoral fractures, retroperitoneal bleeding, and profusely bleeding wounds. Therefore, in hypotensive patients with a pelvic fracture, other potential sites of bleeding must be ruled out. This includes a chest x-ray to look for hemothorax and a focused assessment with sonography for trauma (FAST) exam to look for hemoperitoneum. Pelvic fractures alone can result in lethal internal bleeding. The internal iliac artery and its branches supply the pelvic area, many of which run along the walls of the pelvis and are susceptible to injury. For example, injury to the sacroiliac joint may injure the internal iliac artery that courses

(Continued)

nearby; injury to the pubic rami may injure the nearby pudendal and obturator arteries. Arterial injury, however, is thought to cause hemodynamic instability in only 10% to 20% of patients who have sustained pelvic fractures, with most bleeding from the large pelvic veins and the fracture itself.

Severe pelvic fractures are usually due to large forces (e.g., fall from greater than 15 ft, motorcycle and motor vehicle collisions, pedestrian struck by motor vehicle), and therefore these patients commonly have significant injuries to the head, chest, abdomen, and skeletal system as well. Injuries in the pelvic region that are associated with pelvic fractures may occur to the urethra, vagina, rectum, bladder, and lumbosacral nerve plexus, to name a few. Signs to look for that suggest associated injuries include blood at the urethral meatus, swelling of the scrotum or labia, gross blood or guaiac-positive stool on rectal exam, blood at the vagina, flank ecchymosis, inability to pass a Foley catheter, and gross hematuria. In a recent trauma registry of more than 16,000 patients and more than 1,500 pelvic fractures, the most common abdominal and urogenital injuries associated with pelvic fractures in descending order of frequency were: liver, bladder and urethra, spleen, diaphragm, small bowel, colon, rectum, pancreas, stomach, duodenum.

Once an unstable pelvis has been established on exam, further manipulation should be avoided. Gross stability is assessed by the pelvic rock test, compressing firmly on both anterior iliac spines to see if the pelvis moves as one unit. If the pelvis is unstable and the patient hypotensive, the pelvis should be tightly wrapped and tied with a bedsheet in order to provide compression to close the bleeding fracture sites. The sheet should include the area between the iliac crest and the greater trochanter of the femur. A pelvic sling or external fixator can also be used. An external fixator is usually placed in the OR and thus is not very useful for immediate stabilization in the ED. Pelvic stabilization was previously thought to decrease hemorrhage by a tamponade effect from limiting the volume for blood accumulation in the pelvis, but more recently is thought to promote clotting of the bleeding sources.

CASE CONTINUED

Secondary survey reveals an oriented patient with tenderness and mild instability upon palpation of the pelvis, as well as significant tenderness over the left chest and left upper quadrant. His pelvis is wrapped firmly with a sheet. The FAST exam shows what appears to be a small amount of blood in Morison's pouch. With the patient's blood pressure improved to 105/52 after 2 L of crystalloid fluid, the trauma surgeon now present in the ED elects to take the patient to the CT scanner. CT scan of the head, neck, chest, and abdomen reveal a small anterior hemo-pneumothorax on the left, posterior rib fractures on the left in all 12 ribs, comminuted fractures through the body and neck of the left scapula, shattered spleen, minimally displaced fractures of the inferior and superior pubic rami bones on the left pelvis, pubic symphysis diastasis of 2.1 cm, diastasis of the right sacroiliac joint, and fracture of the right iliac bone posteriorly (Fig. 4-1). The patient's blood pressure

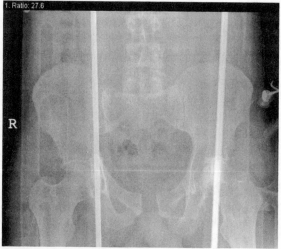

FIGURE 4-1 Trauma series pelvic x-ray showing significant pubic symphysis diastasis; the other pelvic injuries diagnosed by CT scan (diastasis of the right sacroiliac joint, minimally displaced fractures of the inferior and superior pubic rami bones on the left, and fracture of the right iliac bone posteriorly) are difficult to appreciate on this plain film. (*Image courtesy of Massachusetts General Hospital, Boston.*)

drops again to the 80s systolic as he is leaving the CT scanner, at which time a left chest tube is placed and type O+ blood transfused. He is taken to the OR for exploratory laparotomy and splenectomy. Afterwards he is admitted to the ICU. The next day, he returns to the OR for open reduction and internal fixation of his pelvic fractures without incident.

QUESTIONS

4-1. A 22-year-old man is involved in a high-speed motor vehicle collision in which he sustains diffuse subarachnoid hemorrhage, diastasis of the pubic symphysis, bilateral femur fractures, left tibia and fibula fractures, grade II liver laceration, and two nondisplaced right-sided rib fractures. He receives appropriate stabilization and management, but on the next day develops respiratory failure consistent with ARDS. Which of his injuries likely had the greatest contribution to this condition?
   A. Diffuse subarachnoid hemorrhage
   B. Diastasis of the pubic symphysis
   C. Bilateral femur fractures and left tibia and fibula fractures
   D. Grade II liver laceration
   E. Two nondisplaced right-sided rib fractures

4-2. A 16-year-old man involved in an MVC of unknown speed has significant pain upon compression testing of his pelvis. There is a drop of blood present at his urethral meatus. Otherwise his exam is unremarkable. FAST exam is negative. Trauma series x-rays have been taken in the bay, and he remains hemodynamically stable. Besides CT scanning, which of the following would be the next best step?
   A. Exploratory laparotomy
   B. Admit to ICU with serial urinalyses
   C. Obtain pelvis inlet and oulet x-rays to assist operative planning
   D. Retrograde cystourethrography
   E. Pelvic angiography

4-3. A 33-year-old woman is involved in a high-speed MVC and sustains a pelvic fracture that is unstable by exam. You are at a remote hospital without a trauma surgeon but with an orthopedist on-call 45 minutes away. The patient has been hemodynamically stable and can be transferred by air to a trauma center 100 miles away. What is the best approach to stabilizing the pelvis?

A. Fasten two rolled towels, one on each side of the pelvis, and tape to backboard.

B. Use folded bedsheet to wrap around pelvis.

C. Place standard bedpan beneath patient and tape firmly in place.

D. Leave pelvis as is to avoid further injury during transfer to a trauma center.

E. Leave patient as is and await arrival of orthopedist.

4-4. A 19-year-old male pedestrian is struck at moderate speed by a small car. He complains of severe abdominal and pelvic pain. He has an unstable pelvis on your exam, and seems to be somewhat tender in his abdomen, although he is very agitated and the exam is difficult. Of the following organs, which is he most likely to have injured in addition to his pelvis?

A. Spleen

B. Bladder

C. Pancreas

D. Stomach

E. Small bowel

ANSWERS

4-1. C. This polytrauma patient likely developed fat emboli syndrome (FES), a multisystem disorder that results from pulmonary fat embolization and is seen most commonly in patients with long bone fractures. In FES, patients may develop pulmonary or CNS dysfunction, fever, and rash; symptoms usually develop within 12 to 72 hours after initial trauma, but may occur as late as a week. The exact etiology of FES is not clear, but it is thought that pulmonary fat emboli lead to increased pulmonary vascular permeability and hypoxemia.

4-2. D. Some of the findings that may suggest a urologic injury in the setting of pelvic injury from blunt trauma include inability to pass a Foley catheter, bloody urethral discharge, and gross hematuria. Retrograde cystourethrography or retrograde urethrogram (RUG) should be performed to evaluate the

type and location of injury in such cases. This patient has been hemodynamically stable throughout, so pelvic angiography is not currently indicated. Pelvic angiography (and embolization) may be useful for evaluating the trauma patient who has persistent hypotension after other sources of bleeding have been ruled out. Exploratory laparotomy would be indicated if the patient had persistent hypotension with evidence of intraperitoneal blood on the FAST exam.

4-3. B. Stabilization of an unstable pelvis in a blunt trauma patient should be achieved, while acute resuscitative efforts are ongoing, using a sheet wrapped tightly around the pelvis, covering the area between the iliac crests and the greater trochanters of the femurs. By mechanism, this patient likely has associated injuries as well, and should be managed at the trauma center rather than at this small hospital with limited resources, despite the availability of an orthopedist.

4-4. B. Demetriades and associates studied the epidemiology of pelvic fractures using a trauma registry of 16,630 patients sustaining blunt trauma, of whom 1,545 had a pelvic fracture. They found that 16.5% of the patients with pelvic fractures had associated abdominal or urogenital injuries, with the most common organs injured being the liver (6.1%) and the bladder and urethra (5.8%). **In patients with particularly severe pelvic fractures, 31% had associated intraabdominal or urogenital injuries, with the bladder and urethra being most commonly injured (14.6%).**

 ### SUGGESTED ADDITIONAL READINGS

Demetriades D, Karaiskakis M, Toutouzas K, et al. Pelvic fractures: epidemiology and predictors of associated abdominal injuries and outcomes. J Am Coll Surg 2002;195:1–10.

Eastridge BJ, Starr A, Minei JP, et al. The importance of fracture pattern in guiding therapeutic decision-making in patients with hemorrhagic shock and pelvic ring disruptions. J Trauma 2002;53:446–451.

Goulet JA. Hip and pelvic trauma. Orthop Clin North Am 2004;35:ix.

Mirza A, Ellis T. Initial management of pelvic and femoral fractures in the multiply injured patient. Crit Care Clin 2004;20:159–170.

Stab Wound to the Neck

CC: 19-year-old man with stab wound to the neck

HPI: H.B., a 19-year-old man involved in a street fight, gets stabbed in his neck with a 4-inch switchblade. The fight quickly disperses and his friends drive him to the ED where they drop him off at the entrance. He arrives ambulatory to triage holding his left neck. There does not appear to be significant bleeding, but there is swelling on the left side of his neck. His voice is a bit hoarse, but he is not coughing up blood or spitting up blood.

PMHx: None

Meds: None

ALL: None

SHx: Unknown

VS: Temp 37.0°C (98.6°F), HR 96, BP 130/78, RR 18, Sao$_2$ 98% on 15 liters O$_2$ by face mask

PE: *General:* Alert and oriented, some hoarseness. *Airway:* Oropharynx patent; left-sided 2-cm laceration about 3 cm lateral to the midline at the level of the cricothyroid membrane; significant left neck swelling; trachea midline. *Breathing:* Lungs clear bilaterally; mild inspiratory stridor bilaterally. *Circulation:* Heart sounds regular; good radial pulses. *Rapid neuro assessment:* Cooperative; GCS 15; moving all extremities appropriately.

THOUGHT QUESTIONS

- What is the most important immediate intervention for this patient?
- What are the three anatomical zones of the neck and their significance in penetrating neck trauma?

- What are indications for immediate operative exploration versus further workup in the ED?
- Which important structures are at risk and which tests exist to work up potential injuries?

Immediate Actions:
Place on 15 liters O_2 by nonrebreather mask; place on cardiac monitor; establish two large-bore IVs; administer etomidate 20 mg IV and succinylcholine 120 mg IV; intubate using laryngoscope and 7.5 ETT; establish mechanical ventilation; perform secondary survey looking for other wounds; place NG tube and Foley; order CBC, chem 7, tox screen, PT/PTT, urinalysis; type and cross 4 units of PRBCs; activate OR for immediate operative exploration and repair.

Discussion:
A stab wound to the neck is a high-risk injury given the density of important structures present. When considering penetrating trauma, the neck is divided into three zones (Table 5-1). The workup is largely based on the location of the stab wound in one of these three zones. The first consideration in penetrating neck trauma is always airway. Intubation must be performed early if there is any sign of respiratory difficulty or airway narrowing because delay may result in an impossible intubation scenario, as is the case with an expanding hematoma that progressively presses on the trachea, causing total airway obstruction. The next decision is whether to go directly to the OR for operative exploration. An immediate operation is indicated if the patient displays any "hard signs" of significant injury, including airway compromise, circulatory shock, or signs of arterial injury or stroke (Table 5-2).

(*Continued*)

TABLE 5-1 Clinically-Relevant Structures of the Zones of the Neck

Zone I	Zone II	Zone III
Sternal notch and clavicles to cricoid cartilage	Cricoid cartilage to angle of mandible	Angle of mandible to base of skull

Vascular Structures
  Carotid artery
  Vertebral artery
  Subclavian artery
  Subclavian vein
  Internal jugular vein
  External jugular vein
  Anterior jugular vein
  Subclavian vein
Airway Structures
  Trachea
  Domes of the lungs
Digestive System Structures
  Esophagus
Nervous System
  Spinal cord
  Major cervical trunks
  Brachial plexus
Other
  Thyroid gland
  Thoracic duct
	Vascular Structures
	  Common carotid artery
	  Internal carotid artery
	  External carotid artery
	  Vertebral artery
	  Internal jugular vein
	  External jugular vein
	  Anterior jugular vein
	Airway Structures
	  Pharynx
	  Larynx
	  Trachea
	Digestive System Structures
	  Esophagus
	Nervous System
	  Spinal cord
	  Recurrent laryngeal nerve
	  Vagus nerve
		Vascular Structures
		  Internal carotid artery
		  Internal jugular vein
		  External jugular vein
		Airway Structures
		  Oropharynx
		Nervous System
		  Spinal cord
		  Cranial nerves IX–XII
		Other
		  Salivary and parotid glands

Management Angiography first unless hemodynamically unstable	Direct to OR if any hard signs present	Angiography first unless hemodynamically unstable

TABLE 5-2 Hard Signs of Significant Injury in Penetrating Neck Trauma

1. Airway Compromise	2. Circulatory Compromise	3. Uncontrollable Bleeding
Tracheal deviation/stridor Need for intubation Subcutaneous emphysema Air bubbling in wound	Refractory shock Evidence of cerebral stroke Vascular bruit Upper extremity ischemia	Expanding hematoma Pulsatile hematoma Large hemothorax

For patients who are stable, the workup depends on the zone of injury. Injuries in zones I and III that penetrate the platysma muscle require angiography to evaluate for significant arterial injury. This is done whenever possible because surgical access to zones I

(Continued)

and III is difficult, and it is preferable to have the injuries characterized before going in. Injuries to zone II, given the ease of access
to vascular structures, are more often explored in the OR without
prior angiography, especially if there is any indication of vascular
or tracheal injury. However, in stable patients with minimal signs
of serious injury, angiography is often performed, even in zone II
injuries. In addition, bronchoscopy and esophagoscopy should be
done if either tracheal or esophageal injuries are suspected.

CASE CONTINUED

This patient's hoarseness is evidence of laryngeal injury, recurrent
laryngeal nerve injury, or an expanding hematoma pressing on
these structures. With the neck swelling present in this zone II
injury, the last is suspected. The patient requires immediate intubation because his airway will likely close off entirely as the
hematoma progresses. This of course is also a "hard sign" of significant injury and an indication for taking the patient directly to the
OR for exploration. He is intubated using RSI techniques and then
taken to the OR. He is found to have a partial laceration of the
carotid artery that is isolated and repaired. In addition, bronchoscopy and esophagoscopy are performed in the OR, which
reveal no tracheal or esophageal injury, respectively.

QUESTIONS

5-1. A patient is stabbed just below and behind the right ear.
He appears comfortable, his airway and breathing are normal, and
he is hemodynamically stable. The wound is approximately 1 cm
wide and its depth is unclear; there is no surrounding hematoma.
What is the next best step in this patient's managment?
- A. Local wound exploration to determine whether the
  platysma was penetrated
- B. Neck exploration in the operating room
- C. Intubation, given the high likelihood of expanding
  hematoma
- D. CT angiography to identify arterial injury
- E. Simple observation, because this is not considered a neck
  wound

5-2. A patient sustains a stab wound about 2 cm superior to the right clavicle and 3 cm from the midline. He complains of difficulty breathing. His pulse is 120, blood pressure 118/66, respiratory rate 24, and oxygen saturation 92% on room air. His airway is normal and his trachea is midline. It is difficult to hear breath sounds on either side because of the noise in the room, but you feel crepitus above the clavicle extending into the axilla. What is the first step in his management?

A. Place a chest tube on the right side for suspected pneumothorax.

B. Intubate the patient and go directly to the OR for exploration.

C. Obtain an upright chest x-ray to confirm a pneumothorax.

D. Perform angiography to rule out vascular injury.

E. Perform bronchoscopy to evaluate for a tracheobronchial injury.

5-3. A patient is shot with a .22 caliber pistol to the lateral neck about 2 cm below the angle of the jaw. He arrives to the ED alert, able to speak, and with some swelling around the gunshot wound. His airway is normal, his trachea is midline, and breath sounds are equal bilaterally. His vital signs are normal. What is the most appropriate next step in this patient's management?

A. Intubation given blast injury and high likelihood for vascular injury

B. CT angiography

C. Local wound exploration

D. Obtain upright chest x-ray and lateral neck x-ray

E. Go directly to the OR for open exploration

5-4. A patient sustains a stab wound to the midline neck halfway between the top of the thyroid cartilage and the manubrium. He presents to the ED alert but coughing up some blood. His airway is clear, his trachea is midline, and he has clear breath sounds. There is air bubbling out of the wound and there is some crepitus around the wound. His vital signs are normal. What is the appropriate management plan for this patient?

A. Immediate transfer to the OR for open exploration

B. Intubation followed by CXR, then angiography if stable

C. Placement of bilateral chest tubes

D. Place a dressing on the wound, then go to angiography

E. Immediate bronchoscopy

ANSWERS

5-1. D. A wound posterior to the ear is considered a zone III injury. The primary structures at risk are the internal carotid artery and internal jugular vein. There are no "hard signs" that would indicate immediate surgical intervention, such as airway compromise, circulatory shock, or signs of arterial injury (e.g., expanding hematoma, neurologic symptoms, bruits). Local wound exploration is not recommended because it may dislodge a clot and precipitate arterial bleeding. **Given a stable zone III injury, angiography is indicated. In the past, this required formal angiography with femoral artery catheterization, injection of IV contrast, and fluoroscopy. This has been replaced largely by CT angiography. New-generation, multiple-detector CT scanners are able to produce a 3-D reconstruction of the arterial system as dye is introduced, rendering images that rival those of traditional angiography.** CT scan also allows evaluation of other structures of the neck, whereas traditional angiography only evaluated the arterial system.

5-2. A. Zone I injuries are often associated with injuries to the apices of the lungs. A patient with a lateral zone I injury who is short of breath should be assumed to have a pneumothorax and a chest tube should be placed immediately. This diagnosis should not wait for chest x-ray confirmation in a patient who is short of breath with a low oxygen saturation. Injuries to the subclavian artery and vein should also be suspected; these may result in massive hemothorax. If the patient is stable after chest tube placement, then CT angiography can be done to evaluate for a vascular injury. Likewise, bronchoscopy would be indicated after angiography since an injury to the tracheobronchial tree is a possible etiology for the pneumothorax.

5-3. D. A zone II gunshot wound will universally go to the OR whether stable or unstable due to the blast and high potential for significant injury. However, upright chest and lateral neck x-rays are indicated to see where the bullet resides. It is possible, for example, that a bullet entering zone II on the left can traverse the midline and end up in zone I on the right, or that it could travel inferiorly to zone I or even into the thorax. Locating the bullet on plain x-rays is essential for surgical planning. Early intubation should also be a serious consideration in patients with gunshot wounds to the neck and should be done if there is any indication of airway compromise, neck swelling, or circulatory shock.

5-4. B. Air bubbling from a neck wound is a "hard sign" indication for open exploration in the OR. The first priority, however, is to secure the airway. Intubation is a must with someone who has evidence of tracheal injury and bleeding into the airway, despite the fact that the patient may be breathing comfortably with a normal oxygen saturation. After intubation, if the patient is stable, the next step depends on the location of injury. In a zone II injury, most surgeons will take the patient directly to the OR for exploration and tracheal repair. For zone I and III injuries, given the anatomic limitations of open exploration to visualize all vital structures, angiography is preferable before taking the patient to the OR.

 ### SUGGESTED ADDITIONAL READINGS

Abujamra L, Joseph MM. Penetrating neck injuries in children: a retrospective review. Pediatr Emerg Care 2003;19:308–313.

Asensio JA, Chahwan S, Forno W, et al. Penetrating esophageal injuries: multicenter study of the American Association for the Surgery of Trauma. J Trauma 2001;50:289–296.

Munera F, Cohn S, Rivas LA. Penetrating injuries of the neck: use of helical computed tomographic angiography. J Trauma 2005;58:413–418.

Thompson EC, Porter JM, Fernandez LG. Penetrating neck trauma: an overview of management. J Oral Maxillofac Surg 2002;60:918–923.

Crush Injury to the Leg

 CC: 46-year-old construction worker with crush injury to right leg

HPI: B.G. is a 46-year-old construction worker who was working on a new high-rise building. He was guiding the placement of a large steel girder when it suddenly swung around and struck him in the right leg, pinning his leg against another steel girder. It took about 10 minutes for his co-workers to remove the girder. He has extreme pain over the lower leg and is unable to bear weight. He is brought to the ED by ambulance.

PMHx: Hypertension

Meds: Lisinopril

ALL: None

SHx: 1 ppd smoker

VS: Temp 37.0°C (98.6°F), HR 110, BP 165/94, RR 18, Sao$_2$ 100%

PE: *General:* Alert and oriented, uncomfortable. *Extr:* Ecchymosis and swelling of the right lower extremity below the knee; tender over the lateral aspect of the tibia-fibula area; no deformed bone or open laceration; pain to the lateral leg with passive range of motion of the ankle; no tenderness over the knee or the ankle. *Vasc:* Intact dorsalis pedis and posterior tibial pulses, normal distal capillary refill. *Neuro:* Able to dorsiflex and plantarflex at the ankle but very painful, especially with dorsiflexion; intact dorsiflexion of extensor hallucis longus; decreased sensation over the dorsum and lateral aspect of the foot.

THOUGHT QUESTIONS

■ What are the two primary diagnoses to consider with a crush injury to an extremity?

- What is the best explanation for this patient's pain with passive range of motion?
- What are the signs of compartment syndrome?
- How is the diagnosis of compartment syndrome established?

Immediate Actions:
Place an IV and administer morphine 4 mg; elevate leg above the level of the heart; place ice (wrapped in a towel) on leg; order a PA and lateral x-ray of the tibia-fibula.

Discussion:
The first consideration in a crush to an extremity is fracture. An x-ray is always indicated if there is significant tenderness or deformity. The second consideration with a crush injury should be compartment syndrome. This is an often-forgotten diagnosis that has important implications in the long-term function of the limb. Anatomically, the extremities are divided into soft-tissue compartments (Fig. 6-1). These compartments contain muscle-nerve-artery bundles that together provide a specific function (e.g., wrist and hand extension). These compartments are enveloped in fibrous, nontensile fascia, which helps contain each functional bundle. This fascia is taut and does not allow significant swelling to occur within the compartment. Crush injury can result in muscle and soft tissue damage, resulting in cell damage and exudates with subsequent swelling within a compartment. Because the surrounding fascia does not allow for volume expansion, the result is increased pressure within the compartment. If not relieved, this can cause further cellular damage, muscle necrosis, and nerve and artery compression. The result is loss of motor and nerve function, as well as distal ischemia.

This sounds like an easy diagnosis to make but compartment syndrome is often insidious. The hallmark of compartment syndrome is pain out of proportion to the appearance of the limb. Damage within a compartment will not necessarily have outward manifestations, although ecchymosis, abrasions, and swelling are often present due to superficial crush injury as well. The most sensitive sign of

(Continued)

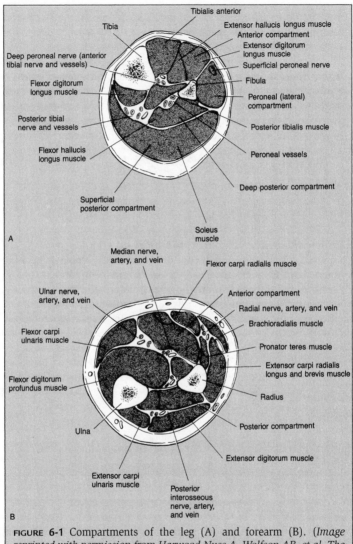

FIGURE 6-1 Compartments of the leg (A) and forearm (B). (*Image reprinted with permission from Harwood-Nuss A, Wolfson AB, et al. The Clinical Practice of Emergency Medicine, 3rd Edition, Philadelphia: Lippincott Williams & Wilkins, 2001.*)

(*Continued*)

compartment syndrome is pain with passive flexion and extension of the muscles within the compartment. This is sometimes difficult to assess due to an associated fracture that will limit range-of-motion testing. Compartment syndrome is classically characterized by the presence of the "6 Ps" (Table 6-1). These are a direct result of muscle, nerve, and/or artery compression; these classic signs, however, are not reliable for making the diagnosis. It is important to realize that arterial compression is a late sign, and the presence of distal pulses certainly does not exclude compartment syndrome.

The diagnosis of compartment syndrome is largely clinical, based on the evidence of muscle, nerve, or artery compression on physical exam. If suspected, compartment pressures need to be measured. This is accomplished with a Stryker device that measures pressure through a hollow-bore needle. This needle is placed through the skin and into the suspected compartment; the importance of knowing the anatomic locations of the different compartments is thus critical. A pressure of 30 to 40 mm Hg is considered positive for compartment syndrome, as pressures are usually below 20 mm Hg. Treatment is operative with an open fasciotomy, which is an incision made longitudinally into the compartment to release the pressure. This must be undertaken immediately if the diagnosis is suspected to prevent long-term disability.

TABLE 6-1 The Traditional "Six Ps" (Not Diagnostic of Compartment Syndrome)

Pain
Pallor
Paresthesias or Paralysis
Pulselessness
Poikilothermia
Pressure (elevated)

 CASE CONTINUED

The tibia-fibula x-ray shows no evidence of fracture. The patient, however, is unable to bear weight on the leg. This raises the suspicion for compartment syndrome, especially given his extreme pain to passive range of motion of the ankle and sensory loss over the distribution of the peroneal nerve. A Stryker device is placed into the anterior compartment of the leg and the pressure is measured at 50 mm Hg. Orthopedics is consulted and the patient is taken directly to the OR for a fasciotomy. One month later, the fasciotomy scar continues to heal, and the patient has regained full motor and sensory function of the lower leg.

QUESTIONS

6-1. A teenager sustains a midshaft fracture of the radius and ulna. In addition to severe pain and swelling, he has decreased sensation over his palm and mottling of his fingers. What is the most sensitive sign of compartment syndrome for this patient?
   A. Numbness in a nerve distribution
   B. Decreased radial artery pulse
   C. Pain with passive range of motion of muscle bundle
   D. Increased distal capillary refill time
   E. Distal muscle weakness

6-2. A pedestrian is struck by a car and sustains a pelvic fracture and soft-tissue injury to the thigh. An x-ray of the femur shows no fracture, but he has extreme tenderness over the lateral aspect of his thigh. He also has extreme pain with passive flexion and extension of his knee. He has normal strength in flexion and extension of the ankle. He is admitted overnight for observation. The next morning he develops dark-colored urine that is dipstick-positive for heme, but with no red blood cells on microscopic examination. What is the most concerning complication associated with this disease process?
   A. Hypokalemia
   B. Acidosis
   C. Sepsis
   D. Vascular insufficiency
   E. Acute renal failure

6-3. A 34-year-old man presents to the ED with a nondisplaced midshaft humerus fracture. He is evaluated by orthopedics and casted from the shoulder to mid-forearm. His distal neurovascular exam is normal. He returns the next day with increased pain, numbness over the medial aspect of the arm and hand, pain with grip, and difficulty manipulating his fingers. What is the most appropriate action?
   A. Obtain x-ray to look for interim displacement
   B. MRI to look for nerve damage
   C. Measurement of upper arm compartment pressures
   D. Removal of cast and re-examination in 30 minutes
   E. Open reduction and fixation of fracture

6-4. An 8-year-old boy falls off his bike onto his right hand. He presents to the ED with elbow pain and swelling. An x-ray shows a supracondylar fracture with 3 mm of posterolateral displacement. He has decreased sensation over the volar aspect of the forearm, a normal radial pulse, and no pain with passive flexion or extension of the fingers. He is able to flex and extend his wrist. What is the most appropriate management?

A. Immediate reduction and casting
B. Splint and admission for observation and reduction by orthopedics
C. Fasciotomy of the anterior arm compartment
D. Splint and discharge with orthopedic follow-up next day
E. Check anterior arm compartment pressures and ORIF if elevated

ANSWERS

6-1. C. Compartment syndrome is evident clinically by signs of muscle, nerve, or artery compression. The signs can be thought of as the "4 Ps": pain, pallor, paresthesias, pulselessness. However, this is inadequate and the diagnosis must always be considered when a patient has pain out of proportion to physical findings. **The most sensitive sign is pain with passive flexion and extension of the involved muscle bundle.** A thorough distal neurologic exam is important that includes motor and sensory testing. Intact distal pulses should not exclude the diagnosis.

6-2. E. This patient has sustained a crush injury of the upper leg with signs of compartment syndrome. Left untreated, this will lead to muscle necrosis and rhabdomyolysis, characterized by the release of intracellular contents such as myoglobin, creatine phosphokinase (CPK), lactate dehydrogenase (LDH), and potassium. This results in spilling of heme-containing myoglobin into the urine, manifesting as brown urine that is heme-positive on dipstick, but which shows no red blood cells on microscopic exam. **The most concerning complication of rhabdomyolysis is acute renal failure, although metabolic acidosis and hyperkalemia can also result.** Treatment is administration of a bicarbonate drip and a search for an etiology. In this case, thigh compartment pressures should be measured and the patient should be taken to the OR for fasciotomy if elevated.

6-3. D. This patient has evidence of ulnar nerve compression, likely due to the cast itself given his initial normal neurologic exam. Midshaft humerus fractures can sometimes be associated with radial nerve injuries, because the nerve runs posteriorly in a groove within the humerus bone. Radial nerve injury would be associated with numbness over the dorsum of the hand and weakness with wrist extension. The ulnar nerve innervates the intrinsic muscles of the hand and thus controls fine-motor movement of the fingers. **Ulnar nerve function should return within minutes of removing a tight-fitting cast.**

6-4. B. Supracondylar fractures in children must be treated very conservatively because of the high association with median nerve and brachial artery injury, and the risk of anterior arm compartment syndrome. Vascular injury results in volar compartment syndrome that can lead to a long-term complication referred to as Volkmann's ischemic contracture, or permanent and disabling flexion of wrist and fingers. This patient has evidence of median nerve injury, although not severe given only sensory deficits. Compartment syndrome is less likely given the painless passive ROM of the fingers and normal wrist strength. Therefore, acute reduction is not necessary. However, given the risk of swelling and subsequent development of compartment syndrome, he should be splinted and admitted to the hospital for observation. Most displaced supracondylar fractures are treated with closed reduction and percutaneous pinning.

 SUGGESTED ADDITIONAL READINGS

Gonzalez D. Crush syndrome. Crit Care Med 2005;33 (1 Suppl):S34–S41.

Greaves I, Porter K, Smith JE, et al. Consensus statement on the early management of crush injury and prevention of crush syndrome. J R Army Med Corps 2003;149:255–259.

Reis ND, Better OS. Mechanical muscle-crush injury and acute muscle-crush compartment syndrome. J Bone Joint Surg Br 2005;87:450–453.

Suzuki T, Moirmura N, Kawai K, et al. Arterial injury associated with acute compartment syndrome of the thigh following blunt trauma. Injury 2005;36:151–159.

Burn

CC: 43-year-old man presents with left lower extremity and left hand burns

HPI: B.B. is a 43-year-old man with a history of HIV who is brought to the ED after having suffered extremity burns. He admits to drinking on the day of presentation, and he last remembers sitting in bed smoking a cigarette. He thinks it possible that the cigarette lit the bed on fire. By the time EMS had arrived, he had already fled the burning bedroom. He denies SOB. His last tetanus shot was 3 years ago. He has had no prior HIV-related infections.

PMHx: HIV, hepatitis C, bipolar disorder

Meds: Stavudine (Zerit) 40 mg PO BID, lamivudine (Epivir) 150 mg PO BID, nevirapine (Viramune) 200 mg PO BID, dronabinol (Marinol) 5 mg PO QHS

ALL: Penicillin causes rash

SHx: Tobacco 1 ppd × 15 years; one to two beers per night; no drugs; lives in own house

VS: Temp 37.2°C (99.0°F), HR 96, BP 142/88, RR 20, Sao_2 98% on RA

PE: *General:* Awake, alert, oriented, cooperative; in no apparent distress. *HEENT:* Conjunctiva clear; no singed nasal or facial hair; no oral burns, oropharynx clear. *CV:* S_1, S_2; regular rate and rhythm; no murmurs, rubs, or gallops; pulses normal. *Chest:* Lungs clear to auscultation bilaterally; no respiratory distress. *Abd:* Soft, nontender, nondistended; bowel sounds present. *Extr:* Left ulnar edge of hand and pinky with blistering, erythema, tenderness to touch; left lower leg from proximal to distal tibia with areas of insensate, leathery, pale burns intermixed with some blistering, tender-to-touch areas; pulses 2+ PT/DP bilaterally; distal sensation intact. *Neuro:* Alert and oriented.

Labs: WBC 5.9 k/mm³, Hct 45.8%, carboxyhemoglobin (COHgb) 18% (normal <10%), chemistries within normal limits

THOUGHT QUESTIONS

- What immediate actions should be taken for this patient?
- How are thermal burns classified?
- How are thermal burns treated?
- How are chemical burns treated?

Immediate Actions:
Remove all clothing and any jewelry; place on 100% oxygen; establish IV and start 1 liter NS; estimate total BSA burned; send CBC, basic chemistries, and carboxyhemoglobin level; obtain CXR; cover burns with a clean, dry sheet.

Discussion:
The first priority for the burn patient is always airway protection. Immediate endotracheal intubation is indicated in the patient with shortness of breath, evidence of soot or swelling to the posterior oropharynx, or infiltrates on CXR. Patients may initially appear well but decompensate rapidly. The most common result of inhalation injury is carbon monoxide poisoning, which elevates blood levels of carboxyhemoglobin. COHgb less than 10% is normal, 10% to 20% is mild (e.g., headache, confusion), 20% to 40% is moderate (e.g., nausea), 40% to 60% is severe (e.g., altered mental status), and greater than 60% is fatal.

Thermal burns are classified traditionally into first-, second-, third-, and fourth-degree burns. First-degree burns affect only the epidermis; these do not require treatment other than cleansing and pain relief. Second-degree burns involve both the epidermis and the dermis, including superficial partial-thickness burns (extending only to the papillary layer of the dermis) and deep partial-thickness burns (extending into the reticular layer of the dermis). Superficial partial-thickness burns can be cleaned, debrided, then dressed with topical antibiotic ointment and gauze. Deep partial-thickness burns need

(Continued)

to be cleaned and may require surgical debridement and/or skin grafting. Third-degree burns are full-thickness burns that involve both the epidermis and dermis; these require surgical repair and skin grafting. Fourth-degree burns additionally involve underlying fat, muscle, or bone, and may require amputation. Extremity burns should be elevated for 24 to 48 hours. Patients who are discharged need their burns reevaluated at 24 hours. Tetanus immunization should be given if not up to date.

Chemical burns, like thermal burns, require immediate action. The chemical should be immediately removed or thoroughly washed away by water, debridement, or neutralization. Alkali substances, which cause liquefaction necrosis that allows deeper penetration of the irritant, generally produce greater damage than the coagulation necrosis caused by acids. Copious irrigation with water is required to remove the offending chemical.

 CASE CONTINUED

The patient is admitted to the hospital and has progressive swelling of his left lower extremity with a very tight, leathery eschar (scab) that is circumferential around the extremity. His pedal pulse decreases and capillary refill becomes sluggish. He is diagnosed with fourth-degree burns of the left lower extremity with impending vascular compromise. He is taken to the OR for fasciotomies of the anterior and lateral tibial compartments, debridement of thermally injured muscle and fascia, and split-thickness skin graft from the ipsilateral hip and thigh. After the procedure, his pedal pulse and capillary refill return to normal. He is managed in the burn unit with a morphine PCA pump for pain control, silver nitrate soaks with dressing changes to the left leg, and bacitracin BID to his left pinky. He is discharged in good condition after 9 days.

QUESTIONS

7-1. A 45-year-old woman is caught in a house fire. She has first- and second-degree burns to both legs anteriorly and the left arm front and back. What is the estimated percent body surface area (% BSA) of her burns?

    A. 9%

    B. 18%

    C. 23%

    D. 27%

    E. 36%

7-2. A 42-year-old man is rescued from a house fire. Upon arrival to the ED, he has facial burns and soot in his oropharynx. On primary survey, he has wheezing but no stridor. He has sustained about 30% BSA second-degree burns. What percentage of fire-related deaths are due to smoke inhalation?

    A. 10%

    B. 30%

    C. 50%

    D. 66%

    E. 75%

7-3. A 42-year-old woman presents to the ED after falling asleep in bed while smoking. She is extricated from her burning house by the fire department. Which of the following findings is most concerning regarding potential inhalation injury and her need for immediate endotracheal intubation?

    A. Soot in the mouth

    B. Stridor

    C. Singed nasal hair

    D. Hoarseness

    E. Expiratory wheezing

7-4. Which patient can be cared for on a regular medical floor instead of the burn unit?
- A. A 24-year-old woman with chemical burn to 5% of her face
- B. A 60-year-old man with a partial-thickness burn involving 12% of his BSA
- C. A 27-year-old man with a partial-thickness burn limited to his upper left arm in a circumferential manner
- D. A 25-year-old woman with a partial-thickness burn involving 12% of her BSA
- E. A 33-year-old man with a full-thickness burn limited to his scrotum

ANSWERS

7-1. D. The rule of 9s (Fig. 7-1) is used to estimate the percent body surface area (% BSA) involved in a burn. This is used to estimate burn severity and also to guide fluid resuscitation. **Each leg is 18% and each arm 9%. Therefore bilateral anterior leg involvement is 18%, plus 9% for the entire left arm.**

7-2. C. Fifty percent of all fire-related deaths are caused by smoke inhalation; it is the primary cause of mortality in burn patients. The three major types of toxic inhalants are tissue asphyxiants (e.g., carbon monoxide, hydrogen cyanide), pulmonary irritants, and systemic toxins. Carbon monoxide poisoning is a serious consequence of smoke inhalation. Clinical pulmonary compromise due to smoke inhalation may be minimal initially; however, the alkaline contents of toxins deposited in the bronchioles and alveoli cause a secondary chemical burn and exudation. Patients can develop ARDS.

7-3. B. Smoke inhalation is characterized by singed nasal hair, facial burns, hoarseness, expiratory wheezing, carbonaceous sputum, and soot in the mouth or nose. **Stridor is evidence of severe airway swelling and is an ominous sign.** Any patient with any of these findings should be considered for endotracheal intubation. Bronchoscopy is typically done to evaluate for bronchial soot and bronchial chemical burn.

7-4. D. Criteria for burn unit admission include second-degree burns over 15% of BSA (10% in children and those over 50 years of age), third-degree burns over 2% to 5% of BSA, second- and third-degree burns to functionally important areas (face, hands, feet,

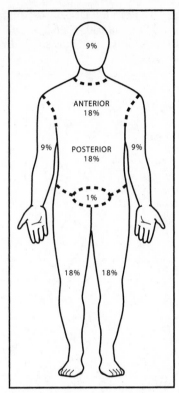

FIGURE 7-1 The Rule of Nines for estimating percentage of body surface area burned. (*Illustration by Shawn Girsberger Graphic Design.*)

genitalia, major joints), inhalation injury, circumferential burns, or any burn in someone with significant comorbid medical conditions.

 ### SUGGESTED ADDITIONAL READINGS

Bishop JF. Burn wound assessment and surgical management. Crit Care Nurs Clin North Am 2004;16:145–177.
Cone JB. What's new in general surgery: burns and metabolism. J Am Coll Surg 2005;200:607–615.

Thomas SJ, Kramer GC, Herndon DN. Burns: military options and tactical solutions. J Trauma 2003;54(5 Suppl):S207–218.
Wasiak J, Cleland H. Minor thermal burns. Clin Evid 2004;(12):2754–2763.

Dog Bite

CC: 79-year-old man presents with a dog bite laceration to the left hand

HPI: D.B. is a 79-year-old man who was bitten by the family dog on his left hand 3 days earlier. On the evening before presentation, his hand became red, slightly swollen, and warm to the touch. He has no pain in the hand or arm. He further denies fever, chills, or any other symptoms. The patient does not remember the date of his last tetanus booster. The dog is up to date on his vaccination shots.

PMHx: Hypertension

Meds: Furosemide (Lasix) 40 mg PO QAM, atenolol 50 mg PO BID

ALL: NKDA

VS: Temp 36.6°C (97.9°F), HR 61, BP 102/60, RR 16, Sao_2 97% on RA

PE: *General:* An older gentleman sitting in a wheelchair in no apparent distress. *Extr:* Dorsum of left hand with 4-cm healing laceration, 6 to 8 mm in width, overlying distal second and third metacarpals; edematous; erythema surrounding wound and streaking from wound toward wrist; no peripheral cyanosis. Mild limitation of index and middle finger flexion due to edema; minimal tenderness over edematous area; two-point discrimination and sensation to light touch intact distally. *Lymph:* No epitrochlear or axillary lymphadenopathy. *Skin:* Otherwise warm and intact elsewhere. *Neuro:* Alert and oriented.

THOUGHT QUESTIONS

- What is the initial management for this patient?
- How are bites managed differently than nonbite lacerations?
- Are lacerations with a delayed presentation managed differently than acute lacerations?
- Which patients with lacerations should get antibiotics?
- When is tetanus prophylaxis indicated?

Immediate Actions:

Obtain IV access; give ampicillin sulbactam (Unasyn) 3 g IV; obtain an x-ray if there is any suspicion of foreign body (e.g., broken tooth), fracture, joint penetration, or osteomyelitis; give tetanus toxoid 0.5 mL IM.

Discussion:

All bites and lacerations on the extremities should be assessed for distal function of tendons, nerves, and vessels before anesthesia is given. The most important factor in preventing infection is debridement of devitalized tissue and adequate wound irrigation (high pressure via syringe and 18-gauge needle with a splash guard using sterile saline, 1% povidone-iodine, or even clean tap water). Bites less than 1 to 2 cm in length and other puncture wounds should be allowed to heal by secondary intention, permitting wound base granulation, wound edge contraction, and re-epithelialization by natural means. Delayed primary closure, or suturing at 24 to 36 hours after the initial injury, can be used for wounds in cosmetically important areas. Larger bite lacerations can be treated like nonbite lacerations; however, primary closure should not be attempted after 12 hours following injury because of increased bacterial counts in the wound and therefore increased likelihood for infection if closed. Large bites in highly vascular areas such as the scalp, face, or neck can be closed up to 24 hours after injury.

(*Continued*)

Routine antibiotic prophylaxis for simple lacerations is not recommended. The following wounds should receive prophylactic antibiotics: any human or cat bite, crush wounds, or deep puncture wounds that cannot be adequately debrided or irrigated, and wounds that are grossly contaminated. Adult tetanus and diphtheria toxoid 0.5 mL IM should be given for any patient with a clean or minor wound whose last tetanus shot was greater than 10 years ago; for all other wounds, Td should be given if last tetanus shot was greater than 5 years ago. For those with unknown or incomplete immunization status, tetanus immunization should be started with Td; for dirty wounds, tetanus immune globulin 250 units should also be given to those with incomplete immunization.

CASE CONTINUED

The patient's dog bite laceration, now 3 days after injury, should not be sutured; it is left open to heal by secondary intention. The bite has led to a hand cellulitis. The patient is admitted to the hospital for treatment with Unasyn 3 g IV every 6 hours for the first 24 to 36 hours or until his cellulitis appears well under control. Treatment also includes warm soaks of the left hand for 15 minutes four times daily for the first 2 to 3 days and elevation of the hand above the level of the heart. After 36 hours of treatment, the swelling and erythema is considerably reduced; he has regained full flexion and extension of his MCP joints. He is discharged on amoxicillin-clavulanate (Augmentin) 875 mg PO BID for 7 days, to be followed up by his primary care doctor in 1 week.

QUESTIONS

8-1. A 56-year-old construction worker who stepped on a long nail at the worksite develops osteomyelitis. Which of the following is the most likely bacterial pathogen involved?

    A. *Staphylococcus aureus*
    B. *Actinobacter*
    C. *Eikenella*
    D. *Klebsiella*
    E. *Pseudomonas*

8-2. A 64-year-old man presents to the ED 1 day after his cat bit him on his right ring finger. Examination leads to the diagnosis of flexor tenosynovitis. Which of the following is a cardinal sign of this condition?

A. Tenderness over the flexor tendon sheath
B. Absence of edema of the finger
C. Pain with passive flexion
D. Extension of the involved digit at rest
E. Erythema of the flexor surface of the involved digit

8-3. A 41-year-old man presents to the ED with a small, jagged laceration on the dorsum of the metacarpophalangeal region after a fistfight. After irrigation and tetanus toxoid, the patient is discharged with a first-generation cephalosporin to cover likely staphylococci or streptococci. What other bacterial species should be covered?

A. *Pasteurella*
B. *Eikenella*
C. *Pseudomonas*
D. *Actinomyces*
E. *Escherichia coli*

8-4. A 28-year-old nurse presents to the ED 15 minutes after a needle-stick accident to her left thumb that occurred while drawing blood from a patient in the OR. Which of the following infections is she at greatest risk of acquiring in this setting?

A. HIV
B. HAV
C. HBV
D. HCV
E. HEV

ANSWERS

8-1. E. Possible sequelae of puncture wounds include cellulitis, abscesses, osteomyelitis, and septic arthritis. Complication rates are higher for puncture wounds than for simple lacerations because the former are difficult to irrigate properly, and the depth of the wound is easily underestimated. Cellulitis is the most common complication of puncture wounds. **Osteomyelitis, when it occurs, is due to *Pseudomonas* organisms in 90% of cases and thus answer choice E is the correct answer.**

8-2. A. The four cardinal signs of flexor tenosynovitis are flexion of the involved digit at rest, tenderness over the flexor

tendon sheath, symmetric or sausage-like swelling of the finger, and pain with passive extension. These cases often require surgical debridement in order to preserve function of the involved digit and hand. IV antibiotics should be started and a hand surgeon consulted.

    8-3. B. The location of this man's wound is classic for "clenched-fist" injury, which occurs when the patient's fist strikes the teeth of another person. Patients may try to conceal the actual cause of their wound obtained from fighting. **Penicillin (or amoxicillin) should be added to this patient's antibiotic regimen to cover *Eikenella*, which has been isolated in up to 15% of clenched-fist injuries and can cause osteomyelitis, septic arthritis, and abscesses of the hand.** For dog and cat bites, *Pasteurella* should be covered with penicillin (or amoxicillin). Coverage for *Pseudomonas* should be included for plantar puncture wounds through athletic shoes and for wounds contaminated by freshwater. *Actinomyces* are one type of anaerobic bacteria isolated from dog bite wounds. *Escherichia coli* are not usually associated with skin wounds.

    8-4. C. Given that the needle-stick exposure is from a contaminated needle, the risks of infection are as follows: 0.3% for HIV, 9% for hepatitis B virus, and 1.8% for hepatitis C virus. The risks of infection for hepatitis A virus and hepatits E virus have been estimated to be negligible after an inadvertent needle-stick injury (these are transmitted by the fecal–oral route). High-risk exposures are needle-sticks with a large-bore hollow needle that had been used for venipuncture in a patient with known infection or someone with HIV risk factors. Prophylactic postexposure treatment can reduce the risk of HIV transmission by 80%. The following agents are currently recommended for this purpose: zidovudine (AZT) and lamivudine (3TC) combination (Combivir), nelfinavir (Viracept), and indinavir (Crixivan).

 ## SUGGESTED ADDITIONAL READINGS

Capellan O, Hollander JE. Management of lacerations in the emergency department. Emerg Med Clin North Am 2003;21:205–231.

Chaudhry MA, Macnamara AF, Clark S. Is the management of dog bite wounds evidence based? A postal survey and review of the literature. Eur J Emerg Med 2004;11:313–317.

Mills AM, Chen EH. Are blood cultures necessary in adults with cellulitis? Ann Emerg Med 2005;45:548–549.

Fall on an Outstretched Hand

CC: 60-year-old woman who fell on her right out-stretched hand

HPI: W.F. is a 60-year-old right-handed woman who decided to take up rollerblading and fell, bracing her fall with her right hand. She heard a snap and had excruciating pain in her right wrist. She did not strike her head and was ambulatory after the fall. Her friend drove her to the ED. Her only complaint is right wrist pain and numbness in her index and middle fingers.

PMHx: None

Meds: None

ALL: NKDA

SHx: No alcohol, drug, or tobacco use

VS: Temp 37.0°C (98.6°F), HR 98, BP 132/88, RR 16, Sao₂ 100% on RA

PE: *General:* Alert, healthy woman in moderate distress. *HEENT:* Atraumatic. *Neck:* Supple; no midline cervical tenderness; full ROM without pain. *CV:* S₁, S₂; regular rhythm; no murmurs. *Chest:* Clear bilaterally; nontender. *Abd:* Soft; nontender. *Extr:* Obvious dorsal deformity of distal right wrist; no lacerations or skin tenting; intact radial pulse and good capillary refill; 5/5 motor strength with flexion/extension of all five digits; able to hold fingers open against resistance; able to oppose thumb and fifth digit; decreased sensation to light touch over palmar aspect of index and middle fingers.

Imaging Studies: See Figure 9-1 for x-ray.

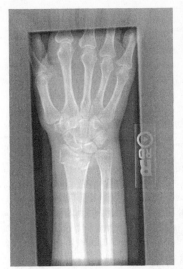 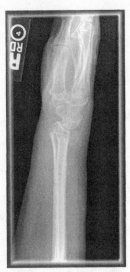

FIGURE 9-1 Anteroposterior (A) and lateral (B) views of the right wrist show a comminuted distal radius fracture with dorsal displacement and angulation of the distal fragment. There is shortening and possible intra-articular involvement, as well as an associated ulnar styloid fracture. (*Image courtesy of Massachusetts General Hospital, Boston.*)

THOUGHT QUESTIONS

- What is the initial management for this patient?
- What are the five components of describing a fracture?
- What are the most important aspects of the physical exam?
- In which situations is an orthopedics consultation required?

Immediate Actions:
Establish IV and administer morphine 6 mg IV; prepare for fracture reduction with finger traps, 10 mL of 2% lidocaine in a syringe with an 18-gauge needle, and splinting materials for a sugar-tong splint.

(*Continued*)

Discussion:

It is very important to be able to describe the nature of a fracture so that you can communicate effectively with your orthopedic consultants over the phone. Fracture description should consist of five identification components (Table 9-1). An open fracture is any fracture exposed to a break in the skin. Anatomic location includes the name of the bone and whether the proximal, middle, or distal third is affected. Simple fractures include transverse, oblique, and spiral fractures; the orientation of the fracture line is described relative to the long axis of the bone. Comminuted fractures have more than two fragments. Displacement is always described by the position of the distal fragment relative to the proximal one, using the anatomic position as a reference. For the wrist, displacement can be dorsal, volar, lateral, or medial. For the femur, displacement can be anterior, posterior, lateral, or medial. Angulation refers to deviation of the distal fragment relative to the proximal one. Instead of lateral and medial, angulation of the distal fragment is termed *valgus* (away from the midline) or *varus* (toward the midline). It is also essential to describe whether the fracture is intra-articular (i.e., involving the joint) or whether it is impacted (i.e., distal fragment jammed into proximal one).

A thorough distal neurovascular exam is essential before manipulation of the fracture is undertaken. This includes sensation to light touch and two-point discrimination in all distal dermatomes, plus motor function of all major muscle groups. Baseline ROM should also be assessed. A vascular exam should consist of distal pulses and capillary refill.

TABLE 9-1 Five Components of Describing a Fracture

Open versus closed	Open includes bone protrusion through skin or laceration over fracture site
Anatomic location	Specific bone and location within proximal, middle, or distal third
Type of fracture	Transverse, oblique, spiral, comminuted
Displacement	Translation of the distal fragment relative to the proximal fragment
Angulation	Deviation of the distal fragment creating an angular deformity

(*Continued*)

Many fracture reductions are done in the ED, including displaced distal radius, ankle, metacarpal, finger, and toe fractures. Displaced long-bone fractures (e.g., humerus, femur, tibia) generally require orthopedic consultation and ORIF in the OR. However, in a setting in which the OR is not readily available and neurovascular compromise is present, these fractures must also be reduced promptly in the ED. Orthopedics consultation is also required for open fractures because they need to be opened in the OR, debrided, and irrigated

CASE CONTINUED

This patient has a comminuted, distal radius fracture (Colles' fracture) with about 50% dorsal displacement, 20% dorsal angulation, and possible intra-articular involvement. There is also an associated ulnar styloid fracture. The patient's right hand is placed in finger traps that serve to elevate the hand over her head and supply traction to the fracture site. The deformity over the dorsum is prepped with Betadine, and an 18-gauge needle (attached to a syringe with 10 mL of 2% lidocaine) is placed into the fracture space. Medullary blood is withdrawn to assure proper location, and 10 mL of lidocaine is injected into the fracture (referred to as a *hematoma block*). This provides excellent anesthesia. The fractured wrist is then manipulated with both hands in order to push the distal fragment back up and into alignment. Once this is achieved, an assistant applies a plaster splint that is molded into position in order to maintain alignment of the fracture fragments. A repeat x-ray shows good alignment. The patient is discharged with a sling and a short course of narcotic analgesics. Orthopedics follow-up is arranged for the next morning because of the comminution and possibility of intra-articular involvement. The orthopedic surgeon is pleased with the fracture alignment and chooses to leave the splint in place and forego surgery.

QUESTIONS

9-1. An 18-year-old woman falls onto her right hand while rollerblading. She presents to the ED with severe distal forearm pain and deformity. She has numbness over the thenar eminence and has difficulty moving her fingers due to pain. Her capillary refill seems somewhat delayed. An x-ray shows a distal radius fracture with about 25% dorsal displacement. Which structure is most commonly injured in association with her fracture?

    A. Radial nerve
    B. Median nerve
    C. Ulnar nerve
    D. Radial artery
    E. Ulnar artery

9-2. An 82-year-old woman with osteoporosis slips and falls onto her right hip. She cannot get up and is brought to the ED by ambulance. As you enter the room you notice her right leg is abducted and externally rotated. What type of injury does she most likely have?

    A. Posterior hip dislocation
    B. Subtrochanteric femur fracture
    C. Intertrochanteric femur fracture
    D. Femoral neck fracture
    E. Acetabular fracture

9-3. An 8-year-old boy falls off his bike onto his outstretched hand with his elbow in extension. He presents to the ED with obvious anterior bowing of his distal humerus. His distal neurovascular exam is intact. The x-ray shows a transverse supracondylar humerus fracture with dorsal displacement and angulation of the distal fragment. Which is the most appropriate treatment?

    A. Fracture reduction and splinting
    B. Fracture reduction and casting
    C. Immediate ORIF in the OR
    D. Splinting, discharge, orthopedic follow-up the next day
    E. Splinting, admission for neurovascular checks

9-4. In the fracture described in the preceding question, the fracture originates in the metaphysis and a portion of it extends into the physis (growth plate) without extending through to the epiphysis. How is this fracture classified?
   A. Salter I
   B. Salter II
   C. Salter III
   D. Salter IV
   E. Salter V

ANSWERS

9-1. B. The median nerve is most often injured with a distal radius fracture of this type (Colles' fracture) because it courses over the volar aspect of the distal radius just before it enters the carpal tunnel into the hand. Dorsal displacement and angulation of the distal fragment can result in stretching of the median nerve and commonly causes sensory deficits over the thumb, index, and middle fingers. The ulnar nerve supplies sensation to the hypothenar eminence, fifth finger, and the ulnar half of the fourth finger. The radial nerve supplies most of the dorsum of the hand. The median nerve supplies musculature for flexion of the thumb, index, and middle fingers, and for opposition of the thumb. The ulnar nerve controls finger abduction and adduction (i.e., fanning fingers out and in). The radial nerve is responsible for wrist extension.

9-2. C. Given the anatomic position of her right leg (abducted and externally rotated), she either has an intertrochanteric femur fracture or displaced femoral neck fracture. Intertrochanteric fractures are much more common and universally result in external rotation because these fractures are located just distal to the fibrous joint capsule that stabilizes the femoral head and neck. Therefore, the powerful gluteus maximus is allowed to externally rotate and abduct the distal fracture fragment (i.e., the femur). The leg is also commonly shortened due to the action of both the hip flexors and extensors. Most hip dislocations are posterior and, as a result, the leg tends to be shortened, adducted, and internally rotated.

9-3. C. Supracondylar humerus fractures occur almost exclusively in children younger than 10 years because at that age the strength of the elbow joint capsule and collateral ligaments is greater than that of the bone. These injuries occur when a child falls onto his or her hyperextended arm. **As the distal humerus**

fractures, it bows forward into the antecubital fossa, which contains the median nerve, the radial nerve, and the brachial artery. Injuries to these structures are very common in this type of fracture; therefore, a supracondylar fracture in children is considered an orthopedic emergency. The best treatment is immediate ORIF in the OR.

9-4. B. The Salter-Harris classification for fractures involving the growth plate (physis) was developed many years ago and is still used as a predictor for subsequent growth delays. The Salter classification can be remembered by the mnemonic SALTeR: **S**ilent—no radiographic evidence of fracture (injury is confined to physis and diagnosis is made clinically based on tenderness); **A**bove—fracture enters metaphysis *above* the physis then extends into it; **L**ower— fracture enters epiphysis from *lower* than (below) the physis (i.e., intra-articular), then extends into it; **T**hrough—fracture extends from metaphysis to epiphysis *through* the physis; **R**ammed—physis is crushed entirely and on x-ray appears *rammed*.

 SUGGESTED ADDITIONAL READINGS

Anderson SJ. Lower extremity injuries in youth sports. Pediatr Clin North Am 2002;49:627–641.

Gomez JE. Upper extremity injuries in youth sports. Pediatr Clin North Am 2002;49:593–626.

Medoff RJ. Essential radiographic evaluation for distal radius fractures. Hand Clin 2005;21:279–288.

Nijs S, Broos PL. Fractures of the distal radius: a contemporary approach. Acta Chir Belg 2004;104:401–412.

Shoulder Pain

CC: 27-year-old woman with right shoulder pain

HPI: S.P. is a 27-year-old woman who was at the gym doing inclined bench presses when she went to put the bar back in place and missed; the bar fell and her right shoulder felt like it "came out." She presents to the ED complaining of severe right shoulder pain, but denies any numbness or tingling in the right arm. She has never had any shoulder problems before.

PMHx: Hemorrhoids

Meds: None

ALL: NKDA

SHx: Denies tobacco, drugs; occasional alcohol

VS: Temp 36.9°C (98.4°F), HR 90, BP 142/86, RR 18, Sao$_2$ 99% on RA

PE: *General:* Thin, healthy-appearing; holding right arm across her chest. *Chest:* Clear bilaterally. *Extr:* Right upper extremity slightly abducted and externally rotated; subcoracoid prominence; subacromial depression; unable to adduct or internally rotate shoulder secondary to pain; normal pinprick sensation over deltoid; neurovascularly intact distally with 2+ radial pulse; warm; good capillary refill at fingers. *Neuro:* 5/5 motor strength at elbow and wrist; 2+ sensory in all dermatomes.

THOUGHT QUESTIONS

- What is the initial management for this patient?
- How does one distinguish anterior from posterior shoulder dislocations?

- Which tests or studies, if any, should be performed if you suspect a dislocation?
- What is the treatment for dislocation?

Immediate Actions:
Establish IV access; give morphine 4–6 mg IV; obtain shoulder x-rays.

Discussion:
Dislocations of the shoulder may be suggested by history (e.g., mechanism of injury) and examination (e.g., presence of obvious deformity and inability to raise arm); confirmation is made by x-rays that include AP and axillary views (isolated view of the glenohumeral joint) of the shoulder. Plain x-rays should be obtained both before and after reduction attempts of any dislocation. In some dislocations (e.g., knee), vascular injury is quite common, and arteriography may be necessary. Treatment of dislocation requires reduction under conscious (procedural) sedation or adequate analgesia. Reduction is carried out by essentially reversing the mechanism of injury. Some dislocations (e.g., hip, knee, ankle) are at substantial risk for complications and will often require orthopedic consultation after the joint has been reduced. Less severe dislocations (e.g., fingers, elbow, shoulder) may only require orthopedic follow-up. For dislocations that cannot be reduced in the ED, surgical intervention is necessary. The presence of distal neurovascular compromise is an indication for immediate reduction.

CASE CONTINUED

Right shoulder films confirm an anterior shoulder (glenohumeral) dislocation without an associated fracture; the AC joint is normal (Figure 10-1). Conscious sedation is achieved with fentanyl 100–300 µg and midazolam (Versed) 4 mg IV, both titrated until the patient is well sedated and able to tolerate dislocation reduction. Traction is applied to the humerus with the arm in slight extension.

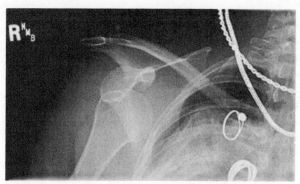

FIGURE 10-1 AP view of the shoulder shows dislocation
with inferior displacement of the humeral head relative to the
glenoid. (*Image courtesy of Massachusetts General Hospital,
Boston.*)

The arm is slowly flexed at the shoulder and externally rotated.
After 5 minutes of traction and slow manipulation, a "thunk" is
felt. The patient feels immediate relief. Repeat shoulder films show
a properly relocated joint. The patient is discharged with ibuprofen
800 mg PO TID, Percocet one to two tablets PO Q4 hr PRN pain, a
shoulder immobilizer, intermittent ice for swelling (not applied
directly to skin), and orthopedics follow-up in 1 week.

 QUESTIONS

10-1. While rollerblading, a 29-year-old man falls onto his out-
stretched left hand. He is wearing wrist guards, helmet, and knee
pads. If he were to dislocate a joint with the described mechanism,
which of the following joints would it likely be?
   A. Ankle
   B. Elbow
   C. Knee
   D. Shoulder
   E. Hip
   F. Sternoclavicular
   G. Lisfranc injury

10-2. A 2-year-old girl is brought to the ED by her mother who says the child had been fine prior to their walk outdoors but now refuses to use her right arm. You see that the girl holds her arm slightly flexed at the elbow; there is no swelling, ecchymoses, or obvious deformity, but she cries when you palpate the radial head. Which of the following terms best describes her condition?

   A. Sprain
   B. Strain
   C. Subluxation
   D. Dislocation
   E. Fracture

10-3. A 15-year-old boy dislocates his shoulder anteriorly after falling during a football tackle. What is the most common complication of this dislocation?

   A. Humeral head compression fracture (Hill-Sachs deformity)
   B. Axillary artery injury
   C. Brachial plexus injury
   D. Recurrent dislocation
   E. Fracture of the anterior glenoid lip (Bankart's fracture)

10-4. A 26-year-old man is involved in a motor vehicle collision and dislocates his left knee. Which of the following is the most likely associated injury?

   A. Popliteal artery injury
   B. Peroneal nerve injury
   C. Compartment syndrome
   D. Posterior tibial nerve injury
   E. Popliteal vein injury

ANSWERS

10-1. B. Elbow dislocations are the second most common type of large-joint dislocations, most often displaced posteriorly from a fall on an outstretched hand. The most common major joint dislocation is at the shoulder (glenohumeral) joint; most are anterior dislocations. The shoulder is susceptible to dislocation because of its wide range of motion and lack of intrinsic bony stability. The least common major joint dislocation is that of the sternoclavicular joint, which occurs with high-mechanism trauma to the chest and is associated with significant thoracic trauma. Ankle dislocations occur universally with associated fractures and neurovascular compromise. All ankle dislocations should be reduced immediately and splinted before x-rays are obtained. Knee and hip dislocations require a significant mechanism of injury and are associated with injuries to the joint capsule, ligaments, soft tissue, and often the neurovascular bundle. Reduction of hip dislocations must be done as soon as possible to prevent complications such as avascular necrosis, traumatic arthritis, and joint instability. Lisfranc injury refers to any dislocation or fracture-dislocation of the tarsometatarsal joints.

10-2. C. The patient has "nursemaid's elbow," or radial head subluxation, which is a common injury in very young children and results from pulling their forearm while in pronated position. Subluxation refers to partial loss of continuity between two articulating surfaces, while dislocation refers to complete loss of continuity between two articulating surfaces. Sprain refers to ligamentous injury resulting from abnormal motion of a joint. Strain refers to injury to muscle or tendon from excessive stretch or contraction. Fracture refers to a break in the continuity of bone or cartilage.

10-3. D. In patients younger than 20 years, recurrent dislocation is the most common complication following anterior shoulder dislocation and occurs with 90% likelihood. The likelihood of recurrent dislocation is much lower for older patients. Humeral head compression fracture (Hill-Sachs deformity) and other bony injuries (e.g., fracture of the anterior glenoid lip or greater tuberosity) are common complications of anterior shoulder dislocation as well. Vascular injury (e.g., axillary artery) is uncommon and happens more often in elderly patients. Nerve injury occurs in about 10% to 25% of cases and usually affects the axillary nerve, though the radial, ulnar, median, and musculocutaneous nerves as well as the brachial plexus can also be injured.

10-4. A. Popliteal artery injury occurs in 50% of patients with knee dislocations. The popliteal artery runs posteriorly in the popliteal fossa; it is immobile because of its attachments proximally to the femur (adductor magnus hiatus) and distally to the tibia (interosseous membrane). The popliteal vein and peroneal nerve, which run with the popliteal artery, can also be injured. All knee dislocations require angiography after reduction to exclude vascular injury. Compartment syndrome and posterior tibial nerve injury are possible but less common.

SUGGESTED ADDITIONAL READINGS

Perron AD, Brady WJ. Evaluation and management of the high-risk orthopedic emergency. Emerg Med Clin North Am 2003;21:159–204.

Quillen DM, Wuchner M, Hatch RL. Acute shoulder injuries. Am Fam Physician 2004;70:1947–1954.

Ufberg JW, Vilke GM, Chan TC, Harrigan RA. Anterior shoulder dislocations: beyond traction-countertraction. J Emerg Med 2004;27:301–306.

Knee Pain and Fever

CC: 28-year-old man with knee pain and fever

HPI: K.P. is a 28-year-old man who has had a sore right knee for 3 days. Today the pain got worse and the knee became mildly swollen. He began to feel ill this morning, with a fever up to 38.9°C (102.0°F) and chills. He now has difficulty bearing weight on his right leg. He has not had penile discharge or burning with urination. He has had no new sexual contacts. He admits to weekly use of IV heroin.

PMHx: Chlamydial urethritis treated 4 years ago

Meds: None

ALL: NKDA

SHx: Occasional IV heroin use; smokes 1/2 ppd; occasional alcohol use

VS: Temp 38.6°C (101.5°F), HR 106, BP 128/88, RR 16, Sao_2 99% on RA

PE: *General:* Alert, healthy man who appears mildly ill. *HEENT:* No pharyngeal lesions; conjunctiva clear. *CV:* S_1, S_2; mildly tachycardic; regular rhythm; no murmurs. *Chest:* Clear bilaterally. *Abd:* Soft; nontender. *GU:* No penile lesions; normal testicles. *Extr:* Right knee swollen, erythematous, warm; ballotable patella; tender to palpation; extreme pain elicited with passive motion. *Skin:* No rashes or lesions. *Neuro:* Alert and oriented.

THOUGHT QUESTIONS

- What is the initial management for this patient?
- What is the differential diagnosis for monoarticular pain?

- How is the joint aspirate analyzed to differentiate septic arthritis from other etiologies?
- Which antibiotics should be used to cover this patient empirically?

Immediate Actions:
Start IV and send blood for CBC with differential, basic chemistries, and blood cultures; obtain urethral swab and send for *Chlamydia* and *Neisseria gonorrhoeae*; obtain knee x-ray; obtain joint fluid aspirate and send for Gram's stain, culture, cell count and differential, crystals, protein, and glucose.

Discussion:
Septic arthritis should be suspected in a patient with monoarticular joint pain and fever, especially in patients with risk factors such as underlying joint disease, arthroplasties, recent joint surgery, IV drug use, and young age with STI risk factors. In adults, monoarticular arthritis is more commonly caused by osteoarthritis, trauma, gout, and pseudogout; these processes can mimic septic arthritis. In children, the differential diagnosis includes JRA, transient synovitis, Legg-Calve-Perthes disease (avascular necrosis of the hip), and slipped capital femoral epiphysis (fractured epiphysis of the femoral head). Less common etiologies include seronegative spondyloarthropathies (Reiter's syndrome, psoriatic arthritis, IBD, ankylosing spondylitis) and reactive arthritis to other bacterial or viral infections (*Chlamydia*, *Salmonella*, *Shigella*, Lyme disease, *Yersinia*, hepatitis B, adenovirus, parvovirus, EBV).

The most important aspect of joint fluid analysis is a Gram's stain and culture to detect microorganisms. Crystal analysis is necessary, although the presence of crystals does not exclude bacterial infection. A leukocyte count greater than 50,000 cells/mm^3 suggests a diagnosis of septic arthritis, although bacterial infection may exist with counts less than 50,000 cells/mm^3. The ratio of joint fluid to serum glucose is typically 1:2 or smaller in septic arthritis. *Staphylococcus aureus* is the most common pathogen, followed by streptococci and *N. gonorrhoeae*. If the Gram's stain is negative, empiric coverage should include nafcillin in addition to ceftriaxone to cover penicillin-resistant *Neisseria*. Joint irrigation by an orthopedic specialist is also necessary in order to remove bacteria and debris.

CASE CONTINUED

The joint aspirate is cloudy and shows 86,000 leukocytes per mm³ with 90% polys, glucose of 48 mg/dL, and a Gram's stain that shows gram-positive cocci in clusters, suggesting *S. aureus*. An x-ray shows an effusion but no evidence of osteomyelitis. Nafcillin 2 g IV Q4 hr is started. Orthopedics is consulted; they perform a joint irrigation at the bedside with three large-bore catheters. The patient is admitted for IV antibiotics and extremity elevation. Blood and fluid aspirate cultures are positive for *S. aureus* that is sensitive to nafcillin. An echocardiogram is done to rule out endocarditis, given that the patient is an IV drug user. The patient recovers uneventfully.

QUESTIONS

11-1. A 22-year-old man presents to the ED with right knee swelling. The knee is swollen and tense, with a ballotable patella. Upon further history he has had urethral discharge that resolved about 2 weeks ago without treatment. On exam, he has no genital lesions or discharge but he does have scattered papules over his abdomen and legs. Which of the following is an accurate statement regarding his condition?

A. Synovial leukocyte count is usually more than 50,000 cells per mm³.

B. Synovial glucose level is usually elevated.

C. Synovial Gram's stain is normal in 75% of cases.

D. Genital, pharyngeal, or rectal cultures are positive in only 20% of cases.

E. Synovial culture is positive in greater than 75%.

11-2. A 53-year-old diabetic man with a history of rheumatoid arthritis and right knee replacement 15 months ago presents with 2 days of right knee swelling. He mentions that he occasionally uses intravenous heroin. He has no fever. He has extreme knee pain with passive range of motion. Which of the following is the greatest risk factor for developing septic arthritis?

A. Rheumatoid arthritis

B. Past joint surgery

C. Adulthood

D. History of IVDA

E. Diabetes mellitus

11-3. A 68-year-old man presents with a swollen, warm knee. Synovial analysis shows 76,000 WBCs per mm³. The Gram's stain is pending. Which of the following would be a poor choice to use as one of a two-drug combination for empiric treatment of this patient's condition?

   A. Ceftriaxone
   B. Oxacillin
   C. Penicillin
   D. Vancomycin
   E. Ciprofloxacin

11-4. A patient presents with knee swelling and is concerned about septic arthritis that he states he has had before and was treated with antibiotics without an operation. Septic arthritis due to which of the following organisms would require IV antibiotic treatment only without joint irrigation?

   A. *Staphylococcus aureus*
   B. *Staphylococcus epidermidis*
   C. *Neisseria gonorrhoeae*
   D. *Escherichia coli*
   E. Joint irrigation is always indicated

ANSWERS

11-1. C. *Neisseria gonorrhoeae* is a common cause of septic arthritis in young, sexually active adults. Primary gonorrheal infection is usually urethral or cervical, although primary rectal and pharyngeal infections must be considered as well. Disseminated gonorrhea can occur within days or weeks of the primary infection; symptoms include fevers, chills, migratory polyarthralgias, and scattered hemorrhagic macules or papules on the trunk and extremities. Disseminated gonorrhea results in purulent arthritis (usually in the knee joint) in 40% of cases. The common finding is sterile purulent joint fluid, which implicates a significant role of the host immune response. Fluid leukocytes are typically less than 50,000 cells/mm³, and the glucose is normal. **The Gram's stain is positive in only 25% of cases, and the culture is positive in only 50% of cases.** Genital, pharyngeal, or rectal cultures are positive in approximately 75% of cases.

11-2.   D. **Underlying joint disease (e.g., rheumatologic disorders, crystal arthropathies, osteoarthritis), recent knee surgery or prosthetic joints, multiple sexual partners, and IV drug**

use are all risk factors for developing septic arthritis. **The most common cause of septic arthritis is believed to be hematogenous spread, making this patient's greatest risk factor his IV drug use.** The immunocompromised, elderly, and diabetics are also at increased risk. Septic arthritis is more common in children than in adults, with most cases occurring in children younger than 2 years. Complications of infection for children are serious, including extension of infection into joint cartilage and bone, disruption of the epiphyseal plate and therefore future growth, and, in hip joint infections, avascular necrosis of the femoral head. Septic arthritis must be considered in any child with a fever and a limp. A thorough joint exam must be done on any infant who presents with a fever.

11-3. C. Penicillin does not cover _Staphylococcus aureus_, and streptococci are often penicillin-resistant. Antistaphylococcal penicillins include methicillin, nafcillin, oxacillin, and dicloxacillin. Methicillin-resistant _S. aureus_ requires coverage with vancomycin. Ceftriaxone is a reasonable choice in addition to an antistaphylococcal penicillin to cover _Neisseria gonorrhoeae_ and gram-negative organisms, which are more common in elderly patients. Similarly, ciprofloxacin can be used as an adjunct to cover gram-negative organisms as well as provide double coverage for _S. aureus_.

11-4. C. Joint irrigation by an orthopedist is essential for cases of septic arthritis except for those caused by _Neisseria gonorrhoeae_. It has been demonstrated that IV ceftriaxone alone is sufficient in treating this condition. This may be due to the low or absent joint bacterial burden found in gonococcal septic arthritis and in part to the excellent joint penetration of ceftriaxone. However, in cases in which the joint fluid leukocyte count is greater than 50,000 cells per mm^3 in the presence of _Neisseria_ infection, joint irrigation is typically performed anyway.

 SUGGESTED ADDITIONAL READINGS

Calmbach WL, Hutchens M. Evaluation of patients presenting with knee pain: Part II. Differential diagnosis. Am Fam Physician 2003;68:917–922.

Shetty AK, Gedalia A. Management of septic arthritis. Indian J Pediatr 2004;71:819–824.

Shirtliff ME, Mader JT. Acute septic arthritis. Clin Microbiol Rev 2002;15:527–544.

Swan A, Amer H, Dieppe P. The value of synovial fluid assays in the diagnosis of joint disease: a literature survey. Ann Rheum Dis 2002;61:493–498.

CASE **12**

Hip and Sternum Pain in a Sickle-Cell Patient

CC: 30-year-old woman with pain in the hips and sternum

HPI: H.S. is a 30-year-old woman with history of sickle-cell anemia (SCA) who complains of pain in her hips and sternum similar to her usual sickle-cell pain crises. She denies fevers, chills, shortness of breath, cough, nausea, vomiting, diarrhea, or abdominal pain. She says she has no chest pain other than her usual sternal pain. Her pain started yesterday, and she has lost her appetite since then.

PMHx: SCA, stroke at age 4 with no residual deficits, pulmonary infarct 10 years ago with acute chest syndrome, asthma, s/p appendectomy, s/p cholecystectomy, seizures at ages 16 and 18. Meds: Albuterol, docusate sodium (Colace), hydromorphone (Dilaudid), hydroxyurea (Hydrea), senna (Senokot), oxycodone (OxyContin)

ALL: Penicillin, meperidine (Demerol), erythromycin

FHx: SCA in several cousins

SHx: Single mother of 6-year-old girl. Denies tobacco, alcohol, or drugs

VS: Temp 38.1°C (100.5°F), HR 120, BP 130/76, RR 26, SaO$_2$ 100% FM

PE: *General:* Well-developed, well-nourished, in mild-moderate distress. *HEENT:* Frontal bossing. *Neck:* Supple; nontender. *CV:* S$_1$, S$_2$; regular; no murmurs; 2+ radial and DP pulses bilaterally. *Chest:* Lungs clear bilaterally. Sternum tender to palpation. Portacath palpable below right upper chest. *Abd:* Soft; nontender, nondistended, no organomegaly. *Extr:* Tenderness to palpation of bilateral hips. *Skin:* No rashes; warm, dry. *Neuro:* Alert and oriented; cranial nerves II to XII intact; normal speech; no motor or sensory deficits.

THOUGHT QUESTIONS

- What are the immediate actions for this patient?
- What are the four types of crises that patients with SCA can develop?
- Which tests can be helpful for evaluating a patient with a sickle-cell crisis?
- What are some of the possible sequelae of SCA and which organ systems are affected?

Immediate Actions:
Administer high-flow oxygen, run normal saline wide open, administer hydromorphone (Dilaudid) 2–4 mg Q15–30 minutes PRN pain or according to schedule agreed upon by primary care provider and patient.

Discussion:
Patients with SCA can develop vaso-occlusive (thrombotic) crisis, hemolytic crisis, sequestration crisis, and/or aplastic crisis. *Vaso-occlusive crises* occur most commonly and are thought to be the cause of acute pain episodes. Sickled red blood cells cause occlusion of small vessels in the bone marrow, leading to bone ischemia and/or infarction, causing severe pain. Precipitating factors are many, including infection, cold, and stress. Pain can be located anywhere, such as the back, chest, long bones, and abdomen. Lab and radiographic tests that may be helpful for determining the type of crisis and for ruling out infection include CBC, reticulocyte count, LFTs, blood bank sample, urinalysis, chest x-ray, and blood cultures. Patients with SCA have a chronic hemolytic anemia with a baseline hematocrit usually between 20% and 30%, but can develop a hemolytic crisis in which their compensated balance is disrupted. *Hemolytic crises* are rare, and usually occur in patients with G-6-PD deficiency as well as SCA; it may also occur due to iron or folate deficiency. Hemolytic crisis causes liver congestion and hepatomegaly, and worsens chronic jaundice. *Sequestration crises* are also rare and are usually seen in young children, who can present with abdominal pain, distention, splenomegaly, lethargy, pallor, or

(Continued)

hypovolemic shock. Sequestration crisis is due to vascular occlusion within the splenic sinusoids, which then leads to entrapment of large volumes of blood within the spleen. Splenectomy is sometimes necessary. Sequestration crisis is the most common cause of death in children with SCA under the age of one year. *Aplastic crises* are characterized by severe marrow depression such that the body does not make enough new RBCs (reticulocyte count <2%) to make up for very low hemoglobin (usually at least 2 g/dL lower than patient's baseline). Aplastic crisis can be precipitated by infection, classically with parvovirus B19, or more rarely by folate deficiency. These patients can present pale, lethargic, or even in shock.

There are numerous sequelae of sickle-cell disease that have been described, involving all organ systems. Examples include acute chest syndrome (superinfection of pulmonary infarction), other infections such as pneumonia and osteomyelitis, stroke, avascular necrosis, "fish-mouth vertebrae" (from marrow hyperplasia, osteopenia, and softening of the vertebral end plates), dactylitis (painful swelling of the hands and feet with fever), bossed skull, skin ulcers, priapism, and cholelithiasis, just to name a few. The patient presented in this case has many features that are classic of SCA patients, including history of stroke, acute chest syndrome, and cholecystectomy, as well as a bossed skull on physical examination.

CASE CONTINUED

In addition to oxygen and IV fluids, H.S. receives 12 mg IV of hydromorphone (Dilaudid) over an hour, a dosing schedule establilshed by her hematologist. She becomes very sleepy, but still complains of pain. Her respirations remain adequate. Her labs are remarkable for WBC 16.3 k/mm³, Hct 28.7% (baseline for her), AST 128 U/L, AP 195 U/L, TB 7.2 mg/dL, DB 3.1 mg/dL, reticulo-cyte count 24.5%, and urinalysis positive for bilirubin. Given her fever, a chest x-ray is obtained, which shows possible early infil-trates in the lower lobes (Figure 12-1). Blood cultures are drawn and she is started on vancomycin, given her indwelling venous catheter. She is admitted for pain control, antibiotics, and observa-tion. During her hospital stay, her hematocrit reaches a nadir of 18%, for which she is given 2 units of PRBCs and a 10-day course

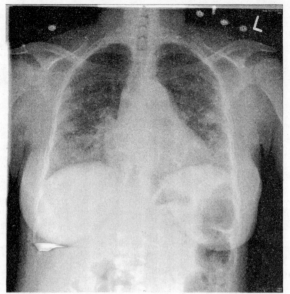

FIGURE 12-1 PA view of the chest shows possible early infiltrates in the lower lobes. (*Image courtesy of Brigham and Women's Hospital, Boston.*)

of hydroxyurea (Hydrea). Her blood cultures grow out methicillin-sensitive *S. aureas* (MSSA), thought possibly due to line infection. She has her Portacath removed in the OR. Her pain is controlled with oxycodone (OxyContin) 240 mg PO TID, hydromorphone (Dilaudid) 14 mg IV Q1–2 hr PRN, and amitryptylline 50 mg PO QHS. She is discharged in good condition on hospital day 13.

QUESTIONS

12-1. A 21-year-old man with SCA complains of 3 to 4 weeks of intermittent unilateral severe headache with contralateral extremity numbness, and now one week of intermittent gait instability, like he is "falling to one side." He also has pain in both arms and both legs today, which is similar to his usual crisis pain. His last pain crisis was a few months ago. His exam is remarkable only for mild tachycardia at 111 bpm and general appearance of mild to moderate discomfort. His neurologic exam is normal. His labs come back with Hgb 3.3 g/dL, Hct 9.7%, plt 48 k/mm^3, retic ct 0.6%, MCV 125 μm^3 (fL) per cell (normal approximately 79-95 μm^3 per cell). In addition to his pain crisis, which of the following best describes his condition?

A. Vaso-occlusive crisis
B. Hemolytic crisis
C. Sequestration crisis
D. Aplastic crisis
E. Malingering

12-2. A 31-year-old woman with sickle-cell trait is most likely to experience which of the following?

A. Frequent pain crises
B. Hematuria
C. Stroke
D. Avascular necrosis
E. Acute chest syndrome

12-3. A 23-year-old man with SCA presents to the ED complaining of bilateral hip pain, similar to his usual pain crises, and a painful erection for the past few hours. He denies penile trauma. Which of the following would be most useful for this condition?

A. Phentolamine
B. Papaverine
C. Packed red blood cells
D. Arterial embolization
E. Fresh frozen plasma

12-4. A 28-year-old woman with SCA presents to the ED complaining of cough, chest pain, and shortness of breath. She is febrile and tachypneic. Which of the following organisms is most likely?
A. *Mycoplasma pneumoniae*
B. *H. influenzae* type b
C. *S. pneumoniae*
D. *Pneumocystis carinii*
E. *Klebsiella* species

ANSWERS

12-1. D. This patient has a very low hematocrit with an inappropriately low reticulocyte count, which reflects bone marrow dysfunction. This is referred to as aplastic crisis. His pain is due to vaso-occlusive, or thrombotic, crisis. His neurologic symptoms are likely transient ischemic attacks due to inadequate cerebral oxygenation from anemia and sickling. Malingering refers to pretending to have symptoms or disease in order to achieve secondary gain other than just being a patient.

12-2. B. Sickle-cell trait refers to the condition of having one normal hemoglobin gene and one sickle cell hemoglobin gene; these patients are largely asymptomatic. Approximately 8% to 10% of African-American babies born in the United States have sickle-cell trait. These persons rarely have sickling crises and only occasionally have splenic infarction. More often, they may experience spontaneous bleeding, such as hyphema and hematuria, or hyposthenuria (inability to concentrate the urine maximally). This patient is thus most likely to experience hematuria. The other options listed are classic complications in persons homozygous for the sickle-cell gene (patients with SCA).

12-3. C. This patient is experiencing priapism, which is a painful, sustained penile erection and a known complication of SCA that can arise due to veno-occlusion by sickled cells in the penis. **Priapism occurs in as many as 10% to 40% of male patients with SCA and can result in impotence. Immediate treatment includes IV fluids, oxygen, pain medication, and urologic consultation; packed red blood cell transfusion may also help.** Some studies show that terbutaline, a β-agonist, may be useful as well. Arterial embolization is only effective in high-flow priapism arising due to a site of arterial bleeding, as may occur following trauma. Phentolamine (an α-antagonist) and papaverine are both agents that cause vasodilation and are used by some patients to induce an erection, which may inadvertently lead to priapism. Intra-cavernous injection of an α-agonist, such as phenylephrine, can reverse the effects of phentolamine and papaverine.

12-4. A. This patient likely has acute chest syndrome, a complication seen in patients with SCA and characterized by fever, cough, chest pain, tachypnea, dyspnea, and leukocytosis. The most likely bacterial pathogen of those listed is *Mycoplasma pneumoniae*; about one-fifth of cases of acute chest syndrome are due to *Mycoplasma pneumoniae* or *Chlamydia pneumoniae*. *S. pneumoniae* and *H. influenzae* are other common pathogens of this condition. *Pneumocystis carinii* is associated with pneumonia in patients with AIDS. *Klebsiella* is classically associated with pneumonia in alcoholics.

 SUGGESTED ADDITIONAL READINGS

Davies SC, Oni L. Management of patients with sickle cell disease. BMJ 1997;315(7109).

De D. Sickle cell anaemia 2: management approaches of painful episodes. Br J Nurs 2005;14:484–489.

O'Connor CE. Recognizing and managing sickle cell crisis in the emergency department. Ir Med J 2003;96:229–230.

II

Patients
Presenting
with Altered
Mental Status
and Neurologic
or Psychiatric
Complaints

Acute Mental Status Change and Headache

CC: 50-year-old man presents with acute onset of confusion and headache

HPI: C.H. is a 50-year-old healthy man who presents to the ED with a coworker who states that the patient had an episode of confusion. The man was driving a pick-up truck with the coworker when he began to swerve off the road. His coworker was able to control the vehicle and bring it to a stop on the side of the road. His coworker describes the patient as being "dazed." He states that the patient didn't know where he was and that he complained of a headache. His coworker drove him to the ED. On arrival to the ED, the patient complains of an occipital headache and mild neck stiffness. He has no recollection of driving earlier. He denies nausea or vomiting. He denies recent trauma, illness, fevers, or chills. He denies recent drug or alcohol use. He denies chest pain or shortness of breath.

PMHx: None

Meds: None

ALL: NKDA

SHx: No alcohol or drugs; 1 ppd smoker

VS: Temp 37.4°C (99.3°F), HR 80, BP 260/130 (MAP 170), RR 16, Sao_2 98% on RA

PE: *General:* Mild pallor and diaphoresis; awake, alert, but mildly confused. *HEENT:* Nonicteric sclerae; pupils 4 mm and reactive bilaterally; no retinal hemorrhages or papilledema; oropharynx moist without exudates; no hemotympanum. *Neck:* Supple; no discomfort to passive flexion. *CV:* S_1, S_2; regular; no murmurs; 2+ radial and DP pulses bilaterally. *Chest:* Clear bilaterally. *Abd:* Soft; nontender. *Rectal:* Guaiac-negative brown stool. *Extr:* No edema, cyanosis, rashes. *Neuro:* Oriented to place, but not time or day; able to answer questions appropriately but states he feels confused; cranial nerves II to XII grossly intact; normal speech; 5/5 motor strength in major muscle groups in upper and lower extremities; normal sensation to light touch and sharp object in all extremities; normal finger-to-nose test.

THOUGHT QUESTIONS

- What interventions need to be done immediately?
- What life-threatening processes need to be considered and ruled out?
- How does the likely etiology of altered mental status (AMS) change with increasing age?
- Does severe hypertension point you to a more specific etiology?

Immediate Actions:
Place oxygen by nasal cannula; check rapid fingerstick glucose; place large-bore antecubital IV; send CBC, basic metabolic panel, PT/PTT, clot to the blood bank; get 12-lead EKG; start nitroprusside drip per dosing protocol to maintain SBP less than 160 or MAP less than 110 mm Hg; take patient immediately to CT scanner.

Discussion:
Hypoxia should be the first consideration in any patient who presents to the ED with AMS. Check breathing and oxygen saturation immediately, then give oxygen. Hypoglycemia should be the second consideration. All patients with AMS require either a rapid fingerstick, or empiric glucose given orally or intravenously. Myocardial infarction should be the next consideration; therefore, obtain a 12-lead EKG, especially if the patient is older than 50 years. These three etiologies are often missed on initial evaluation because it is not intuitive to associate these with AMS. Now a differential diagnosis for AMS can be formulated by systematically starting from top to bottom. Common etiologies for AMS are listed in Table 13-1.

(Continued)

The combination of sudden onset of AMS with a headache, stiff neck, and hypertension are strongly suggestive of a subarachnoid hemorrhage. A hemorrhagic stroke, whether subarachnoid or intraparenchymal, typically causes acute systemic hypertension. As blood accumulates within the closed cranium, the ICP rises, which triggers an autoregulatory increase in mean arterial pressure. This acute rise in blood pressure can exacerbate intracranial bleeding; thus, rapid blood pressure control is essential.

TABLE 13-1 Etiologies for Altered Mental Status

Primary CNS	Ischemic or hemorrhagic stroke, meningitis, seizure, space-occupying lesion
Toxic	Stimulants, anticholinergics, sedatives, alcohol withdrawal, and many others
Metabolic	Hypoglycemia, hypercalcemia, uremia, hyponatremia
Infectious	Meningitis, pneumonia, UTI
Cardiovascular	Acute myocardial infarction
Pulmonary	Hypoxia due to pneumonia, pulmonary edema, or other pulmonary process
Shock	*Hypovolemic* due to massive GI bleeding or exsanguination, *cardiogenic* due to myocardial infarction, *septic* due to bacteremia

CASE CONTINUED

Intravenous nitroprusside is started with a goal to maintain a MAP of about 100 mm Hg. The patient is rolled immediately to the CT scanner, which shows a subarachnoid hemorrhage without any mass effect or evidence of transtentorial herniation (Figure 13-1). The head of the bed is elevated to 30 degrees to minimize increased ICP. Phenytoin (Dilantin) 1 g IV is given to prevent seizures. Neurosurgery is consulted and a CT angiogram (CT scan after intravenous contrast injection) is obtained, which shows a ruptured MCA berry aneurysm. The patient is taken to the OR for a craniotomy and aneurysm clipping.

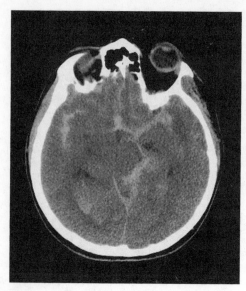

FIGURE 13-1 Non-contrast head CT shows large subarachnoid hemorrhage (hyperdense regions) in the basal subarachnoid spaces of the brain, suggesting a ruptured berry aneurysm. (*Image courtesy of Massachusetts General Hospital, Boston.*)

QUESTIONS

13-1. A 75-year-old man with history of poorly controlled hypertension presents to the ED with complaint of sudden onset severe headache. His BP is 220/140. He rapidly becomes combative and confused. What is the best first step in this patient's management?

A. Administer mannitol 10 mg IV in order to increase the cerebral-serum osmolar gradient.

B. Rapid-sequence intubation and subsequent hyperventilation.

C. Call neurosurgery to take the patient to the OR.

D. Administer furosemide 20 mg IV to decrease ICP.

E. Administer 1 liter NS bolus IV in order to increase the cerebral perfusion pressure.

13-2. A 91-year-old woman is diagnosed with a subarachnoid hemorrhage due to an arteriovenous malformation seen on CT angiography after presenting to the ED with the worst headache of her life. She is a nursing home resident with multiple medical problems but is mentally sharp and declines neurosurgery. She is therefore started on several new medications, including nimodipine. Nimodipine is given to prevent which of the following complications?

  A. Seizure
  B. Cerebral artery vasospasm
  C. Rebleeding
  D. Hydrocephalus
  E. Tachycardia

13-3. A 30-year-old woman presents to the ED with a history of sudden-onset severe headache and nausea. She has a history of migraine headache but states that the quality of this headache is different from her usual migraine. She is afebrile, with no signs of meningismus (e.g., neck stiffness, photophobia, positive Kernig's sign), and has a normal neurologic exam. A CT scan of her head is normal. What is the next step in her management?

  A. Discharge home with rectal prochlorperazine (Compazine) and close instructions to return if her symptoms worsen.
  B. Observe for 6 hours, administer another liter of normal saline, and discharge home if she continues to feel better.
  C. Perform a lumbar puncture to exclude subarachnoid hemorrhage.
  D. Consult a neurologist for evaluation of atypical migraines.
  E. Observe for 6 hours and then obtain a repeat CT scan; if normal, discharge home.

13-4. A 72-year-old woman with history of orthostatic hypotension, Barrett's esophagus, polycystic kidney disease, gout, endometriosis, and remote head trauma s/p MVC 30 years prior is diagnosed with a subarachnoid hemorrhage after presenting with an unrelenting headache of the past two days. Which of the following is a risk factor for subarachnoid hemorrhage?

  A. History of orthostatic hypotension
  B. History of Barrett's esophagus
  C. History of polycystic kidney disease
  D. History of gout
  E. History of endometriosis
  F. History of head trauma
  G. Old age

ANSWERS

13-1. B. This patient has clinical signs concerning for an acute intracranial hemorrhage, likely subarachnoid or intraparenchymal given the history. Because his mental status is quickly deteriorating, rapid-sequence intubation (RSI) should be performed first. RSI provides airway protection for a patient who is at extremely high risk for vomiting and aspiration, which often leads to chemical pneumonitis and sepsis. RSI also allows for chemical sedation, which eliminates anxiety and agitation, thus decreasing ICP. It further allows for mechanical ventilation and blowing off of carbon dioxide; this has also been shown to decrease ICP. Neurosurgery should ideally see a patient before paralytic agents are used in order to obtain a baseline neurologic exam; however, RSI should never be delayed in a patient who is rapidly deteriorating. Answer choices A and D are reasonable steps but should follow RSI. Calling neurosurgery is also critical, but again, RSI should not be delayed.

13-2. B. Seizure, cerebral artery vasospasm, rebleeding, and hydrocephalus are complications of SAH, as well as increased ICP. Rebleeding accounts for 25% of deaths related to SAH. Therefore, operative repair of the bleeding source, either a berry aneurysm or arteriovenous malformation, is important. Patients are started on an anticonvulsant, such as phenytoin, to prevent seizures. **Vasospasm of affected cerebral arteries is a significant cause of morbidity within the first 3 weeks after SAH, which can lead to an ischemic territorial stroke. To prevent this, patients are started on a calcium channel blocker, typically nimodipine 60 mg PO every 6 hours, to maintain cerebral vasodilation.**

13-3. C. Recent literature suggests that in patients with a good story for subarachnoid hemorrhage (i.e., sudden onset of the "worst headache of my life"), a CT scan will be normal in 15% of those with SAH. Therefore, the current standard of care is to follow a normal CT scan with a lumbar puncture if there is any suspicion for SAH. Xanthochromia, or a yellow tinge in the cerebrospinal fluid, will appear if the hemorrhage is greater than 12 hours old. Xanthochromia is detected in most labs by mass spectrometry and is suggestive of SAH. If the symptoms are less than 12 hours old, SAH is diagnosed by the same or increased number of red blood cells in tube 4 as compared with tube 1. If red cells are present, further studies must be performed to exclude the possibility of a leaking aneurysm (e.g., CT angiogram, MR angiogram, or angiography).

13-4. C. History of polycystic kidney disease is a risk factor associated with subarachnoid hemorrhage, as are fibromuscular dysplasia, hypertension (especially severe), history of aneurysms or vascular lesions in other areas of the body, and family history of SAH. Spontaneous SAH tends to occur more in those between 30 and 50 years old. The other choices listed are not known to be risk factors for SAH.

 ## SUGGESTED ADDITIONAL READINGS

Ward TN, Levin M, Phillips JM. Evaluation and management of headache in the emergency department. Med Clin North Am 2001;85:971–985.

Wijdicks EF, Kallmes DF, Manno EM, et al. Subarachnoid hemorrhage: neurointensive care and aneurysm repair. Mayo Clin Proc 2005;80:550–559.

Wilson SR, Hirsch NP, Appleby I. Management of subarachnoid hemorrhage in a non-neurosurgical centre. Anaesthesia 2005;60:470–485.

Acute Mental Status Change and Fever

CC: 42-year-old man presents with acute onset of confusion and fever

HPI: C.F. is a 42-year-old healthy man who presents to the ED with new-onset confusion and agitation. He was seen earlier in the ED for a complaint of facial pain and green nasal discharge. He was diagnosed with acute sinusitis and discharged home on a 14-day course of amoxicillin-clavulanate (Augmentin). He returns 4 hours later with his wife, who states he was behaving strangely and seemed confused. He is having sweats and a worsening headache, but he denies neck or back pain. He has no nausea or vomiting. He has no complaints of focal numbness or weakness, and he has no difficulty walking.

PMHx: None

Meds: None

ALL: NKDA

SHx: No alcohol, drugs, or tobacco

VS: Temp 39.6°C (103.3°F), HR 110, BP 190/90, RR 16, Sao$_2$ 98% on RA

PE: *General:* Ill-appearing, diaphoretic; awake, confused, agitated. *HEENT:* Nonicteric sclerae; pupils 4 mm and reactive bilaterally; moderate papilledema; oropharynx dry without exudates; no hemotympanum. *Neck:* Stiff with passive flexion. *CV:* S$_1$, S$_2$; regular; tachycardic; no murmurs; 2+ radial and DP pulses bilaterally. *Chest:* Clear bilaterally. *Abd:* Soft; nontender. *Rectal:* Guaiac-negative brown stool. *Extr:* No edema, cyanosis, or rashes. *Neuro:* Oriented to hospital, but not time or day; does not answer questions appropriately or cooperate with exam; cranial nerves II to XII grossly intact; no dysarthria; 5/5 motor strength in major muscle groups in upper and lower extremities; normal sensation to light touch and sharp object in all extremities.

THOUGHT QUESTIONS

- Which interventions need to be done immediately?
- Which life-threatening diagnoses must be considered with fever and altered mental status (AMS)?
- Which organisms are most common in meningitis for neonates? For children and adults?
- Which empiric antibiotic coverage should be used in suspected meningitis before Gram's stain or culture results are available?

Immediate Actions:
Protect yourself by wearing a mask (see Case 41 for details about respiratory and other types of precautions); perform rapid fingerstick glucose; place large-bore antecubital IV; send CBC, basic metabolic panel, PT/PTT, clot to the blood bank, blood cultures; hang ceftriaxone 2 g IV; perform 12-lead EKG; take patient immediately to head CT, followed by an LP if the scan is normal.

Discussion:
As with any patient with AMS, one must first think of abnormalities in oxygenation, perfusion, or serum glucose. Therefore, oxygen saturation, peripheral pulses, 12-lead EKG, and fingerstick glucose should be done. The next concern is for an acute intracranial process such as subarachnoid or intraparenchymal bleeding; the patient needs a head CT immediately. Fever and AMS should raise concern for acute bacterial meningitis. This disease is rapidly progressive and uniformly deadly, so when it is suspected, the patient needs IV antibiotics *before* imaging or LP are performed. Concern about sterilizing the CSF and altering the results of the LP are unfounded and pose great danger to the patient. Other disease processes that could cause fever and AMS include brain abscesses, more commonly seen in IV drug abusers

(*Continued*)

or those with endocarditis. Toxoplasmosis or cysticercosis is more prevalent in immunocompromised patients. Viral encephalitis caused by HSV or varicella-zoster can also present similarly. Viral meningitis is difficult to distinguish clinically from bacterial meningitis and is a diagnosis of exclusion after CSF culture results are negative for bacterial growth.

The most common organisms in neonates are group B *Streptococcus* and *Neisseria meningitidis*. In children and adults, the most common organisms are *Streptococcus pneumoniae*, *Neisseria meningitidis*, and *Listeria monocytogenes*. Ceftriaxone is commonly the first-line empiric agent because of its broad coverage of gram-negative and gram-positive organisms. It also readily crosses the blood–brain barrier. Ampicillin is added for coverage against *Listeria*. Vancomycin should also be added to cover cephalosporin-resistant strains of streptococcus. Acyclovir is given empirically to cover against herpes encephalitis. For patients with confirmed meningococcal (*Neisseria*) meningitis, all close contacts must receive prophylactic antibiotics because of the high incidence of transmission. Prophylaxis includes rifampin 600 mg (10 mg/kg) PO every 12 hours for four doses or ciprofloxacin 500 mg PO in a single dose (for adults only). Prophylaxis is not required for other types of meningitis.

CASE CONTINUED

Ceftriaxone 2 g IV is given and the patient goes directly to head CT, which is normal. He becomes more disoriented and agitated, and is thus intubated for airway protection and anesthesia for the LP. The LP reveals cloudy CSF with an opening pressure greater than 40 cm of water. The cell count reveals 11,000 white cells/mm^3, 400 red cells/mm^3, protein 740 mg/dL, and glucose 24 mg/dL (see Table 14-1 for interpretation of CSF results). Vancomycin 1 g IV and ampicillin 2 g IV are given. The Gram's stain shows gram-positive cocci in pairs, consistent with *S. pneumoniae*. The patient is admitted to the medical ICU.

TABLE **14-1** Differentiation Between Bacterial and Viral Meningitis Based on CSF Results

	Normal	Bacterial	Viral
Cell count (WBC)	<5 cells/mm³	*Usually* >500 cells/mm³	*Usually* <500 cells/mm³
Cell differential	<1 PMN/mm³	*Usually* PMN predominant	Nearly 100% lymphocytes
Red cells	None	Elevated	Elevated
Protein	15–45 mg/dL	*Often* >100 mg/dL	50–100 mg/dL
Glucose	45–65 mg/dL	*Often* <40 mg/dL	Normal
Opening pressure	5–20 cm H₂O	*Often* >20 cm H₂O	Usually normal
Gram's stain	No organisms	Organisms seen 80% of time	No organisms

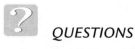

QUESTIONS

14-1. An 18-year-old boy presents to the ED with a fever, headache, and neck stiffness over the past day. His temperature is 40.2°C (104.4°F), pulse 106, and blood pressure 116/74. On physical exam he looks ill and his neck is stiff. He has a normal neurologic exam. A lumbar puncture reveals 5 WBC/mm³ and 1,240 RBC/mm³ in tube 1, and 6 WBC/mm³ and 1,360 RBC/mm³ in tube 4. The CSF protein is 68 mg/dL and the glucose is 78 mg/dL. This boy most likely has:

    A. Subarachnoid hemorrhage

    B. *Listeria* meningitis

    C. HSV encephalitis

    D. Pneumococcal meningitis

    E. Subdural hematoma

14-2. A 76-year-old woman presents with altered mental status and fever. A lumbar puncture shows 1,600 WBC/mm³ with 94% PMNs. She is started on ceftriaxone, vancomycin, ampicillin, and acyclovir and admitted to the ICU. Which of the following is associated with Waterhouse-Friderichsen syndrome?

    A. Seizure disorder

    B. Focal paralysis or sensory loss

    C. Intellectual impairment

    D. Sensorineural hearing loss

    E. Bilateral adrenal hemorrhage

14-3. A 16-year-old girl presents to the ED with fever, headache, and neck stiffness. On exam, she has flexion of the hips and knees in response to passive flexion of the patient's neck. What name is associated with this sign?
A. Kernig
B. Cullen
C. Psoas
D. Brudzinski
E. Rovsing

14-4. A 32-year-old man presents with headache and subjective fever for 4 days. Which of the following CSF results would be reassuring, suggesting a diagnosis other than bacterial meningitis?
A. WBC greater than 5 cells/mm^3 in an adult
B. WBC greater than 30 cells/mm^3 in a neonate
C. Decreased CSF protein
D. Opening pressure greater than 20 cm H$_2$O
E. Decreased CSF glucose

ANSWERS

14-1. C. HSV is the most common cause of encephalitis in the United States. HSV-1 is the causative agent in 95% of cases, and the patient often has simultaneous mucocutaneous manifestations of HSV infection. HSV encephalitis typically concentrates in the temporal lobes and can be identified by MRI. **Characteristic CSF findings are elevated RBCs without significant elevation in WBC. Protein is also mildly elevated.** Given the elevated CSF erythrocyte count, this entity may be difficult to distinguish from subarachnoid hemorrhage, and further imaging may be indicated to exclude a ruptured aneurysm or arteriovenous malformation. Treatment for HSV encephalitis is IV acyclovir.

14-2. E. Acute bacterial meningitis is a devastating illness with a mortality of up to 20% even with treatment. Mortality is significantly higher in those who do not receive early treatment and in those who present with altered mental status or focal neurologic findings. Complications are common and include intellectual impairment, seizure disorder, focal neurologic impairment, hydrocephalus, hearing loss, and others. **The Waterhouse-Friderichsen syndrome describes bilateral adrenal hemorrhage, which is more common with meningococcal meningitis.**

14-3. D. Brudzinski's sign refers to flexion of the hips and knees in response to passive flexion of a patient's neck, indicative of meningeal irritation. Kernig's sign in meningitis is elicited while the patient's hip is flexed by extending the knee—contraction, pain, or resistance of the hamstrings is a positive result. The psoas sign is used to help diagnose appendicitis, while Cullen's sign refers to periumbilical ecchymosis or bluish discoloration and may be seen in hemorrhagic pancreatitis or with other retroperitoneal hemorrhage. Rovsing's sign refers to pain in the RLQ elicited by palpation or pressure in the LLQ, indicative of acute appendicitis.

14-4. C. Increased, rather than decreased, CSF protein would be expected in meningitis. The other options listed, including WBC greater than 5 cells/mm³ in an adult or greater than 30 cells/mm³ in a neonate, opening pressure greater than 20 cm H_2O, and decreased glucose, would be findings consistent with meningitis. See Table 14-1 for a description of CSF results for bacterial versus viral meningitis. However, it is important to realize that these guidelines are not absolute and that bacterial meningitis must be considered in anyone with more than 5 WBC/mm³ in the CSF. Bacterial meningitis typically has greater than 500 WBC/mm³, with a predominance of PMN cells. Viral meningitis, which has a benign clinical course, is usually characterized by fewer than 500 WBC/mm³, almost all of which are lymphocytes. However, bacterial meningitis may also have a lymphocytic predominance, especially if the WBC count in the CSF is less than 1,000 cells/mm³. Any patient with a suspicion for bacterial meningitis must be admitted and treated at least until the CSF cultures show no bacterial growth and the patient is clinically improving.

 ## SUGGESTED ADDITIONAL READINGS

Chavez-Bueno S, McCracken GH Jr. Bacterial meningitis in children. Pediatr Clin North Am 2005;52:795–810.

De Gans J, van de Beek D. Dexamethasone in adults with bacterial meningitis. N Engl J Med 2002;347:1549–1556.

Gendelman HE, Persidsky Y. Infections of the nervous system. Lancet Neurol 2005;4:12–13.

Peate I. An overview of meningitis: signs, symptoms, treatment and support. Br J Nurs 2004;13:796–801.

Weakness and Malaise

 CC: 82-year-old man with weakness and malaise

HPI: W.M. is an 82-year-old man with widely metastatic prostate cancer status post palliative chemotherapy who complains of being weak and not feeling himself for the last few days. He reports that he had the "shakes" and felt cold with malaise, but denies fevers, nausea, or vomiting. He has a history of bilateral ureteral obstruction and is status post bilateral nephrostomy tube placements. He also has an indwelling suprapubic tube, which was last changed 2 weeks ago due to hematuria and obstruction. He suffers from chronic diarrhea but has had negative *C. difficile* testing. He denies chest pain, shortness of breath, palpitations, headache, cough, abdominal pain, dysuria, hematuria, or any other specific complaints.

PMHx: Metastatic prostate cancer with bilateral ureteral obstruction; metastases to lung, right pelvis, lumbar spine, and liver; s/p multiple chemotherapies, currently undergoing mitoxantrone chemotherapy. Spinal stenosis, hypertension, hyperlipidemia, nephrolithiasis, Ogilvie syndrome, s/p bilateral orchiectomy, s/p back surgery, GERD, DVT right leg s/p IVC filter.

Meds: ASA 81 mg PO QD, atorvastatin (Lipitor) 20 mg PO QD, levofloxacin 250 mg PO QOD, MVI 1 tab PO QD, iron polysaccharide (Niferex), KCl, dexamethasone (Decadron) 4 mg PO QD, esomeprazole (Nexium) 20 mg PO QD

ALL: NKDA

SHx: Lives with wife, denies tobacco and alcohol use

VS: Temp 37.2°C (99.0°F), HR 125, BP 90/palp, RR 30, S_aO_2 93% on room air

PE: *General:* Pale-appearing elderly gentleman, sallow but in no apparent distress. *HEENT:* Nonicteric sclerae; pupils 3 mm and reactive bilaterally; oropharynx with dry mucous membranes, without erythema or exudates; normal tympanic membranes. *Neck:* Supple; full range of motion, no bruits, no thyromegaly, no lymphadenopathy. *CV:* S_1, S_2; regular, mildly tachycardic, III/VI systolic murmur at apex; 2+ radial and carotid pulses bilaterally, 1+ DP pulses bilaterally. *Chest:* Clear bilaterally. *Abd:* Soft; nontender; moderately distended abdomen; no hepatosplenomegaly; hypoactive bowel sounds, suprapubic tube in proper position. *Back:* Bilateral nephrostomy tubes with no evidence of skin infection surrounding sites. *Skin:* Few areas of ecchymosis and dry scaling on extremities and trunk. *Neuro:* Alert and oriented; cranial nerves II to XII intact; normal speech; 5/5 motor strength in major muscle groups in upper and lower extremities; normal sensation to light touch and sharp object in all extremities; no pronator drift.

THOUGHT QUESTIONS

- What are the immediate actions for this patient?
- What is the likely source of this patient's presenting problem?
- What is early goal-directed therapy (EGDT)?
- Who should receive "stress-dose" steroids?

Immediate Actions:
Place large-bore antecubital IV; send CBC, basic metabolic panel, PT/PTT, two sets of blood cultures, urinalysis, and urine culture; place oxygen by nasal cannula; place on cardiac monitor and obtain 12-lead EKG; obtain portable chest x-ray; give dexamethasone (Decadron) 10 mg IV; administer levofloxacin 500 mg IV, vancomycin 1 g IV, and metronidazole (Flagyl) 500 mg IV; administer 2 L normal saline over 30 minutes and reassess blood pressure.

Discussion:
Sepsis, or septic shock, is due to overwhelming infection in the bloodstream by endotoxin-producing bacteria, classically gram-negative bacteria but very frequently *Streptococcus* and *Staphylococcus* species as well. Circulating endotoxins lead to

(Continued)

release of inflammatory mediators that in turn dilate peripheral capillary beds. This causes leaking of intravascular fluids into surrounding tissue, or third-spacing, causing hypotension and decreased end-organ perfusion. The end-result is a precipitous illness, multi-organ failure, and impending death. Symptoms and signs to be wary of include fever or hypothermia, tachypnea, tachycardia, altered mental status, rigors, gray or mottled appearance, hypotension, or decreased urine output. Labs may show leukocytosis with bandemia, acidosis, or elevated lactate.

Early goal-directed therapy (EGDT) is a stepwise approach to treating sepsis, instituted upon presentation to the ED and continued for the first 6 hours until the patient can be admitted to the intensive care unit (ICU). The EGDT protocol was studied by Rivers and associates who were able to demonstrate a 16% decrease in absolute mortality. Inclusion criteria for EGDT are patients with suspected infection (e.g., fever, tachycardia, increased respiratory rate, leukocytosis) and systolic blood pressure less than 90 mm Hg after a 1- to 2-liter bolus of normal saline. The cornerstone of EGDT is broad-spectrum antibiotic coverage after two sets of blood cultures have been drawn. Endotracheal intubation should be considered early in sepsis since breathing itself can account for 30% of the basal metabolic energy demand. A central venous catheter is placed in the internal jugular (IJ) or subclavian vein, which allows for measurement of central venous pressure (CVP). CVP is a surrogate for overall intravascular fluid status. Normal saline should be administered rapidly until a CVP of 8 to 12 mm Hg is reached, thus "filling the tank." Vasopressors should only be added once the target CVP is reached, and the goal is to maintain a mean arterial pressure (MAP) greater than 65 mm Hg. Once CVP and MAP goals are achieved, central venous oxygen saturation (S_vO_2) is measured, which is a surrogate for tissue oxygenation, or tissue perfusion. The latter is a function of blood oxygen carrying capacity (i.e., hemoglobin level) and cardiac output. If the S_vO_2 is less than 70% and hematocrit is less than 30%, then blood transfusion is initiated. Once the hematocrit is greater than 30% and the S_vO_2 remains below 70%, dobutamine is added to increase cardiac output up to a maximum dose of 20 μg/kg.

There are many factors to consider when treating patients with sepsis, not the least of which is trying to determine and adequately treat the underlying precipitant. Often a source of infection is obvious

(*Continued*)

either by physical exam, blood work, chest x-ray, or urinalysis. An abdominal process should also be considered as this may require surgical intervention. Septic patients are often too unstable to go to CT scan, which places high importance on the abdominal exam. Another consideration in sepsis and refractory hypotension is adrenal insufficiency. Patients who take oral steroids (e.g., prednisone) have chronic adrenal down-regulation and are therefore adrenally-insufficient. These patients should receive "stress-dose" steroids, typically dexamethasone 10 mg IV, during a time of infection or other physical stress when one's own body would normally respond with release of endogenous cortisol. Another medicine currently under investigation is drotrecogin alfa (Xigris), an agent that acts to inhibit the massive inflammatory cascade that plays a large role in the pathophysiology of sepsis.

 ## CASE CONTINUED

Two large-bore IVs are placed and aggressive fluid resuscitation started as the patient is placed on oxygen and a cardiac monitor. Broad-spectrum antibiotics are given after blood and urine cultures are sent. The patient develops a fever to 38.9°C (102°F), and his systolic blood pressure is 85 mm Hg as the first liter of fluid finishes. A right-sided subclavian line is placed and initial CVP is 4 mm Hg. A goal CVP of 8 to 12 mm Hg is achieved after 3,300 mL of IV normal saline. His labs are remarkable for WBC 14.2 k/mm^3 with 60% polys and 11% bands, Hct 31.5%, and 10 to 20 WBCs/hpf on urinalysis. EKG shows sinus tachycardia but no ST or T-wave abnormalities. A chest x-ray reveals low lung volumes but no obvious infiltrates. A KUB shows dilated bowel loops. He receives a single dose of gentamicin 80 mg IV to double-cover gram-negative organisms. He also receives acetaminophen (Tylenol), ibuprofen (Motrin), and dexamethasone 10 mg IV, and is started on norepinephrine given persistent hypotension with a MAP less than 65 mm Hg. His blood pressure responds to treatment and he is transferred to the MICU in stable condition. His urine culture later grows *E. coli* and his antibiotics are tailored to susceptibility.

QUESTIONS

15-1. A 78-year-old woman is brought in by family who says she is weak, febrile, and not eating. On exam, her blood pressure is 85/palp with a fever of 38.9°C (102°F). An EKG is unremarkable. Which of the following indicates a correct ordering of steps in her management?

    A. Central venous line, vasopressors, PRBC, crystalloid, S_vO_2 measurement

    B. S_vO_2 measurement, PRBC, vasopressors, central venous line, crystalloid

    C. Crystalloid, PRBC, central venous line, S_vO_2 measurement, vasopressors

    D. Vasopressors, central venous line, S_vO_2 measurement, crystalloid, PRBC

    E. Crystalloid, central venous line, vasopressors, S_vO_2 measurement, PRBC

15-2. A 79-year-old nursing home resident presents with high fevers and abdominal pain. His temperature is 39.4°C (102.9°F) and blood pressure is 80/palp; he has a diffusely tender abdomen. What is an appropriate choice of antibiotics?

    A. Vancomycin

    B. Ceftriaxone and azithromycin

    C. Ampicillin, gentamicin, metronidazole

    D. Vancomycin, levofloxacin, metronidazole

    E. None; await results of blood and urine and other tests

15-3. A 54-year-old woman presents to the ED with high fever, hypotension, dysuria, urinary frequency, and packed WBCs on urine sediment. She has a history of hypertension, severe COPD, and high cholesterol, and takes lisinopril, prednisone, and atorvastatin (Lipitor), The MICU resident wants to do a "cort stim" test (cosyntropin stimulation test) tomorrow morning. In addition to gram-negative coverage, which of the following should you give her tonight?

    A. Hydrocortisone

    B. Dexamethasone

    C. ACTH

    D. Cortisol

    E. None of the above, to avoid interfering with the results of the cort stim test

15-4. A 69-year-old man with a history significant only for diabetes and arthritis presents with confusion, fever, and hypotension. His chest x-ray shows a lobar pneumonia. After giving 2 L normal saline and IV antibiotics, a CVP is transduced at 9 mm Hg. The patient's blood pressure remains 85/45 (MAP 58 mm Hg). Which of the following is the vasopressor of choice?

    A. Epinephrine
    B. Dobutamine
    C. Phenylephrine (Neo-Synephrine)
    D. Vasopressin
    E. Norepinephrine (Levophed)
    F. No vasopressor is needed at this time

ANSWERS

15-1. **E.** **This woman is hypotensive and febrile; she is likely septic.** **Initial treatment consists of a rapid fluid bolus of 1 to 2 liters of crystalloid and broad-spectrum antibiotics after sending blood and urine cultures. If hypotension persists, then EGDT is initiated, starting with placement of a central venous line and measurement of CVP. Crystalloid is continued rapidly until a goal CVP of 8 to 12 mm Hg is reached, always staying aware of the potential need to intubate. Vasopressors are added only after this goal is reached and the patient remains hypotensive. Central venous oxygen saturation level then guides the need for PRBC transfusion or dobutamine administration.**

15-2. **D.** This patient presents with likely sepsis due to an abdominal source, possibly bowel perforation. Broad-spectrum IV antibiotics should be given immediately after IV access is obtained and blood drawn for labs and culture. The coverage should include gram-positive, gram-negative, and anaerobic organisms. Vancomycin is administered to cover methicillin-resistant *S. aureus* (MRSA), given the increasing prevalence of resistance, especially in nursing home residents. **Vancomycin provides good gram-positive coverage including MRSA, levofloxacin provides good gram-negative coverage, and metronidazole provides anaerobic coverage.** Choice B is treatment for community-acquired pneumonia requiring hospitalization. Choice C is a reasonable choice for abdominal sepsis, although it does not cover MRSA.

15-3. **B.** Stress-dose steroids should be given to any patient with possible adrenal insufficiency or any patient with persistent hypotension despite aggressive fluid and vasopressor resuscitation.

This patient is adrenally insufficient given his chronic prednisone use. **Dexamethasone (Decadron) is a synthetic analog of cortisol that will not interfere with the cosyntropin test as it does not result in down-regulation of the release of adrenocorticotropic hormone (ACTH).** Cosyntropin is a synthetic version of ACTH, which is secreted from the anterior pituitary in response to CRH (corticotropin-releasing hormone) from the hypothalamus, secreted in response to stress. Both hydrocortisone and cortisol would themselves down-regulate the production of ACTH from the anterior pituitary and thus interfere with the cort stim test.

15-4. E. After the initial fluid bolus and IV antibiotics are given, and the goal CVP of 8 to 12 mm Hg has been reached, a vasopressor is indicated to achieve a MAP of greater than 65 mm Hg. **Norepinephrine and dopamine are two commonly used vasopressors in hypotensive patients with sepsis. Norepinephrine increases blood pressure primarily by potent vasoconstriction, whereas dopamine has potent inotropic effects, increasing stroke volume and heart rate. Norepinephrine is the preferred agent in sepsis according to the Surviving Sepsis Campaign guidelines published in 2004.** Epinephrine has greater likelihood of causing tachycardia and decreased splanchnic circulation. Dobutamine is the *inotropic* agent of choice for patients with low cardiac output despite adequate fluid resuscitation and pharmacologic vasoconstriction. Phenylephrine, a pure α-agonist, is the least likely to produce tachycardia, but it decreases stroke volume. Vasopressin is not considered first-line in septic shock, but rather an adjunct to the other vasopressors in patients with refractory hypotension.

 SUGGESTED ADDITIONAL READINGS

Dellinger RP, Carlet JM, Masur H, et al. Surviving Sepsis Campaign guidelines for management of severe sepsis and septic shock. Crit Care Med 2004;32:858–873.

Landry DW, Oliver JA. The pathogenesis of vasodilatory shock. N Engl J Med 2001;345:588–595.

Rivers E, Nguyen B, Havstad S, et al. Early goal-directed therapy in the treatment of severe sepsis and septic shock. N Engl J Med 2001;345:1368–1377.

Shapiro NI, Howell M, Talmor D. A blueprint for a sepsis protocol. Acad Emerg Med 2005;12:352–359.

Confusion and Hot Skin in an Elderly Man

CC: 82-year-old man with confusion and hot skin

HPI: C.H. is an 82-year-old man who was found this afternoon in his apartment lying on the couch lethargic and confused. His son tried to get him up but could not; C.H. was mumbling incomprehensibly. He lives alone in a poorly ventilated apartment, and the fan to the air conditioner had broken the previous night. The temperature outside is 102°F and his apartment was very hot per the EMS report. His fingerstick glucose was 110 mg/dL. His son had seen him yesterday and states that he had been doing well.

PMHx:. Hypertension, CVA, gout

Meds: Aspirin 81 mg PO QD, atenolol 50 mg PO QD, hydrochlorothiazide 25 mg PO QD, allopurinol 200 mg PO BID

ALL: NKDA

SHx: Remote history of tobacco use; no alcohol

VS: Temp 41.5°C (106.7°F) rectally, HR 118, BP 74/42, RR 24, Sao_2 96% on RA

PE: *General:* Elderly, thin man; awake but staring off; mumbling. *HEENT:* No evidence of trauma; conjunctiva clear; oropharynx dry. *Neck:* Supple; no adenopathy; no meningismus. *CV:* S_1, S_2; tachycardic; no murmurs. *Chest:* Clear bilaterally. *Abd:* Soft, nondistended, nontender; normal bowel sounds. *Rectal:* Brown stool, heme-negative; normal prostate. *Extr:* Well-perfused; no edema. *Skin:* Dry, flushed, and hot. *Neuro:* Awake but lethargic and not following commands; cranial nerves appear grossly intact; moving all extremities; no rigidity or myoclonus.

THOUGHT QUESTIONS

- What is the initial management for this man?
- What is the differential diagnosis for altered mental status and hyperthermia?
- Which organ systems are most vulnerable to hyperthermia?
- How is hyperthermia best treated?

Immediate Actions:
Place on cardiac monitor and 100% oxygen by face mask; fully expose the patient, spray with room-temperature water, and start fanning; establish IV access; send blood for CBC, chem 7, LFTs, lipase, CK, TnI, lactate, TSH, PT, PTT, fibrin split products, blood cultures; give NS 1 liter bolus; obtain 12-lead EKG; place Foley catheter and send for urinalysis; obtain arterial blood gas; obtain portable chest x-ray; order head CT.

Discussion:
Hyperthermia is due either to an elevated thermoregulatory set point (e.g., febrile illness, certain drugs) or the inability to adequately dissipate heat. The latter results in heat exhaustion (dehydration, fatigue, malaise, vomiting, headache) and eventually heat stroke (altered mental status, seizures, hypotension, centrilobular liver necrosis, renal failure). Other considerations given hyperthermia and altered mental status should include CNS infection, CVA, thyroid storm, drug-induced heat illness (e.g., anticholinergic agents, sympathomimetics), neuroleptic malignant syndrome (muscular rigidity, dyskinesia, hyperthermia induced by neuroleptic medication), and malignant hyperthermia. In classic heat stroke, when the core body temperature rises above 40°C (104°F), the brain and liver are the most vulnerable to irreversible damage. Even if treated, seizures and long-term neurologic sequelae are common. Centrilobular liver necrosis occurs, resulting in elevated transaminases, and can lead to coagulation abnormalities and DIC. Peripheral vasodilation leads to hypotension and high-flow

(Continued)

cardiac failure. The best method of cooling is by ice water immersion, although this is not usually practical in the ED. The best alternative is to expose the patient, spray with room-temperature water, and set up fans to facilitate convective and evaporative cooling.

CASE CONTINUED

EKG, chest x-ray, and CT scan are unremarkable. The patient is diagnosed with classic heat stroke. A rectal probe is placed to follow the patient's core body temperature. After convective cooling is employed for 45 minutes, the rectal temperature decreases to 39.0°C (102.2°F). At this point, active cooling is stopped to prevent overshoot hypothermia. The patient's mental status improves. Abnormal labs include BUN 36 mg/dL, Cr 2.6 mg/dL, ALT 456 U/L, AST 520 U/L, CK 860 U/L. The patient is diagnosed with heat stroke, renal failure, and mild rhabdomyolysis. He is admitted for IV hydration and observation.

QUESTIONS

16-1. On a very hot summer day, a 90-year-old mildly demented woman is found by a neighbor to be confused in her small non-air-conditioned apartment. There is no evidence of trauma, but her skin is hot and her rectal temperature is found to be 40.6°C (105.1°F). In addition to other methods, which of the following choices would be best for helping to lower her core body temperature?
   A. Acetaminophen
   B. Ibuprofen
   C. Aspirin
   D. Cooled blankets
   E. Water spray and electric fan

16-2. A young girl is playing in the Arizona desert under a hot summer sun. Which of the following mechanisms of heat dissipation plays the most important role in preventing her from getting heat exhaustion?
   A. Conduction
   B. Convection
   C. Radiation
   D. Evaporation
   E. Sublimation

16-3. A 20-year-old man runs a marathon on a hot sunny day. In the last stretch before the finish line, he collapses. Which of the following distinguishes his condition from classic heat stroke?

A. Hyperpyrexia (temp >41°C or 105.8°F)
B. Altered mental status
C. Lactic acidosis
D. Hot, dry skin
E. Transaminase elevation

16-4. A 79-year-old man with minimal medical history is brought to the ED by his niece who found him lying on a couch in his basement apartment, lethargic and confused. The niece says his apartment was so hot and humid that she could barely breathe. The patient's vitals are T 40.8°C (105.5°F), HR 112, BP 82/44, RR 24, Sao_2 97% on room air. What is the most effective means of correcting this patient's hypotension?

A. Correcting hyperpyrexia
B. Aggressive fluid rehydration
C. Colloid suspension
D. Inotropic agents
E. Vasopressors

ANSWERS

16-1. E. Antipyretics are contraindicated in environmental heat illness. Antipyretics act to lower the thermoregulatory set point, which is elevated in fever. Endogenous pyrogens are thought to increase prostaglandin synthesis in the preoptic area of the anterior hypothalamus, the area responsible for thermoregulation. Aspirin and other NSAIDs inhibit prostaglandin synthesis, and thus lower the set point. Environmental heat illness is not associated with an altered set point; rather, it is caused by the inability to dissipate heat. Therefore, NSAIDs play no role in this disease. Furthermore, aspirin uncouples oxidative phosphorylation, which exacerbates liver necrosis. NSAIDs and acetaminophen can also contribute further to liver and kidney damage. **In heat stroke, which this patient likely has, core body temperature can be lowered with the use of electric fans, ice water immersion, bowel irrigation, and cooled IV fluids. Cool mist spray and electric fans are considered the most effective means of passive cooling, utilizing the concept of convective cooling.**

16-2. D. Conduction is the transfer of heat from a warm to a cool body through direct contact. Water has a thermal conductivity 32 times that of air; therefore, ice water immersion is the most effective means of heat dissipation. Convection is heat transfer from the body to the surrounding air and is proportional to the air temperature and wind velocity. A cool air fan is an effective means of convective heat dissipation. Radiation is the transfer of heat via electromagnetic energy. It accounts for about 65% of heat loss in cold environments, whereas it is a major source of heat gain in hot environments. **Evaporation is the conversion of liquid to gas, which consumes heat energy. Evaporation of sweat from the skin is the major source of heat dissipation in a hot environment.**

16-3. C. Heat stroke is classified as either classic or exertional. Both types are characterized by hyperpyrexia (temperature >41.0°C or 105.8°F), altered mental status, dehydration, hot dry skin, and transaminase elevations. Classic heat stroke is caused by inadequate dissipation of environmental heat and typically occurs in the elderly, or in infants, who are exposed for a prolonged period to a hot, humid environment. Underlying medical or psychiatric illness, immobility, alcoholism, lower socioeconomic class, poorly ventilated homes, and certain medications predispose to this condition. Lactic acidosis, rhabdomyolysis, and acute renal failure are not prominent in classic heat stroke unless the patient has been incapacitated for a long period of time. **Exertional heat stroke occurs typically in healthy young people and is related to strenuous exertion and excessive endogenous heat production. In this condition, lactic acidosis, acute renal failure, rhabdomyolysis, and DIC are more prominent features.**

16-4. A. This patient has heat stroke causing his hypotension. Hyperpyrexia results in peripheral vasodilatation in an effort to maximize peripheral blood flow for heat dissipation. In turn, splanchnic and renal vascular beds vasoconstrict, which leads to end-organ damage. Loss of peripheral vascular tone leads to hypotension and high-output cardiac failure. **Typically, CVP is normal, meaning that hypovolemia is often not the primary factor in the hypotension. Cooling results in constriction of peripheral vascular beds and normalization of blood pressure.** Rehydration is also indicated, although overaggressive rehydration should be avoided. Vasopressors, especially α-agonists such as norepinephrine, will cause further splanchnic and renal vasoconstriction and should also be avoided if possible.

SUGGESTED ADDITIONAL READINGS

Hadad E, Rav-Acha M, Heled Y, et al. Heat stroke: a review of cooling methods. Sports Med 2004;34:501–511.

Heled Y, Rav-Acha M, Shani Y, et al. The "golden hour" for heat-stroke treatment. Mil Med 2004;169:184–186.

Smith JE. Cooling methods used in the treatment of exertional heat illness. Br J Sports Med 2005;39:503–507.

Homeless Alcoholic Found Unresponsive and Cold

CC: 52-year-old man found unresponsive and cold

HPI: A.H. is a 52-year-old man who was found in the park face-down in the snow by a police officer. The man is known to local police and usually stays in a shelter. He was found tonight in −7°C (20°F) weather lying next to an empty pint of vodka. He was unarousable upon EMS arrival, although he had a faint pulse at 42/min and a blood pressure of 74 by palpation. His fingerstick glucose was 152 mg/dL.

PMHx: Alcohol-withdrawal seizures

Meds: None

ALL: Unknown

SHx: One to two pints per day of vodka; heavy smoker

VS: Temp 27.0°C (80.6°F) rectally, HR 42, BP 68/42, RR 6, Sao$_2$ unable to obtain

PE: *General:* Disheveled, unresponsive, cyanotic, cold. *HEENT:* No evidence of trauma; conjunctiva clear; oropharynx dry. *Neck:* Supple; no adenopathy. *CV:* S$_1$, S$_2$; bradycardic; no murmurs. *Chest:* Faint breath sounds bilaterally. *Abd:* Soft, nondistended; no bowel sounds. *Rectal:* Brown stool, heme-negative; no rectal tone. *Extr:* Poorly perfused; mottled; no edema. *Skin:* Cold, dry; no rashes. *Pulses:* Faint carotid and femoral pulses; absent radial and pedal pulses. *Neuro:* Unresponsive to voice or pain; not moving any extremities; pupils 3 mm and fixed.

THOUGHT QUESTIONS

- What is the initial management for this man?
- Which underlying conditions must be considered?
- At which minimal core temperature is ACLS medication effective?
- What is the most effective method for rewarming this patient?

Immediate Actions:

Intubate with 8.0 ETT without medications and initiate mechanical ventilation with warm, humidified oxygen; place on cardiac monitor; place two large-bore IVs and central venous catheter; obtain 12-lead EKG; remove all wet clothes and cover with heated blankets or place under heat lamps; place a rectal probe; send blood for CBC, chem 7, LFTs, lipase, CK and TnI, serum tox screen, Ca, Mg, phosphate, and blood cultures; start 2 liters of warmed NS; place a Foley catheter and send urinalysis and urine tox; obtain portable chest x-ray.

Discussion:

Hypothermia is defined as a core body temperature less than 35.0°C (95.0°F) (Table 17-1). Moderate hypothermia is considered less than 32.0°C (89.6°F), and severe hypothermia less than 24.0°C (75.2°F). Hypothermia is usually a result of exposure to a cold or wet environment with inadequate clothing or shelter. Infants and the elderly are particularly at risk. Underlying conditions must also be considered in someone found down and cold, such as hypoglycemia, acute stroke, AMI, sepsis, intoxication or poisoning, metabolic abnormalities, or hypothyroidism. Hypothermia is heralded at 35.0°C (95.0°F) by shivering, confusion, and impaired judgment. Below 32.0°C (89.6°F) shivering stops, and below 30.0°C (86.0°F) a person loses consciousness. At temperatures below 25.0°C (77.0°F), brady- and tachydysrhythmias are common. Cardioversion and ACLS medications are ineffective until the body is rewarmed to around 30.0°C (86.0°F). For severe hypothermia, active core rewarming is indicated, including gastric, intrathoracic, and intraperitoneal lavage. The most effective means of rewarming is cardiopulmonary bypass.

(Continued)

TABLE 17-1 Categories of Hypothermia		
Hypothermia	**Temperatures**	**Comments**
Mild	<35.0°C (95.0°F)	Shivering present; impaired judgement
Moderate	<32.0°C (89.6°F)	Shivering ceases
	<30.0°C (86.0°F)	LOC; ACLS meds and cardioversion ineffective
	<25.0°C (77.0°F)	Brady- and tachydysrhythmias
Severe	<24.0°C (75.2°F)	Active core rewarming indicated

 ## CASE CONTINUED

After the initial evaluation is completed, the patient loses all pulses and the monitor shows ventricular fibrillation. He is shocked with 200 J, 300 J, and then 360 J, all without success. Chest compressions are started. Bilateral chest tubes are placed and an intraperitoneal catheter is placed. Intrathoracic and intraperitoneal lavage with warm sterile saline is started. Warm saline lavage is also performed through an orogastric tube. After 20 minutes, his rectal temperature is 29.0°C (84.2°F). Cardioversion is repeated, and his rhythm reverts to sinus bradycardia with Osborne J waves (Figure 17-1), a classic finding in hypothermia. Active rewarming is continued. The patient is admitted to the MICU, where his body temperature eventually normalizes. He recovers full neurologic function and is discharged from the hospital.

 ## QUESTIONS

17-1. A lost hiker is found in subzero temperatures after 2 days. Which of the following findings would point toward a milder degree of hypothermia?
   A. Shivering
   B. Core temperature less than 32.0°C (89.6°F)
   C. Altered mental status
   D. Cold diuresis
   E. Respiratory alkalosis

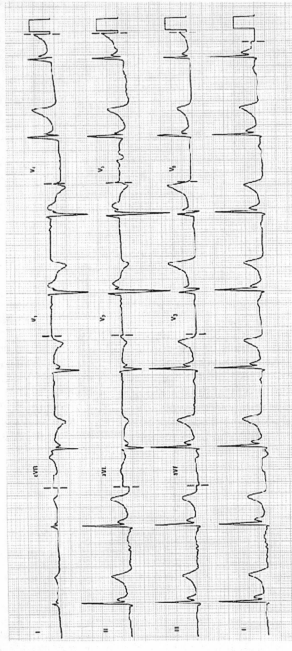

FIGURE 17-1 Twelve-lead EKG shows Osborne J waves (notched upward deflection following the QRS complex), characteristic of severe hypothermia. (*Image courtesy of Massachusetts General Hospital, Boston.*)

17-2. A commercial fisherman is brought to the ED after standing watch for 8 hours on a boat in a snowstorm. His boatmates were having difficulty arousing him and called 911. He is breathing spontaneously but feels very cold to the touch. His core temperature is 31°C (87.8°F). An EKG is obtained. Which finding is considered pathognomonic for hypothermia?

    A. Osborne J waves
    B. Atrial fibrillation
    C. QT prolongation
    D. Ventricular fibrillation
    E. Sinus bradycardia

17-3. A 58-year-old homeless man is found in the snow unresponsive. He is placed on a monitor and found to be in ventricular fibrillation. He is shocked with 150 J monophasic into a sinus bradycardia. He is then intubated and transported to the ED. Which of the following is the most effective means of active core rewarming for him?

    A. Hemodialysis
    B. Warm body cavity fluid lavage
    C. Heated, humidified oxygen
    D. Cardiac bypass
    E. Warmed intravenous fluids

17-4. A mountain climber is stranded unexpectedly above 12,000 feet overnight in a snowstorm. The next day, he is able to make it down the mountain but no longer has sensation in his hands or feet. He states that they feel like "dead weight." His fingers and toes appear pale and waxy. He cannot move his fingers or toes and has no sensation to light touch. Which one of the following would likely be harmful to his condition?

    A. Administer penicillin IV
    B. Treat similar to thermal burn after rewarming
    C. Immersion in warm water bath to rewarm
    D. Debridement of hemorrhagic blisters
    E. Debridement of clear blisters

ANSWERS

17-1.   A. Shivering is a physiologic response to mild hypothermia in an effort to generate endogenous heat. This response ceases at about 32.0°C (89.6°F), which is the temperature at which hypothermia is considered to be moderate. Significant EEG slowing occurs at 33.5°C (92°F), and consciousness is lost at temperatures less than 30.0°C (86.0°F). At 20.0°C (68.0°F), EEG activity as well as cardiac electromechanical activity stop. However, neuronal death does not immediately occur. At temperatures less than 20.0°C (68.0°F), patients can tolerate total circulatory arrest for longer than 1 hour without neurologic sequelae upon rewarming. Hence the saying, "A patient isn't dead until he is warm and dead." Hypothermia also causes peripheral vasoconstriction in order to minimize heat loss. This results in increased renal blood flow and diuresis. Therefore, upon rewarming, patients require fluid resuscitation to restore intravascular volume. Hypothermia is initially marked by hyperventilation and a respiratory alkalosis. As the core temperature falls, the respiratory rate falls as well, and a respiratory acidosis will result.

17-2. A. EKG changes in hypothermia are common because cold temperatures inhibit conduction tissue as well as alter the myocardial depolarization threshold. **Osborne J waves, or hypothermic humps, are pathognomonic for hypothermia and can occur at temperatures less than 32.0°C (89.6°F). They consist of upward deflections, or humps, directly following the QRS complex, and are most pronounced in the inferior and lateral leads.** Atrial fibrillation is also common when the temperature falls below 32.0°C (89.6°F). Conduction delays can cause PR and QRS prolongation, but QT prolongation is more often described with hypothermia. Below 25.0°C (77.0°F), VF and asystole are common. Malignant arrhythmias are refractory to cardioversion and cardiac resuscitative medication until the core temperature approaches 30.0°C (86.0°F).

17-3. D. Active *external* rewarming exposes the body to an external heat source. Examples include warm baths, heat lamps, and warmed blankets. Active *core* rewarming refers to techniques that allow for internal heat exchange. Active core rewarming can be as simple as heated, humidified oxygen or warmed IV fluids. More invasive methods include warm fluid lavage (e.g., peritoneal, thoracic, gastrointestinal) and extracorporeal rewarming (e.g., hemodialysis, arteriovenous or venovenous bypass, and cardiac bypass). **Cardiac bypass is the most effective means of active core rewarming, achieving a core temperature increase of about 10.0°C (18.0°F) per hour.**

17-4. D. Frostbite occurs in hands, feet, nose, and ears when exposed for a prolonged period to extremely cold temperatures. Tissue ice crystal formation is required for frostbite to occur, which requires tissue temperatures below −4.0°C (24.8°F). Rewarming results in blood vessel damage, plasma leakage, thrombosis, ischemia, and eventually gangrene. Frostbite severity is classified in a manner similar to that for thermal burns. First-degree frostbite is superficial and consists of skin erythema and a firm plaque over the area of injury. Second-degree frostbite consists of superficial vesicles filled with clear or milky fluid and surrounded by erythema. Third-degree frostbite extends into the deep dermis and is characterized by hemorrhagic blisters. Fourth-degree frostbite involves underlying muscle and bone, which leads to mummification and gangrene. **Treatment consists of rapid rewarming with warm water. Clear vesicles should be drained, but hemorrhagic vesicles should be left intact. Tetanus and prophylactic IV penicillin G are both indicated.**

 SUGGESTED ADDITIONAL READINGS

Biem J, Koehncke N, Classen D, et al. Out of the cold: management of hypothermia and frostbite. CMAJ 2003;168:305–311.

Kempainen RR, Brunette DD. The evaluation and management of accidental hypothermia. Respir Care 2004;49:192–205.

Long WB 3rd, Edlich RF, Winters KL, et al. Cold injuries. J Long Term Eff Med Implants 2005;15:67–78.

Rice R. Hypothermia—potentially deadly year round. JAAPA 2005;18:47–52.

Fever, Confusion, and Seizure in a Prisoner

CC: 42-year-old man with fever, agitation, hallucinations, and seizure

HPI: D.S. is a 42-year-old man who entered prison 2 days ago. This morning he woke up with drenching sweats, was tremulous, and vomited three times. He appeared hypervigilant and agitated. He had a witnessed tonic-clonic seizure that lasted about 3 minutes. He was postictal for 15 to 20 minutes. When EMS arrived, he was squirming and picking at his shirt, complaining that there were bugs all over him. He admits that he usually drinks one to two pints of vodka daily, but has never had difficulty quitting and has never had a seizure before.

PMHx: None

Meds: None

ALL: None

SHx: 1 ppd tobacco; one to two pints vodka daily; occasional IV heroin and cocaine use

VS: Temp 38.5°C (101.3°F), HR 132, BP 188/110, RR 24, Sao$_2$ 100% on RA

PE: *General:* Thin, anxious man; looking around wildly; diaphoretic, flushed; coarse tremors. *HEENT:* Pupils 6 mm and reactive; no icterus; oropharynx clear and dry. *Neck:* Supple; no adenopathy; no meningismus. *CV:* S$_1$, S$_2$; tachycardic; no murmurs. *Chest:* Clear bilaterally. *Abd:* Soft, nondistended, nontender; hyperactive bowel sounds. *Rectal:* Brown stool, heme-negative; normal prostate. *Extr:* Well-perfused; no edema. *Skin:* Warm, moist; no rashes or lesions. *Neuro:* Hyperalert, disoriented to place and time; confabulating; follows simple commands; CN II to XII intact; 5/5 motor strength in all extremities; unable to do finger-to-nose test; ataxic gait; hyperreflexic in all extremities.

THOUGHT QUESTIONS

- What is the initial management for this man?
- What is the differential diagnosis for fever, delirium, and seizure?
- Which classes of medication are used to treat this disorder?
- Which level of care does this patient require?

Immediate Actions:
Place on cardiac monitor and 100% oxygen by face mask; establish IV access; check fingerstick glucose; send blood for CBC, chem 7, LFTs, Ca, Mg, phosphate, tox screen, PT, PTT, blood cultures; give NS 2-liter bolus; obtain 12-lead EKG; give ceftriaxone 2 g IV, lorazepam (Ativan) 2 mg IV, haloperidol (Haldol) 5 mg IV, thiamine 100 mg IV, magnesium 2 g IV; obtain head CT; perform lumbar puncture.

Discussion:
Fever, delirium, and seizure usually accompany serious illness. CNS infection (e.g., meningitis, encephalitis, or brain abscess) should be the primary concern and treated immediately with antibiotics before any diagnostics are done. Hypoglycemia can cause delirium and seizure, which in turn can lead to fever. Other concerns are intracranial hemorrhage, sepsis, toxic ingestions (e.g., anticholinergics, sympathomimetics, aspirin, phenothiazines), thyrotoxicosis, heat stroke, fulminant hepatic failure, and benzodiazepine or barbiturate withdrawal.

With a history of heavy alcohol use and recent cessation, alcohol withdrawal syndrome is a likely etiology. Alcohol use leads to changes in neurotransmitter activity in the brain, such as activation of the major inhibitory brain neurotransmitter, γ-aminobutyric acid (GABA). In alcohol withdrawal, the relative lack of GABA activity leads to a state of hyperarousal. Other neurotransmitters believed to play a role in the manifestations of alcohol ingestion and alcohol withdrawal include norepinephrine,

(Continued)

serotonin, dopamine, and glutamate. Delirium tremens (DTs), a severe manifestation of alcohol withdrawal, occurs 2 to 3 days after alcohol cessation and is characterized by gross tremor, profound confusion, fever, incontinence, visual hallucinations, and mydriasis. Treatment consists of large amounts of benzodiazepines, which occupy the upregulated GABA receptors and suppress withdrawal symptoms. Other useful agents include butyrophenones (e.g., haloperidol, droperidol), β-blockers (e.g., propranolol, atenolol), and α-agonists (e.g., clonidine). Patients with delirium tremens require care in the ICU because of their requirement for large amounts of benzodiazepines and their propensity for seizures.

CASE CONTINUED

The patient receives lorazepam 4 mg IV, haloperidol 10 mg IV, and clonidine 0.2 mg PO in the first hour with some relief of symptoms. His labs, tox screen, head CT, and lumbar puncture are all essentially normal; based on his history, a diagnosis of severe alcohol withdrawal is made. During the second hour, he requires additional lorazepam 4 mg IV and haloperidol 10 mg IV for agitation and hallucinations. He is admitted to the MICU for frequent benzodiazepine and butyrophenone dosing and close observation. On the third day, he is tapered to lorazepam 1 to 2 mg every 4 to 6 hours PO and is discharged back to prison.

QUESTIONS

18-1. A 49-year-old chronic alcoholic is struck by a small car at low speed while crossing an intersection. He sustains an open femur fracture for which he is taken emergently to the OR. Postoperatively, he initially does well with stable vital signs. On the second hospital day, however, he is agitated, tachycardic, and hypertensive. Which of the following would be useful in his management?

A. β-Agonists
B. α_1-Agonists
C. α_2-Agonists
D. Naloxone
E. Flumazenil

18-2. A college freshman is brought to the ED after passing out in his bedroom after attending a party earlier in the evening. A serum tox screen is significant for an alcohol level of 400 mg/dL. How many hours will it likely take until he sobers up enough to legally be able to drive?

- A. 2 hours
- B. 4 hours
- C. 8 hours
- D. 12 hours
- E. 16 hours

18-3. A 76-year-old man has a history of chronic alcoholism, ischemic stroke, MI, cardiomyopathy, hypercalcemia, and thrombocytosis. Which of his problems is associated with chronic alcohol abuse?

- A. Ischemic stroke
- B. MI
- C. Cardiomyopathy
- D. Hypercalcemia
- E. Thrombocytosis

18-4. A 62-year-old woman with heavy EtOH history is brought in by friends who say she is confused and unable to walk straight. On exam, she has a sixth nerve palsy on left lateral gaze. Which of the following is most likely deficient?

- A. Vitamin B_1
- B. Vitamin B_2
- C. Vitamin B_3
- D. Vitamin B_6
- E. Vitamin B_{12}

ANSWERS

18-1. C. This patient has symptoms of alcohol withdrawal. Even though alcohol acts directly on central GABA receptors and results in their upregulation, it also has indirect effects on central adrenergic and dopamine receptors. Intravenous benzodiazepines are the mainstay of therapy and are often needed in large quatities to prevent delirium tremens. **Alcohol cessation is associated with increased levels of catecholamines, which results in the hyperadrenergic symptoms of hypervigilance, diaphoresis, tachycardia, hypertension, and mydriasis. Both β-antagonists (e.g., propranolol, atenolol) and α_2-agonists (e.g., clonidine) act to**

blunt this adrenergic surge. In addition, dopaminergic receptors are activated and result in psychosis and hallucinations. Butyrophenones (e.g., haloperidol, droperidol) block dopamine receptors and are also useful in treating these symptoms. Naloxone and flumazenil are not useful in treating acute alcohol withdrawal.

18-2. D. Alcohol clearance depends on many factors, including age, sex, body weight, speed of consumption, food in the stomach, smoking, and chronic alcoholism. Alcohol is metabolized in the liver to acetaldehyde by the enzyme alcohol dehydrogenase and then to acetic acid by the enzyme aldehyde dehydrogenase. Chronic alcohol intake activates an alternate pathway, the microsomal ethanol-oxidizing system (MEOS), which results in more rapid metabolism by alcoholics. A clearance rate of 25 mg/dL/hr is a good rule of thumb for estimating time to sobriety for an intoxicated patient in the ED given an initial alcohol level. The significance of this point for working in the ED is being able to predict when your intoxicated patient will be sober. **On average, a patient will clear 100 mg/dL every 4 hours. In most states, the legal driving limit for blood alcohol is 100 mg/dL, or 0.1 mg%. It will therefore take approximately 12 hours until this patient's alcohol level decreases from 400 mg/dL to 100 mg/dL.**

TABLE 18-1 Adverse Effects Associated with Chronic Alcohol Abuse

System	Effect
Psychologic	Dependence, depression
Cardiovascular	Atrial and ventricular tachyarrhythmias, congestive cardiomyopathy
Gastrointestinal	Peptic ulcer disease, esophageal and gastric cancer, hepatitis, cirrhosis, pancreatitis, chronic diarrhea
Neurologic	Symmetric sensorimotor polyneuropathy, Wernicke's encephalopathy, Korsakoff's amnesia, myopathy, intracranial hemorrhage, movement disorders, cerebellar degeneration
Infectious	Pneumonia, tuberculosis, spontaneous bacterial peritonitis, bacterial endocarditis
Endocrinologic/ metabolic	Male hypogonadism, gynecomastia, hypoglycemia, hypertriglyceridemia, hyperuricemia, hypokalemia, hypomagnesemia, hypocalcemia, hypophosphatemia, ketoacidosis
Hematologic	Anemia, leukopenia, thrombocytopenia, clotting factor deficiencies

18-3. C. Chronic alcohol abuse is at the root of many social and medical problems. The long-term effects of alcohol use are multisystemic. Alcohol-related illness includes cardiovascular, gastrointestinal, neurologic, infectious, endocrinologic and metabolic, and hematologic problems, not to mention psychiatric and cognitive effects. **Of the problems that this patient has, his cardiomyopathy (congestive) is associated with chronic alcohol abuse.** See Table 18-1 for a list of associated ailments by system.

18-4. A. Wernicke's encephalopathy is an illness described in alcoholics that is thought to be due to thiamine (vitamin B$_1$) deficiency. The classic features of this disorder include ophthalmoplegia (typically sixth-nerve palsy), ataxia, and altered mental status (usually confusion, lethargy, or stupor). Ophthalmoplegia usually precedes gait and mental status changes. Korsakoff's psychosis is also a component of this disorder and is described as an amnesic state, or loss of short-term memory. Korsakoff's psychosis is typically elicited as the patient's mental status clears during treatment with thiamine. This entire symptom complex is referred to as the Wernicke-Korsakoff syndrome.

 SUGGESTED ADDITIONAL READINGS

Bayard M, McIntyre J, Hill KR, et al. Alcohol withdrawal syndrome. Am Fam Physician 2004;69:1443–1450.

Foster JH. The recognition and treatment of acute alcohol withdrawal. Nurs Times 2004;100:40–43.

Kosten TR, O'Connor PG. Management of drug and alcohol withdrawal. N Engl J Med 2003;348:1786–1795.

CASE **19**

Young Woman Found Down

CC: 26-year-old woman found down

HPI: F.D. is a 26-year-old woman who was found on the floor of her apartment by her boyfriend. She was lying next to an empty, unlabeled pill bottle and an empty bottle of whiskey. Upon EMS arrival, she was breathing spontaneously but would only moan to deep painful stimulus. Her pulse was 126 and blood pressure 92/62. EMS placed her on oxygen and started an 18-gauge antecubital IV with 1 liter of normal saline wide open. En route to the ED, she was placed on a cardiac monitor and noticed to have a wide QRS complex.

PMHx: Unknown

Meds: Unknown

ALL: Unknown

VS: Temp 36.0°C (96.8°F), HR 122, BP 88/64, RR 12, Sao$_2$ 96% on 4-liter nasal cannula

PE: *General:* Obtunded; no spontaneous eye opening or purposeful movement. *HEENT:* Pupils 2 mm and reactive; no nystagmus; oropharynx dry; no gag to pharyngeal stimulation; no scalp lacerations or facial contusions. *Neck:* Supple. *Chest:* Clear bilaterally; no crepitus; no contusions. *CV:* Tachycardic; regular; no murmurs; thready radial pulses. *Abd:* Soft; no masses. *Rectal:* Normal tone; heme-negative brown stool. *Extr:* No edema; no needle tracks. *Skin:* Cool and moist; no cyanosis. *Neuro:* Unresponsive; withdraws all extremities to deep painful stimulus; 2+ reflexes all extremities; negative Babinski reflex (downgoing toes).

THOUGHT QUESTIONS

- Which actions should be taken immediately?
- What are the four major toxidromes to consider in the acutely poisoned patient?
- What is the general management approach to the poisoned patient?

Immediate Actions:
Establish a second 18-gauge IV; place on cardiac monitor; check fingerstick glucose; intubate the patient using succinylcholine 100 mg and a 7.5-mm ETT; get a 12-lead EKG; give 50 mEq bicarbonate IV bolus, then continue bicarbonate drip until QRS is less than 100 ms (mix 100–150 mEq in 1 liter D5W); give 2-liter bolus of NS; place an orogastric (OG) tube; give activated charcoal 1 g/kg through the OG tube; place a Foley catheter; send labs for CBC, chem 7, LFTs, Ca, Mg, Phos, and serum and urine tox screens.

Discussion:
For young patients with altered mental status, toxic ingestion should be high on the differential diagnosis. Hypoglycemia is also a major cause of AMS; therefore, a fingerstick glucose must be checked or IV glucose administered. Other causes of AMS should also be considered (refer to cases in this section). Four major clinical toxidromes include opioid/sedative, sympathomimetic, cholinergic, and anticholinergic (see Table 19-1). Opioids/ sedatives cause CNS and respiratory depression, hypothermia, and bradycardia. In addition, opioids cause miosis. Sympathomimetics cause psychomotor agitation, diaphoresis, tachycardia, hypertension, hyperthermia, and seizures. Cholinergics cause excessive secretions, diaphoresis, vomiting, miosis, urination, muscle fasciculations, and weakness. Anticholinergics cause delirium, mydriasis, dry flushed skin, dry mouth, urinary retention, decreased bowel sounds, and hyperthermia.

(Continued)

TABLE **19-1**   Major Toxidromes

Toxidrome	Toxins	Symptoms
Opioid/sedative	Opioids (heroin, morphine, codeine), barbiturates, benzodiazepines, ethanol	CNS/respiratory depression, miosis (opioids), hypotension, bradycardia, hypothermia, decreased GI motility
Sympathomimetic	Cocaine, amphetamines, decongestants (phenylpropanolamine, ephedrine, pseudoephedrine), theophylline	Tachycardia, hypertension, hyperpyrexia, diaphoresis, mydriasis, delirium, seizures, tachyarrhythmias
Cholinergic	Insecticides, sarin nerve gas, physostigmine, edrophonium, acetylcholine	"SLUDGE" (salivation, lacrimation, urination, diarrhea, GI cramping, emesis); or "DUMBELS" (diarrhea, urination, miosis, bronchospasm/bronchorrhea, emesis, lacrimation, salivation); also diaphoresis, bradycardia, seizures
Anticholinergic	Antihistamines, tricyclic antidepressants, phenothiazines, belladonna alkaloids (atropine, scopolamine), antiparkinsonian agents	Delirium, tachycardia, dry flushed skin, mydriasis, hyperpyrexia, decreased GI motility, urinary retention, seizures, dysrhythmias

Treatment of all toxic ingestions should begin with assessment of airway, breathing, and circulation. Endotracheal intubation should be done for any obtunded patient who cannot drink charcoal or tolerate a nasogastric tube. Ventricular dysrhythmias or bradydysrhythmias should be treated according to ACLS protocols. Tachycardia and hypotension should be treated with aggressive fluid resuscitation. Comatose patients should receive a "coma cocktail" consisting of glucose 50 mL of D50, naloxone (Narcan) 0.4 mg IV, and thiamine 100 mg IV. Seizures should be treated immediately with benzodiazepines and phenobarbital if necessary. Phenytoin (Dilantin) has no role in the poisoned patient. Decontamination is the mainstay of all toxic ingestions. All patients should receive activated charcoal 1 g/kg. This is often mixed with an osmotic cathartic, such as sorbitol 1 g/kg of 70% solution, in order to promote GI motility. After these measures have been taken, certain antidotes can be considered for specific toxins (see Table 19-2).

(Continued)

TABLE 19-2 Antidotes to Specific Toxins	
Toxin	**Antidote**
Opiates	Naloxone
Acetaminophen	N-Acetylcysteine (NAC)
Salicylates	Sodium bicarbonate, dialysis
Anticholinergics	Physostigmine
Tricyclic antidepressants	Sodium bicarbonate
Methanol, ethylene glycol	Ethanol, fomepizole (4-MP), dialysis
Insecticides (organophosphates)	Atropine, pralidoxime (2-PAM)
β-Blockers	Glucagon
Calcium channel blockers	Calcium chloride, glucagon
Cyanide	Sodium nitrite, sodium thiosulfate
Digoxin	Digoxin-specific Fab fragments (Digibind)
Benzodiazepines	Flumazenil
Iron	Deferoxamine
Lead	EDTA, dimercaprol (BAL), DMSA, d-penicillamine

CASE CONTINUED

Two large-bore IVs are established and NS is started wide open, the patient is intubated, an orogastric tube is placed, and activated charcoal 50 g diluted in water is placed down the OG tube. A 12-lead EKG shows a QRS duration of 150 ms (normal < 100 ms). The patient has signs of a tricyclic antidepressant (TCA) overdose, so she is given sodium bicarbonate 50 mEq IV bolus followed by a bicarbonate drip until QRS is less than 100 ms (mix 100–150 mEq in 1 liter D5W). Her blood pressure increases to 105/80 mm Hg after 2 liters of NS. She is admitted to the ICU, where she is continued on a sodium bicarbonate drip for the next 12 hours. The drip is weaned with no further widening of her QRS complex, and she becomes more responsive and follows commands. She is extubated and transferred to a psychiatric unit.

QUESTIONS

19-1. A young woman presents to the ED after an unknown overdose. As she is brought into the treatment bay, she begins to have tonic-clonic activity. Which of the following in overdose is most commonly associated with seizures?

A. Opioids
B. Antihistamines
C. Antidepressants
D. Anticholinergics
E. Sympathomimetics

19-2. A 34-year-old man presents to the ED after taking all of his amitryptiline in a suicide attempt. He is confused, tachycardic, and vomiting. What causes large pupils, dry mucous membranes, and delirium in this type of overdose?

A. α-Receptor blockade
B. β-Receptor blockade
C. Muscarinic receptor blockade
D. Inhibition of serotonin and norepinephrine reuptake
E. Sodium channel blockade

19-3. A 46-year-old woman ingests a whole bottle of aspirin with a fifth of whiskey and calls EMS. She is found alert, with vitals signs significant for a pulse of 126. She is given syrup of ipecac to induce vomiting in order to evacuate gastric contents. By the time she reaches the ED, she is drowsy and is therefore intubated for airway control. Her blood pressure is 88/42 and she is administered normal saline wide open. An NG tube is placed, through which activated charcoal is given. Which of the following is no longer recommended in the management of the poisoned patient?

A. Aggressive airway management
B. Circulatory resuscitation
C. Gastric emptying with ipecac
D. Gastrointestinal decontamination by activated charcoal
E. Whole-bowel irrigation

19-4. The administration of activated charcoal (AC) has been the standard of care in the treatment of the poisoned patient. Recently this practice has been brought into question given its uncertain benefit in many cases and the associated risk for vomiting and aspiration. AC would be useless immediately following ingestion of which of the following agents?

    A. Digoxin
    B. Diphenhydramine
    C. Amitriptyline
    D. Lithium
    E. Acetaminophen

ANSWERS

19-1. E. A number of drugs in overdose are known to precipitate seizures, but there are several classes of agents that are notorious for doing so. As a class of drugs, sympathomimetics (e.g., amphetamines, cocaine) are most commonly associated with seizures. Anticholinergic agents are also known to cause seizures. The classic anticholinergic agent is atropine, which blocks muscarinic receptors. Many other agents have anticholinergic effects, including antihistamines (e.g., diphenhydramine), phenothiazines (e.g., chlorpromazine), and tricyclic antidepressants (e.g., amitriptyline, doxepin). Heroin overdose does not typically cause seizures, although opioids in general have an initial excitatory effect on the CNS and are associated with seizures in children. Propoxyphene and meperidine are two opioids that can cause seizures in adults.

19-2. C. Tricyclic antidepressants are probably the most dangerous prescription medication because they are rapidly lethal in overdose. TCAs result in toxicity by a number of different means. Sodium-channel blockade causes QRS widening, QT prolongation, and subsequent ventricular arrhythmias. **Muscarinic receptor blockade results in anticholinergic effects such as tachycardia, large pupils (mydriasis), dry mucous membranes and skin, and delirium ("mad as a hatter, blind as a bat, dry as a bone, hot as hades").** α-receptor blockade causes vasodilation and hypotension. Inhibition of serotonin and norepinephrine reuptake results in catecholamine depletion and also contributes to hypotension. The cardinal signs of TCA overdose are ventricular arrhythmias, hypotension, and decreased mental status. Sodium bicarbonate is a life-saving intervention in TCA overdose because an alkaline pH combined with a sodium load increases conduction through cardiac fast sodium channels and prevents ventricular arrhythmia.

19-3. C. The general approach to the poisoned patient is the same regardless of the specific ingestion or exposure. The first priority is airway management, which includes ensuring adequate oxygenation and ventilation. Patients need to be intubated if they have significantly decreased mental status or if they have airway compromise secondary to a caustic ingestion. It is important to prevent aspiration, which is a common occurrence during aggressive orogastric decontamination. The next priority is cardiovascular support, which includes treating arrhythmias and hypotension. The cornerstone of managing the poisoned patient is decontamination, which can include cutaneous, ocular, pulmonary, or gastrointestinal decontamination. The last is achieved by administration of activated charcoal (AC). AC works by adsorbing the toxin onto its large surface area, creating a reverse concentration gradient and drawing toxin from the bloodstream into the gut, thereby diluting the toxin by acting as an osmotic agent. **Induced vomiting with ipecac has not been shown effective and leads to aspiration with chemical pneumonitis.**

19-4. D. Activated charcoal is indicated in any toxic ingestion because of its decontaminating properties and its minimal potential for harm. However, a number of substances do not bind to AC. In general, these include alcohols (e.g., methanol, ethylene glycol, isopropyl alcohol), hydrocarbons (e.g., gasoline, kerosine), and metals (e.g., iron, mercury, lead). Lithium, which is an alkali metal, is also not adsorbed by AC. The clinical signs of lithium toxicity are CNS-related, most notably decreased mental status, ataxia, and nystagmus. Cardiac conduction abnormalities can also be seen because lithium is a sodium analogue and blocks cardiac sodium channels. Lithium is cleared by the kidneys and can result in renal failure. Whole bowel irrigation with polyethylene glycol can help to decrease gastrointestinal absorption; however, peak serum levels occur within 2 hours of ingestion. Dialysis is indicated to remove lithium from the serum if the patient has evidence of severe neurologic, cardiac, or renal toxicity.

 SUGGESTED ADDITIONAL READINGS

Abbruzzi G, Stork CM. Pediatric toxicologic concerns. Emerg Med Clin North Am 2002;20:223–247.

Chu J, Wang RY, Hill NS. Update in clinical toxicology. Am J Respir Crit Care Med 2002;166:9–15.

Kerr GW, McGuffie AC, Wilkie S. Tricyclic antidepressant overdose: a review. Emerg Med J 2002;19:596.

Ricaurte GA, McCann UD. Recognition and management of complications of new recreational drug use. Lancet 2005;365: 2137–2145.

CASE **20**

Gas Bomb in the Hospital Lobby

 CC: Terrorist attack in the hospital lobby

HPI: On a busy Monday afternoon in the lobby of a large urban hospital, a gas grenade is detonated. There is sudden chaos as people are scattering. Within seconds, a number of people are seen falling to their knees and flat onto the floor. Security is mobilized immediately, and within minutes two security personnel and one emergency physican have donned decontamination suits with respirators. There are five people who are lying unconscious on the floor. Two have vomited. One is approached and examined quickly.

PMHx: Unknown

VS: HR 132

PE: *General:* Unconscious, apneic, twitching of face and extremities. *HEENT:* Pupils pinpoint. *Neck:* Rapid faint carotid pulse. *CV:* S_1, S_2; tachycardic; no murmur. *Neuro:* Flaccid muscle tone.

THOUGHT QUESTIONS

- What specific toxidrome is involved?
- What is the first priority in the management of these patients?
- Is there an antidote for this condition?
- Is there concern for people exposed to the gas but who have safely fled?

Immediate Actions:
Intubate and bag ventilate in lobby; before entry into ED, remove all clothing; establish IV access; administer atropine 6 mg IV; administer pralidoxime chloride (2-PAM) 600 mg IV over 30 minutes; administer diazepam (Valium) 5 mg IV; administer further atropine doses 2 mg IV every 5 to 10 minutes as needed for continued bronchospasm.

Discussion:
The patients in this scenario display signs of anticholinergic toxicity, with stimulation of both muscarinic and nicotinic receptors. This is characteristic of organophosphate toxicity, which exists in volatile form as sarin gas, the substance used in the Tokyo subway bombing in the early 1990s. Sarin gas is classified as a nerve agent, similar to the liquid organophosphate VX. Both act by inhibiting acetylcholinesterase, an enzyme that degrades acetylcholine (ACh) at the postsynaptic membrane. Overstimulation of postsynaptic muscarinic receptors results in a syndrome of miosis, bronchospasm, and generalized oversecretion (e.g., lacrimation, bronchorrhea, rhinorrhea, vomiting, diarrhea, urination). Overstimulation of nicotinic receptors, located in the postsynaptic neuromuscular junction, results in muscle fasciculations and flaccid paralysis, similar to the effects of succinylcholine. In contrast to exposure to agricultural organophosphates, nerve gas tends to cause tachycardia, not the bradycardia that might be expected with unopposed ACh activity. Of these symptoms, the two classic findings associated with nerve gas are miosis and muscle fasciculations; these findings should prompt immediate and specific action.

The first priority in management is airway control and mechanical ventilation, as the patient is paralyzed and apneic. The antidote for nerve gas exposure is very specific and consists of three agents: atropine, pralidoxime chloride, and diazepam. Atropine is an antimuscarinic agent that has an important effect of reversing bronchospasm and hypersecretion. In agricultural organophosphate exposure, atropine is titrated to resolution of miosis and large quantities can be required. In nerve gas exposure, miosis is somewhat refractory to atropine, and its administration is titrated to resolution of bronchospasm. 2-PAM blocks the nicotinic receptors and reverses paralysis.

(*Continued*)

Diazepam is given to prevent seizures, which are common with organophosphate poisoning. Mark I is an FDA-approved IM autoinjector kit available for use by environmental hazard-response teams in the field. Each injection contains atropine 2 mg and 2-PAM 600 mg. Sarin gas is absorbed through the pulmonary capillary beds and distributed within seconds; its peak effect is within 5 minutes. Those who escaped from the scene and are asymptomatic after 20 or 30 minutes will remain unaffected. Mild exposure can result in rhinorrhea, wheezing, nausea or vomiting, muscle weakness, or blurred vision.

CASE CONTINUED

The five victims are quickly lined up, intubated in succession, and provided with mechanical ventilation. The hospital is alerted of a likely sarin gas exposure and all the atropine and 2-PAM is mobilized from the pharmacy. The patients' clothing is removed before entrance into the ED, where IV access is established and each is given atropine 6 mg IV, along with diazepam 5 mg IV. Fifteen minutes later, 2-PAM is available and each patient is administered 600 mg IV. Within several minutes, all five patients are awake and require deep sedation with propofol. This allows further administration of atropine as needed in order to allow bronchospasm and airway edema to resolve.

QUESTIONS

20-1. A laboratory worker in a top-secret military installation is inadvertently exposed to aerosolized anthrax spores. He is decontaminated with soap and water and taken to the clinic. He is entirely asymptomatic with a normal physical exam, including a clear oropharynx, normal breath sounds, and no rash. This particular worker had not been vaccinated against anthrax. What is the most appropriate intervention?

    A. Full-body wash with anti-bacterial cream

    B. Oral amoxicillin for 60 days

    C. Oral ciprofloxacin for 60 days

    D. IV ciprofloxacin due to risk of inhalation

    E. No treatment required because disease requires exposure to bacilli

20-2. Twenty members of a Russian government delegation travel together on a flight from Kiev to the United States. Within 2 weeks, they develop high fevers, chills, and severe headaches. This is followed several days later in some by a maculopapular rash that progresses to vesicles and pustules, mostly on the face and arms. What is the most appropriate treatment?

- A. No treatment, as this illness is self-limiting
- B. Ciprofloxacin 400 mg IV twice daily for a month
- C. Vaccinia immune globulin (VIG) intravenously
- D. Intravenous immune globulin (IVIG)
- E. Quarantine and expectant care

20-3. A vapor is released in a New York subway station in a crowd of people. A yellowish cloud envelops 20 to 30 people, who scatter from the scene coughing and gagging. A decontamination team arrives at the scene and determines the vapor to be mustard gas. The exposed people seem to be mostly asymptomatic with the exception of a few who have a dry cough and wheezing. They are all transported by police van to the nearest large ED. In a decontamination room, their clothes are removed and they are washed with water and diluted bleach (1:10 hypochlorite solution). Which of the following statements regarding this exposure is accurate?

- A. Decontamination will not change the extent of disease.
- B. Significant exposure will manifest within minutes as diffuse erythema.
- C. There is no delayed systemic toxicity after 2 days.
- D. The clinical hallmark is second-degree burns with vesicles 4 to 8 hours after exposure.
- E. Mustard gas antidote is the most important aspect of treatment.

20-4. A terrorist group is developing a weapon for use in aerosolized form. They use a human subject for testing and force him to breathe the substance. Within several days he develops fevers, chills, and a flu-like illness. Shortly thereafter he develops fulminant pneumonia, systemic toxicity, and a coagulopathy that results in clotting and subsequent gangrene in the nose, fingers, and toes. He subsequently dies. Which of the following statements about this disease is accurate?

A. It was known in medieval times as "black death" but no longer seen as a natural disease.

B. It is amenable to antibiotic treatment.

C. It has a bubonic form that is transmitted from a rodent reservoir via mosquito bites.

D. It caused a worldwide epidemic during World War I, resulting in the death of millions.

E. Human-to-human transmission is not possible.

ANSWERS

20-1. C. Anthrax is an illness that results from exposure to the spores, not the actual bacilli, of *Bacillus anthracis*. It is primarily a disease of farm animals, but is uncommon in developed countries because of farm animal vaccination programs. Vaccination exists for humans as well. Exposure to spores can be of three types: inhalation, ingestion, and cutaneous. Inhalation of spores results in phagocytosis by macrophages, transport to tracheobronchial lymph nodes, and multiplication of bacilli. In about a week after exposure, a nonspecific illness will ensue, including fevers, malaise, and dry cough. The classic chest x-ray finding is a widened mediastinum and hilar adenopathy. If untreated, this quickly leads to septic shock, ARDS, and hemorrhagic mediastinitis. Mortality is over 90%. GI anthrax can result from ingesting undercooked, contaminated meat, or simply ingesting the spores themselves. Symptoms include severe abdominal pain, hematemesis, and bloody diarrhea; mortality is about 50%. Cutaneous anthrax results from direct contact with spores, and mortality is about 20% if untreated. Within several days from exposure, papules develop that become vesicular. After another week, the lesions rupture causing a black eschar, hence the name "anthrax" (Greek for coal). **Treatment for anthrax with toxicity is intravenous ciprofloxacin, doxycycline, or penicillin G, although most weapons-grade anthrax is resistant to penicillin. Simple cutaneous anthrax and asymptomatic**

exposure is treated with oral ciprofloxacin or doxycycline for 60 days, while the patient simultaneously undergoes vaccination.

20-2. E. Smallpox was deemed no longer a naturally occurring disease in 1980 because of worldwide immunization programs; however, reservoirs of variola virus still exist in the United States and Russia. Variola virus is transmitted via aerosol and is highly infectious, making it an ideal biological weapon. After inhalation, the virus is transported to regional lymph nodes, where it replicates and spreads to spleen, bone marrow, liver, and other lymphoid tissue. Within 2 weeks, constitutional symptoms appear with fevers, chills, malaise, and headaches. Several days thereafter the virus localizes to skin, resulting in a maculopapular rash, followed by vesicles and pustules starting on the head, face, and arms and spreading downward. People are highly contagious from the time the rash appears until the scabs fall off, about 2 weeks. **Once the disease is present, there is no treatment except for quarantine and expectant care.** Mortality is about 30% for variola major. Vaccinia immune globulin (VIG) is effective for people at risk for exposure.

20-3. D. Mustard gas is classified as a vesicant, which is an agent that induce burns and blister formation after direct skin contact. Mustard gas is considered an ideal agent for terrorists because it is liquid at room temperature and can be easily vaporized. Its mechanism of action is unclear, but it damages cellular DNA and causes cell death. **The classic injury is similar to second-degree burns with vesicle formation. Symptoms do not occur until 4 to 8 hours after exposure; rapid decontamination with water or hypochlorite solution will significantly decrease injury.** There is no antidote for mustard gas. Inhalation injury can be significant, resulting in airway edema and hemorrhagic necrosis of bronchioles. Delayed systemic effects occur 3 to 5 days after exposure and include stem cell death with neutropenia, which can result in fatal infection, especially in the setting of extensive skin damage.

20-4. B. Pneumonic plague is similar in presentation to the influenza outbreak of 1918 that resulted in the death of millions. One distinguishing characteristic of pneumonic plague is the action of a bacterial coagulase enzyme that affects cooler areas of the body, resulting in black gangrene (hence the term "black death" from medieval times). The plague is currently pandemic in many underdeveloped regions of the world; it is endemic in the western United States. Rodents are the reservoir and fleas the vector, although cats are also a potential reservoir. Infected flea bites result in *Yersinia pestis*, a gram-negative bacillus, migration to local lymph nodes, and then proliferation. This causes inflammation and necrosis, resulting in extremely tender, enlarged nodes, known as buboes (as in bubonic plague). This can progress to septicemic plague with endotoxemia, shock, DIC, and death. Both bubonic and septicemic plagues are noncommunicable. Bubonic plague, however, can also result in pneumonic plague, which is highly contagious because bacilli are released through the respiratory tract. This is how "black death" became widespread in medieval times and this is similarly how *Yersinia pestis* can be used as a biological weapon in modern times. **The plague is susceptible to antibiotic therapy, including intravenous gentamicin, doxycycline, and ciprofloxacin. Oral therapy, including doxycycline, ciprofloxacin, or chloramphenicol, is used for mild bubonic plague or exposure prophylaxis.**

SUGGESTED ADDITIONAL READINGS

Agarwal R, Shukla SK, Dharmani S, et al. Biological warfare—an emerging threat. J Assoc Physicians India 2004;52:733–738.

Gosden C, Gardener D. Weapons of mass destruction—threats and responses. BMJ 2005;331:397–400.

Lee EC. Clinical manifestations of sarin nerve gas exposure. JAMA 2003;290:659–662.

Newmark J. Nerve agents. Neurol Clin 2005;23:623–641.

Shaking Convulsions

CC: Young man presents with shaking convulsions

HPI: S.S. is a young man who collapses in the lobby of the hospital and is noted by bystanders to have "shaking convulsions," during which his eyes roll into his head and his arms and legs shake. He does not strike his head on the ground. A nurse is on the scene quickly and checks his pulse, which is regular at about 100 beats per minute. He vomits a small amount. He is put on a stretcher and rolled into the ED. There is no family with him and no medical identification tag on his body. He has already stopped seizing when he arrives in the ED, and he does not appear to have lost control of his bladder. He is still unresponsive.

PMH: Unknown

Meds: Unknown

ALL: Unknown

VS: Temp 36.6°C (97.9°F), HR 108, BP 122/88, RR 20, Sao$_2$ 96% on RA

PE: *General:* Young man in his 20s or 30s; unresponsive but breathing spontaneously. *HEENT:* Pupils 4 mm and reactive bilaterally; 3-mm bite laceration to right side of tongue; no head contusions or lacerations. *CV:* S$_1$, S$_2$; tachycardic without murmurs; 2+ radial and 2+ DP pulses. *Chest:* Lungs clear to auscultation bilaterally. *Abd:* Soft; nondistended; bowel sounds present. *Extr:* No ecchymosis or deformity. *Skin:* Warm; mild pallor; no rashes. *Neuro:* Opens eyes, moans, and localizes pain with deep sternal rub; moves all extremities.

THOUGHT QUESTIONS

- What is the initial management for this patient?
- What is the differential diagnosis for seizure?

- What is the most common cause of seizure in a patient with a known seizure disorder?
- Which tests can be useful in aiding the diagnosis?

Immediate Actions:
Assure airway patency, spontaneous breathing, and peripheral pulses; place on 15 liters oxygen by face mask; place a bite block and nasopharyngeal airway (nasal trumpet) if still seizing; obtain an 18-gauge antecubital IV; check a fingerstick glucose and correct if necessary; administer lorazepam (Ativan) 2 to 4 mg IV bolus if still seizing and not hypoglycemic.

Discussion:
Hypoglycemia should always be the first thought in a patient with altered mental status or seizure, especially if the patient's history is unknown. Once hypoglycemia is established, sugar must be administered, preferably intravenously. If IV access is difficult or unavailable, sublingual sugar paste is an option. Glucagon 1 mg can also be injected IM (0.1 mg/kg in children), which will stimulate glycogenolysis and elevate serum glucose in 15 to 20 minutes.

For a patient who is normoglycemic and still seizing, benzodiazepines are the first-line treatment. Fast-acting agents such as diazepam (Valium), lorazepam (Ativan), or midazolam (Versed) are typically used. If the seizure is refractory to several doses of benzodiazepines and lasts 30 minutes or longer, referred to as status epilepticus, then phenobarbital should be used at 20 mg/kg IV at a rate of 60 mg/min. A patient in status epilepticus should also receive phenytoin (Dilantin) 20 mg/kg at a rate of 1 mg/kg/min. The drug phenytoin contains a diluent, propylene glycol, which can cause hypotension and cardiac arrhythmias; therefore, the patient requires a cardiac monitor.

The differential diagnosis for new-onset seizure is large, but a practical approach to diagnosis should focus on three possible etiologies: CNS, toxic, and metabolic (Table 21-1). CNS causes include a space-occupying lesion (e.g., tumor or abscess),

(Continued)

intracranial hemorrhage (e.g., subdural or subarachnoid blood), and infection (e.g., meningitis or encephalitis). Tricyclic antidepressant overdose is rapidly lethal and can be inferred by EKG findings of a widened QRS complex and prolonged QT interval. This is important to recognize because large doses of sodium bicarbonate can be cardioprotective and save the patient's life. Many other toxins can cause seizures, including amphetamines and cocaine, PCP, salicylates, heavy metals, toxic alcohols, and inhaled hydrocarbons (e.g., sniffing glue). Alcohol withdrawal is a more common cause of seizure compared with any other toxic ingestion. Metabolic disturbances that most commonly cause seizure include hypoglycemia, hyponatremia, and calcium and magnesium disturbances. In pregnancy, a seizure is assumed to be caused by eclampsia and is treated with magnesium.

Most patients who present to the ED with seizure will have an identifiable cause (e.g., hypoglycemia, epilepsy, alcohol withdrawal) and do not require head CT or LP to pursue further diagnostic possibilities. It is important to note that many events can be misinterpreted as seizures, especially those related to hypoxia due to poor oxygenation or poor perfusion. Therefore, it is essential to confirm normal vital signs, oxygen saturation, peripheral perfusion (e.g., warm and pink extremities, good radial and DP pulses), and EKG.

TABLE 21-1 Differential Diagnosis of New-Onset Seizure

CNS	Toxic	Metabolic	Other
Space-occupying lesion	TCA	Hypoglycemia	Eclampsia
Tumor	Amphetamines	Hypernatremia	
Abscess	Cocaine	Hypocalcemia	
Infection	PCP	Hypomagnesemia	
Meningitis	Salicylates	Hyponatremia	
Encephalitis	INH	Hypothyroidism	
ICH	Heavy metals		
CVA	Toxic alcohols		
AVM	Inhaled hydrocarbons		
Acute hydrocephalus	Alcohol withdrawal		

CASE CONTINUED

The patient is given supplemental oxygen by nasal cannula, and IV access is obtained. His bedside glucose is measured at 32 mg/dL. He is given one ampule of D50W intravenously, after which he becomes more alert and cooperative. He further drinks a glass of orange juice. A repeat fingerstick glucose 30 minutes later is 119 mg/dL. As the patient becomes more lucid, you learn that he is a 27-year-old, insulin-dependent diabetic who forgot to eat breakfast that morning. After 1 hour of observation in the ED, he has a normal neurologic exam and eats a turkey sandwich. His repeat fingerstick blood glucose level is 174 mg/dL. He is discharged home with his girlfriend, who will stay with him over the next 24 hours.

QUESTIONS

21-1. A 62-year-old woman with type II diabetes on glyburide presents after a hypoglycemic seizure lasting approximately 1 minute. She is otherwise healthy, taking no other medications, with no known drug allergies. She is afebrile with normal vital signs. Her physical examination is significant only for mild confusion. Which of the following statements is correct?

    A. Patients on oral hypoglycemic agents are more susceptible to hypoglycemic episodes than those who are taking insulin.

    B. The glucose-lowering effect of glyburide is independent of insulin secretion from pancreatic β-cells and is more a function of stimulating peripheral glucose utilization.

    C. Glyburide, a second-generation sulfonylurea, has an extended duration of action for up to 24 hours; therefore, this patient must be admitted to the hospital for observation.

    D. An insulin-dependent diabetic patient must be hospitalized for medication adjustment after an episode of hypoglycemia associated with altered mental status or seizure.

    E. Patients without a history of epilepsy who present after a seizure need to have a head CT and LP performed in the ED.

21-2. A 47-year-old man with a history of alcohol abuse presents to the ED after having a seizure. He has had both seizures and blackouts in the past. His last alcoholic drink was the evening before. This morning he experienced palpitations, diaphoresis, and a feeling of dizziness before losing consciousness and having a seizure lasting under a minute. Which of the following accurately describes alcohol and seizures?

    A. Excessive alcohol intake is not a risk factor for seizure.

    B. Alcohol intake itself can precipitate seizures due to the neurotoxic effects of alcohol and its metabolites.

    C. Cessation of alcohol rarely precipitates seizures.

    D. Hypotension and anxiety are symptoms of alcohol withdrawal.

    E. DTs typically occur 1 to 2 weeks after cessation of alcohol intake.

21-3. A 29-year-old man is brought to the ED by his family after he started to seize 35 minutes earlier. His fingerstick blood glucose level is 102 mg/dL. He vomits and continues to have generalized tonic-clonic movements. What is the best management for this patient?

    A. Supplemental oxygen, IV access, and IV lorazepam boluses, followed by rapid-sequence intubation and pentobarbital coma if the patient continues to seize.

    B. Supplemental oxygen, IV access, 50 mL (25 mg) of 50% dextrose in water IV, thorough history and physical exam, basic electrolyte panel, and observation until patient is able to tolerate food intake and repeat glucose measurement is in the normal to high range.

    C. Supplemental oxygen, IV access, and IV phenytoin titrated until patient stops seizing, followed by an EEG.

    D. Supplemental oxygen, IV access, and EEG to confirm epileptiform activity prior to infusion of anticonvulsant agents as indicated.

    E. Supplemental oxygen, IV access, and IV diazepam titrated until patient stops seizing, followed by an EEG.

21-4. A 5-year-old previously healthy girl presents after having a witnessed seizure at home. Her temperature is 40.2°C (104.1°F). Which of the following is characteristic of febrile seizures?

    A. Usually a partial (focal) seizure

    B. Usually lasts more than 20 minutes

    C. Usually occurs after the first 48 hours of a febrile illness

    D. Usually occurs in children aged 5 to 10 years

    E. Usually not associated with postictal state

ANSWERS

21-1. C. Type II diabetes, although not fully understood, is associated more with an abnormality in peripheral utilization of insulin as opposed to an absolute deficiency of insulin. Therefore, type II diabetic patients are more tolerant to excess levels of insulin without subsequent hypoglycemic episodes, whereas type I diabetic patients will become rapidly hypoglycemic when insulin is high without adequate blood glucose levels. Glyburide is a second-generation sulfonylurea, which acts in part to increase insulin secretion from β-cells. This agent is typically used in adult-onset diabetes when insulin therapy is not yet required. The action of biguanides (e.g., metformin) is independent of insulin secretion and enhances glucose utilization in peripheral tissues. These agents are typically used as an adjunct to sulfonylureas in type II diabetes. **Glyburide, unlike other sulfonylureas (e.g., glipizide), has a very long duration of action; therefore, hospital admission is indicated after an episode of hypoglycemia. Occasionally a glucose drip is required to maintain adequate serum glucose levels in a patient on glyburide.** Insulin-dependent diabetic patients can be discharged home after a hypoglycemic episode provided they do not have a serious etiology for their hypoglycemia (e.g., myocardial infarction, CVA, serious infection) and that they are able to eat. The primary doctor should be contacted regarding changes in insulin dosing and close follow-up. Admission should be considered in elderly patients and those who are unable to reliably manage their insulin at home.

21-2. B. Alcohol-related seizures are precipitated by alcohol intake, whereas alcohol-withdrawal seizures occur after reduction or cessation of alcohol intake (anywhere from within 6 to 48 hours and up to 1 week after reduction or cessation of intake). **Excessive alcohol intake is a risk factor for seizure due to increased likelihood of head injury, predisposition to metabolic disorders, and lowering of the seizure threshold in people with an underlying seizure disorder.** When evaluating an alcoholic patient, one must also consider head injury, toxic co-ingestions, missed medications, sleep deprivation, and electrolyte imbalances as a potential source for seizure. Symptoms of alcohol withdrawal include hypertension, anxiety, nausea, tremulousness, tachycardia, insomnia, and delirium tremens. DTs are characterized by disorientation, visual and tactile hallucinations, paranoid ideation, and delirium. DTs typically occur 48 to 72 hours after cessation of alcohol intake.

21-3. A. Treatment of a normoglycemic seizure begins with airway control, assessment of circulation, and benzodiazepines. Priorities are first to give supplemental oxygen, assure good peripheral pulses and blood pressure, gain IV access, and give either IV lorazepam (4–8 mg) or IV diazepam (10–20 mg). **Status epilepticus is defined as repeated seizure activity without interictal recovery, or as continuous seizure activity for more than 30 minutes. If several boluses of benzodiazepine fail to stop the seizure, the patient needs to be paralyzed, intubated, and started on a phenobarbital drip.** IV phenytoin is also indicated; however, its onset of action is 30 to 45 minutes. Prolonged, untreated seizure activity eventually leads to metabolic acidosis and neuronal death. A patient can continue to have a seizure even though paralyzed. Therefore, the patient needs to be admitted to the neurologic ICU for continuous EEG monitoring and titrated phenobarbital to control the seizure.

21-4. E. Febrile seizures are seizures that occur in children between the ages of 3 months and 5 years, typically within the first 24 hours after onset of a febrile illness. These seizures are usually generalized, tonic-clonic, occur after a rapid rise in temperature, and last no longer than 15 minutes. **There is usually a rapid return to normal mentation after the seizure has stopped (i.e., there is no postictal phase).**

 SUGGESTED ADDITIONAL READINGS

ACEP Clinical Policies Committee. Clinical policy: critical issues in the evaluation and management of adult patients presenting to the emergency department with seizures. Ann Emerg Med 2004;43:605–625.

Bazakis AM, Kunzler C. Altered mental status due to metabolic or endocrine disorders. Emerg Med Clin North Am 2005;23:901–908.

Huff JS, Morris DL, Kothari RU, et al. Emergency department management of patients with seizures: a multicenter study. Acad Emerg Med 2001;8:622–628.

Smith PE, Cossburn MD. Seizures: assessment and management in the emergency unit. Clin Med 2004;4:118–122.

Left-Sided Paralysis

CC: 73-year-old man presents with difficulty speaking and left-sided paralysis

HPI: L.P. is a 73-year-old left-handed man with diabetes and hypertension who woke up in the morning unable to get out of bed and with difficulty speaking. He was found in bed by his son, who lives in the apartment upstairs. He had last been seen at 11:00 the previous evening in good health.

PMHx: IDDM × 25 years, hypertension, diabetic neuropathy, right total knee replacement

Meds: Insulin 20 U NPH QAM, 40 U NPH QPM

ALL: NKDA

FHx: Mother with CAD; sister with stroke at age 65

SHx: Lives alone; past tobacco history of <1 ppd, stopped 30 years ago; occasional alcohol use

VS: Temp 38.0°C (100.4°F), HR 76, BP 133/60, RR 17, Sao$_2$ 98% on RA

PE: *General:* Awake and interactive. *HEENT:* Atraumatic; oropharynx clear. *Neck:* Supple, nontender; no bruits. *CV:* S$_1$, S$_2$; regular rate and rhythm; no murmurs, rubs, or gallops; pulses normal. *Chest:* Lungs clear to auscultation bilaterally; no respiratory distress. *Abd:* Soft, obese, nontender, nondistended; bowel sounds present. *GU:* Guaiac-negative brown stool; nontender; normal tone. *Extr:* Warm; 2+ pulses throughout. *Neuro:* PERRL; left visual field loss (i.e., left hemianopsia); left lower facial droop; able to name objects but with difficulty getting words out; 0/5 strength left upper extremity and 2/5 left lower extremity; 5/5 strength right upper and lower extremities; sensation and reflexes normal; normal finger-to-nose test on the right; left hemineglect.

Labs: WBC 13.0 k/mm³ (88% polys, 0% bands, 9% lymphs), Hct 35.0%, plt 337 k/mm³, Na 139 mEq/L, K 4.4 mEq/L, Cl 106 mEq/L, CO_2 26 mEq/L, BUN 14 mg/dL, Cr 0.9 mg/dL, Glu 226 mg/dL, Ca 9.0 mg/dL, PT 12.9, PTT 25.7, INR 1.1, UA neg

THOUGHT QUESTIONS

- Which immediate actions should be taken for this patient?
- Why is it important to get an immediate head CT?
- Which patients with acute stroke should receive thrombolytic therapy?

Immediate Actions:
Place on oxygen; establish IV; send CBC, basic chemistries, cardiac enzymes, coags, blood-bank sample; get 12-lead EKG; obtain STAT head CT.

Discussion:
Acute neurologic deficits are caused by either an ischemic or hemorrhagic stroke. A noncontrast head CT scan will diagnose a hemorrhagic stroke but is often normal in early ischemic stroke. If the scan is normal, IV contrast is injected and the scan is repeated in order to look for cerebral artery occlusion. Large-territory strokes (i.e., ACA, MCA, PCA) can have devastating effects (Table 22-1). Occlusion of the MCA is common and causes contralateral motor and sensory deficits; usually the upper extremities and facial nerves are affected more than the lower extremities (ACA territory). Speech deficits are also common. The majority of people have speech centers located in the left parietal lobe and will experience either expressive or conductive aphasia with a left MCA stroke. A greater percentage of left-handed people than right-handed people have speech centers located in the right parietal lobe. Large MCA strokes are also associated with hemineglect and visual field deficits.

(*Continued*)

TABLE 22-1 Ischemic Stroke Symptoms Based on Affected Vessel

Origin of Blood Supply	Vessel Affected	Part of Brain Supplied	Symptoms
Carotid arteries	ACA	Basal + medial cerebral hemispheres Ant. 2/3 parietal lobe Ant. caudate nucleus Parts of IC + putamen Ant. hypothalamus	Contralateral leg > arm weakness/numbness Gait clumsiness Altered mentation Impaired judgment and insight
Carotid arteries	MCA	Lateral cerebral cortex (ant. frontal to postero-lateral occipital lobe) Parts of IC + putamen Lentiform nucleus External capsule	Contralateral face and arm > leg weakness/numbness Agnosia Hemianopsia Aphasia if dominant hemisphere Gaze preference toward lesion side
Vertebral arteries	PCA	Brainstem Cerebellum Thalamus Auditory and vestibular centers of ear Medial temporal lobe Visual occipital cortex	Cranial nerve deficits, diplopia Nausea, vomiting Vertigo, ataxia Altered consciousness Crossed findings (decreased pain + temp. sensation ipsilateral face and contralateral body

Stroke has been found to be treatable in a select group of patients if IV thrombolysis (e.g., recombinant tissue plasminogen activator) is given within 3 hours of symptom onset. Thrombolysis is used in patients who have large-territory ischemic strokes who will likely be severely debilitated without intervention. Absolute contraindications to thrombolysis include rapidly improving symptoms, prior history of hemorrhagic stroke, any evidence or suspicion for current hemorrhagic stroke, significant GI bleed or major surgery within 1 month, previous ischemic stroke within 3 months, inability to maintain blood pressure lower than 185/110 mm Hg, or current anticoagulation.

CASE CONTINUED

The initial head CT shows mild cortical blurring in the right parietal region. A CT angiogram (i.e., with IV contrast) shows a large filling defect of the proximal right MCA and oligemia (underperfusion) of the right MCA territory, with likely PCA involvement as well (Figure 22-1). Because the onset of symptoms is unknown and the noncontrast CT already shows evidence of cortical swelling (usually not evident until 6 to 12 hours after stroke onset), it is decided to withhold thrombolysis because of the risk of causing a hemorrhagic conversion of the stroke. The patient's EKG shows atrial fibrillation, which is new for him. The patient is admitted to the neurosurgical ICU for further management. An echocardiogram shows an atrial thrombus, and the patient is started on heparin. He is discharged to a rehabilitation facility on warfarin (Coumadin).

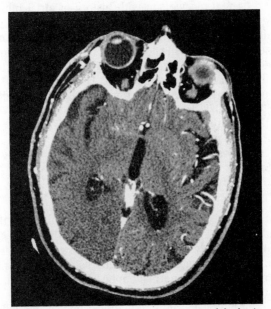

FIGURE 22-1 Contrast-enhanced CT image of the brain showing right-sided hypoperfusion (arterial vessels are enhanced on the opposite side) in a large area involving parietal and occipital regions. (Note that when reading a CT scan, the right side of the patient corresponds with the left side of the image.) (*Image courtesy of Massachusetts General Hospital, Boston.*)

QUESTIONS

22-1. An elderly woman presents with sudden-onset of aphasia and right-sided hemiparesis. Upon arrival to the ED she is awake but unable to speak. Her airway, breathing, and circulation are intact. On exam she can squeeze her left hand and press with her left foot to command. You are unable to ascertain whether or not she has a headache. You send her for a noncontrast CT scan of the head while you consider possible etiologies. In general, what is the most common etiology of acute stroke?

A. Hemorrhage
B. Thrombosis
C. Embolus
D. Hypoperfusion
E. Infection

22-2. An 84-year-old woman with history of atrial fibrillation presents to the ED with diplopia that began acutely 2 hours earlier, accompanied by dizziness and nausea. She takes warfarin, KCl, and diltiazem (Cardizem); she does not smoke. Vital signs are temp 37.0°C (98.6°F), BP 180/100, HR 120–150 AF, RR 16, saturation 98% on 4-liter NC. Her labs include WBC 11.4 k/mm³, Hct 39.0%, plt 299 k/mm³, Na 140 mEq/L, K 4.0 mEq/L, BUN 23 mg/dL, INR 1.1, and SGOT 63 U/L. Head CT shows no signs of bleed. What is the most likely cause of her stroke?

A. Hemorrhage
B. Thrombosis
C. Embolus
D. Hypoperfusion
E. Infection

22-3. A 53-year-old man presents with eyelid drooping that he has noticed for the past few days. He also noticed that when he was outside in the heat, only the left side of his face was perspiring. On exam, his pupils are unequal, the right being very small. His extraocular movements are normal but he has drooping of the right eyelid. Otherwise he has a normal neurologic exam. Without any more history or physical exam information, which of the following can be ruled out as a cause for his findings?

A. Tumor
B. Vertebral artery dissection
C. Herpes zoster
D. Stroke
E. Trauma

22-4. A 74-year-old man with a history of TIAs presents with acute-onset left-sided hemiparesis. What is the most likely etiology of his stroke?
A. Hemorrhagic
B. Thrombotic
C. Embolic
D. Hypoperfusion
E. Unable to know

ANSWERS

22-1. B. Eighty to eighty-five percent of strokes are ischemic in nature, while the remainder are hemorrhagic. Ischemic strokes include those due to thrombosis, embolus, and hypoperfusion. The majority of strokes are caused by thrombosis of atherosclerotic cerebral vessels leading to inadequate blood flow to a region of the brain. Lacunar strokes are micro-occlusions of small subcortical perforating vessels that supply the basal ganglia and brainstem. Lacunar strokes occur more commonly in patients with underlying hypertension or diabetes. Lacunar strokes, since they involve small subcortical territories, often involve purely motor or sensory deficits. Approximately one-fourth of ischemic strokes are embolic events, most commonly originating from the heart. Common conditions that lead to cardiac mural thrombus are atrial fibrillation, recent myocardial infarction, and cardiomyopathy.

22-2. C. This patient has a subtherapeutic INR on warfarin for AF (INR therapeutic range 2.0–3.0); her stroke with this history is most likely due to an embolic event in the posterior circulation (vertebrobasilar stroke). The vertebrobasilar system supplies the brainstem, cerebellum, and posterior cerebral artery. Posterior circulation strokes present in a wide variety of ways and involve cranial nerves, cerebellar function, and long motor and sensory tracts. Symptoms may be subtle, including unsteady gait, vertigo, nausea and vomiting, visual field cuts, and diplopia. Posterior circulation strokes may also cause unconsciousness, unlike anterior circulation strokes, due to the location of the reticular activating system in the medulla.

22-3. B. Internal carotid artery dissection, not vertebral artery dissection, is a cause of Horner's syndrome. Horner's syndrome is caused by interruption of sympathetic nerve fibers that originate from thoracic spinal nuclei and course up the mediastinum around the aorta and up the internal carotid arteries. Disruption of these fibers leads to ipsilateral miosis, ptosis, and anhydrosis. Internal carotid artery dissection results in hematoma formation in the wall of the artery, which stretches the sympathetic nerve fibers. Local tumor or neck trauma may also cause Horner's syndrome. Stroke would be an uncommon cause of Horner's syndrome.

22-4. B. TIAs are associated most often with thrombotic strokes. TIAs cause symptoms that resolve within 24 hours. These symptoms typically correlate to a specific vascular distribution, pointing to an underlying atherosclerotic source. Patients with TIAs have a 5% to 6% chance per year of having a stroke. Patients with TIAs warrant an admission to find a reversible source for thrombosis or embolism. The work-up includes a carotid Doppler study or MRA of the anterior circulation, including the carotid arteries. High-grade stenosis of the carotid arteries warrants surgical carotid endarterectomy. A patient with high-grade stenosis of a cerebral artery is a good candidate for anticoagulation or antiplatelet therapy. Cardiac echocardiography is done to look for an embolic source (e.g., mural thrombus) for the TIA.

 SUGGESTED ADDITIONAL READINGS

Adams HP Jr, Adams RJ, Brott T, et al. Guidelines for the early management of patients with ischemic stroke. Stroke 2003;34: 1056–1083.

Goldstein LB, Simel DL. Is this patient having a stroke? JAMA 2005;293:2391–2402.

Lewandowski C, Barsan W. Treatment of acute ischemic stroke. Ann Emerg Med 2001;37:202–216.

Sa de Camargo EC, Koroshetz WJ. Neuroimaging of ischemia and infarction. NeuroRx 2005;2:265–276.

Dizziness

CC: 48-year-old woman with dizziness

HPI: D.Z. is a 48-year-old woman who had a sudden onset of dizziness today while sitting at her desk. The room began to violently spin around her, and after several minutes she vomited and became diaphoretic. She tried to get up from her desk but was unable to do so. She put her head down, and after 10 minutes her symptoms resolved. Two hours later she had another episode as she tilted her head to the left to write. She denies hearing loss or tinnitus. She denies any prior history of dizziness. She denies any recent illness. She is now asymptomatic.

PMHx: None

Meds: None

ALL: NKDA

SHx: No alcohol, tobacco, or drug use

VS: Temp 37.0°C (98.6°F), HR 78, BP 122/84, RR 16, Sao₂ 100% on RA

PE: *General:* Healthy-appearing; comfortable. *HEENT:* Conjunctiva clear; oropharynx clear; TMs clear. *Neck:* No adenopathy; no bruits. *CV:* S₁, S₂; no murmurs. *Chest:* Clear bilaterally. *Abd:* Soft, nondistended, nontender. *Extr:* Well-perfused; no edema. *Neuro:* Alert, oriented; CN II to XII intact; no nystagmus, no diplopia, no visual field deficits, normal corneal reflexes; 5/5 motor strength in all extremities, no pronator drift; normal sensation throughout; normal finger-to-nose test and rapid alternating movements; normal gait including heel-to-toe walking.

THOUGHT QUESTIONS

■ What is the differential diagnosis for dizziness?

- Which features distinguish peripheral from central vertigo?
- What are etiologies for both peripheral and central vertigo?

Discussion:

Patients use the word *dizzy* to describe a number of different sensations, including a sense of motion or spinning, lightheadedness, weakness, unsteadiness, or simply malaise or depression. It is important to have the patient describe the sensation without using the word *dizzy* to elicit the specific symptom. Given the wide interpretation of the word *dizzy*, the differential diagnosis is also wide. Symptoms of lightheadedness or weakness can be consistent with dysrhythmias, hypovolemia, anemia, electrolyte disturbances, or viral illnesses. Unsteadiness can be a sign of cerebellar dysfunction, vertebrobasilar insufficiency, or posterior circulation stroke.

Vertigo, or the sensation of the world spinning around, is caused by either a peripheral or central process. Peripheral vertigo is typically sudden in onset, transient or fatigable, suppressed by visual fixation, and associated with nausea, vomiting, and horizontal or rotatory nystagmus. Central vertigo is associated with milder symptoms, is more sustained, is not fatigable or suppressed with visual fixation, and is associated with nystagmus that can be horizontal, rotatory, or vertical. Peripheral vertigo is often caused by benign positional vertigo (BPV), a process whereby otoliths precipitate from the endolymph in the semicircular canals and stimulate the hair cells of the crista ampullaris, causing vertigo. This is a benign illness that will eventually resolve as the otolith is cleared from the semicircular canal. Other causes of peripheral vertigo include labyrinthitis (e.g., reactive to nearby otitis media, ototoxic drugs, head trauma, perilymphatic fistula), vestibular neuronitis (i.e., inflammation of the eighth cranial nerve), and Ménière's disease. Causes of central vertigo are more serious and include CNS infection, vertebrobasilar artery insufficiency, subclavian steal syndrome, cerebellar stroke, vertebrobasilar migraine, tumor, acoustic neuroma, and multiple sclerosis. For any patient in which a central etiology of vertigo is a concern, an MRI of the brain should be obtained.

CASE CONTINUED

A Dix-Hallpike maneuver is performed, in which the patient drops rapidly onto her back from a sitting position with her head turned to one side and her neck extended slightly. Ten seconds after dropping her onto her back with her head extended over the end of the bed, she begins to develop symptoms. Horizonto-rotatory nystagmus develops, and she feels as if she will vomit. An IV is started, 1 liter NS given, and lorazepam (Ativan) 1 mg IV administered. Her symptoms improve significantly, and she is discharged with a prescription for meclizine (Antivert) 25 mg PO every 6 hours as needed for her diagnosis of BPV.

QUESTIONS

23-1. A 45-year-old woman presents to the ED with complaint of nausea and dizziness. She describes the dizziness as "the room is spinning," and she has had a couple previous episodes of these symptoms in the past. Her vital signs are normal. Her neurologic exam is normal, including tandem gait. She has mild decreased hearing on the left side. Which of the following does she most likely have?
   A. Multiple sclerosis
   B. Benign positional vertigo
   C. Labyrinthitis
   D. Vertebrobasilar ischemia
   E. Vestibular neuronitis

23-2. A 58-year-old man with history of BPH develops urosepsis for which he is admitted to the hospital, treated, and subsequently discharged. A couple of months later, he is noted to have mild sensorineural hearing loss in both ears. Which of the following medications was likely used to treat him during his hospitalization?
   A. Trimethoprim-sulfamethoxasole (Bactrim)
   B. Levofloxacin
   C. Nitrofurantoin
   D. Gentamicin
   E. Ceftriaxone

23-3. A 70-year-old woman complains of dizziness and vomiting since waking up this morning. She has no prior history of vertigo. Which of the following historical features or physical examination findings might suggest central rather than peripheral vertigo?

A. Sudden onset
B. Decreased corneal reflex
C. Horizonto-rotatory nystagmus
D. Transient and episodic
E. Vomiting and diaphoresis

23-4. A 52-year-old woman with a past medical history of high cholesterol and arthritis complains of episodes of dizziness over the past several days. She describes that the room spins and she gets nauseated, though she has not vomited. Not moving at all seems to help. Each episode lasts under a minute. On your examination, she has a positive Dix-Hallpike test. Which of the following agents has been shown useful in the treatment of her condition?

A. Caffeine
B. Diazepam
C. Aspirin
D. Pseudoephedrine
E. Heparin

ANSWERS

23-1. C. This patient describes multiple episodes of vertigo and has hearing loss, which is consistent with labyrinthitis, an inflammation or dysfunction of the vestibular labyrinth. True labyrinthitis involves both the semicircular canals and the cochlea; therefore, sensorineural hearing loss is expected. Other etiologies of vertigo associated with sensorineural impairment include Ménière's disease and acoustic neuroma. The Weber and Rinne tests are used to differentiate between sensorineural and conductive hearing loss. For the Weber test, the tuning fork is placed in the middle of the forehead; if sensorineural hearing loss is present, the sound will localize to the good ear. For the Rinne test, the butt of the tuning fork is first placed on the mastoid, followed by the vibrating ends placed beside the head at the ear. If the sound is louder when placed over the mastoid, then a conductive hearing loss, or middle ear process, exists. Since central hearing nuclei are spread widely throughout the brainstem, focal central lesions such as multiple sclerosis or brainstem stroke do not typically affect hearing.

23-2. D. A number of therapeutic medications have toxic side effects related to the inner ear structures and may result in sensorineural hearing loss or vertigo. The most commonly used agents include aminoglycosides (e.g., gentamicin), vancomycin, erythromycin, phenytoin (Dilantin), loop diuretics (e.g., furosemide), and salicylates. The other medications listed (levofloxacin, nitrofurantoin, ceftriaxone, trimethoprim-sulfamethoxazole) are not typically associated with causing hearing loss.

23-3. B. Peripheral vertigo is characterized by sudden onset, transient duration, fatigability, an episodic nature, suppressibility with visual fixation, horizonto-rotatory nystagmus, and intense associated symptoms such as vomiting and diaphoresis. **Decreased corneal reflexes are often the first sign of a brainstem lesion. Other signs of a central process for which one must test include cranial nerve deficits (e.g., diplopia, dysarthria, facial droop, facial numbness), cerebellar dysfunction (e.g., ataxia, dysmetria), and extremity motor or sensory deficits.**

23-4. B. Benzodiazepines (e.g., diazepam, lorazepam) are extremely effective for acute vertigo because of their sedative action on the limbic system, the thalamus, and the hypothalamus. Neurons involved in vestibular stimulation are mediated by acetylcholine; therefore, anticholinergic agents (e.g., meclizine, diphenhydramine, promethazine, scopolamine) are very effective as well. Patients should be told to avoid stimulants (e.g., caffeine, nicotine, pseudoephedrine) because they can exacerbate vertigo.

 SUGGESTED ADDITIONAL READINGS

Halmagyi GM. Diagnosis and management of vertigo. Clin Med 2005;5:159–165.
Kanagalingam J, Hajioff D, Bennett S. Vertigo. BMJ 2005;330:523.
Lempert T, von Brevern M. Episodic vertigo. Curr Opin Neurol 2005;18:5–9.
Swartz R, Longwell P. Treatment of vertigo. Am Fam Physician 2005;71:1115–1122.

Suicide Attempt

CC: 72-year-old man who cut his wrist

HPI: S.T. is a 72-year-old man who had an argument this morning with his wife. After the argument he went to the garage and cut his wrist with a wood-carving knife. He sat there for about 10 minutes bleeding on the floor before his wife found him and called EMS. EMS transported him without incident to the ED while holding direct pressure to the wound. The man denied lightheadedness en route. In the ED he states that he has never liked his wife, has had enough, and just wants to end it all. He has never had a psychiatric illness or attempted suicide before. He states that he would have let himself bleed to death if his wife hadn't found him. He states that his life is lousy because he has so many medical problems and he can't tolerate his wife. He has had difficulty sleeping, he has a poor appetite, and he doesn't have any activities he enjoys doing anymore. He states that there is no way the situation can ever improve and that next time he'll use a gun instead. He denies homicidal thoughts or hallucinations.

PMHx: Ischemic cardiomyopathy, NIDDM, hypertension, h/o CVA, chronic renal insufficiency, gout, peptic ulcer disease, s/p AAA repair, s/p cholecystectomy

Meds: Aspirin 325 mg PO QD, ticlopidine 250 mg PO BID, atenolol 50 mg PO QD, captopril 50 mg PO TID, glyburide 5 mg PO QD, isosorbide dinitrate 40 mg PO BID, allopurinol 300 mg PO QD

ALL: NKDA

SHx: Quit smoking 10 years ago; occasional alcohol; lives with wife of 46 years

FHx: Father died of unknown cause at young age; mother died of MI at age 74

VS: Temp 36.5°C (97.7°F), HR 74, BP 132/74, RR 16, Sao_2 100% on RA

PE: *General:* Chronically ill-appearing; distant but cooperative; flat affect. *HEENT:* Conjunctiva clear; oropharynx clear. *Neck:* Supple; no adenopathy. *CV:* S$_1$, S$_2$; II/VI SEM at apex. *Chest:* Mild bibasilar crackles. *Abd:* Soft, nondistended, nontender; normal bowel sounds. *Extr:* Well-perfused; trace edema; volar aspect of left wrist with 3-cm laceration from midline extending to ulnar side, mild oozing without direct pressure; 5/5 motor strength with wrist flexion, finger flexion, grip strength, and thumb opposition; normal sensation in hand. *Neuro:* Alert and oriented; CN II to XII intact; 5/5 motor strength all extremities; normal reflexes throughout; normal gait.

THOUGHT QUESTIONS

- What is the initial step in evaluating a patient following a suicide attempt?
- What are some parameters used to evaluate a patient's risk for future suicide attempts?
- Which patients with major depression or suicidal thoughts can be safely discharged?

Discussion:
The first priority in evaluating a patient following a suicide attempt is medical stabilization and assessment of injuries or poisoning. The second priority is to identify any underlying medical conditions that may be predisposing to the patient's mood or actions (e.g., primary CNS process, hypoxia, delirium). In most cases, all the necessary information can be obtained through a thorough history and physical exam.

It is challenging in the ED, with the limited time available, to evaluate a patient who has made a suicide attempt or gesture and to decide whether it is safe for that patient to go home. The mnemonic SAD PERSONS identifies several high-risk features that should be considered when making this decision: **S**ex; **A**ge; **D**epression or hopelessness; **P**revious suicide attempts or psychiatric admissions; **E**xcessive alcohol or drug use; **R**ational thinking loss (psychotic features that are affecting ability to

(*Continued*)

think rationally); **S**eparated, divorced, or widowed; **O**rganized or serious attempt; **N**o social supports; **S**tated future intent. White males over age 65 are by far the highest risk group for suicide (85% of all suicides), although suicide among males younger than 30 has dramatically increased. It is important to understand the circumstances surrounding the events and determine whether a suicide attempt was truly lethal or whether it was a gesture or call for help. A clear plan or possession of a firearm raises serious concern. The patient's insight into the future is also important, regarding whether there is perceived hope or whether they feel there is no way of escaping their problems. Substance abuse and lack of social support are also risk factors that should be considered.

Patients can be discharged home following a suicide attempt provided the following are true: 1) The crisis has been identified and addressed; 2) the patient is at lower risk based on SAD PERSONS criteria; 3) there is a verbal "contract" to return to the ED if the condition worsens; 4) family or friends are available to stay with the patient; and 5) specific follow-up has been arranged for within 48 hours. If there is any doubt as to the safety of the patient or others, admission and acute psychiatric consultation should be arranged.

CASE CONTINUED

The patient's wound is explored for major vascular or tendon injuries, then closed with interrupted sutures; he also receives a tetanus booster. It is determined that he meets a number of the SAD PERSONS high-risk criteria, including being a white male over age 65, stating the intent of killing himself and carrying through only to be stopped by his wife, relaying a real sense of hopelessness and anhedonia (loss of pleasure in activities), and conveying a plan to carry out suicide with a gun. He agrees to be admitted to the hospital for psychiatric evaluation and treatment.

QUESTIONS

24-1. A 36-year-old woman who was recently divorced presents to the ED with profound depression and feelings of hopelessness. She feels that she has no reason left to live. Upon further questioning, you learn that she has recently increased her alcohol intake and that she has access to a firearm. Which of the following is the most concerning when assessing the risk of potential suicide?

A. Divorced
B. Possession of firearm
C. Sense of hopelessness
D. Female 30 to 40 years of age
E. Alcohol use

24-2. A 29-year-old woman with psychiatric history presents to the ED following a suicide attempt. Which of the following psychiatric illnesses is associated with the highest rate of suicide?

A. Major depression
B. Borderline personality disorder
C. Antisocial personality disorder
D. Bipolar disorder
E. Schizophrenia

24-3. A 66-year-old man is found dead on arrival by EMS at his home, with a nearby suicide note. What is the most commonly reported method of completed suicide?

A. Medication overdose
B. Jumping from heights
C. Firearms
D. Poison ingestions
E. Stab wounds

24-4. A 34-year-old black man is brought to the ED from jail where he was found trying to hang himself. As part of your assessment you take a social and family history and find that he recently lost his job, which he claims led him to commit armed robbery. You discover that he was beaten by his father during childhood before his father shot himself in the head. Which of the following social factors is associated with low prevalence of suicide?

A. Family violence or sexual abuse
B. Unemployment
C. Family history of suicide
D. Minority
E. Incarceration

ANSWERS

24-1. C. There are many risk factors for suicide, and each case must be considered on an individual basis. **Four factors from the SAD PERSONS criteria are given greatest weight: depression or hopelessness, rational thinking loss, organized or serious attempt, and stated future intent.** These criteria represent the emotional state of patients, their ability to think through the problem rationally, and their intent or plan to carry out suicide or resolve their problems.

24-2. A. Patients with major depression are at the highest risk (15% to 20%) for committing suicide. Other high-risk psychiatric illnesses include schizophrenia, bipolar disorder, borderline personality disorder, and panic disorder. Antisocial personality disorder has not been associated with a high rate of suicide.

24-3. C. Firearms account for 70% of completed suicides, mostly in elderly and adolescent men. Firearms have recently surpassed drug overdose as the leading cause in women as well. The presence of a firearm in the household increases an adolescent's risk for suicide by 5 to 10 times. The use of firearms in suicide is usually associated with alcohol or drug use. Ingestion of drugs or poison accounts for 72% of suicide *attempts*; these are carried out mostly by women. Tricyclic antidepressants are responsible for the most deaths among patients attempting suicide by toxic ingestions.

24-4. D. Social factors and family history should be considered when evaluating a patient's risk for future suicide attempts. Probably the most important factor for a good prognosis is the presence of a support network from family, friends, social organizations, or church. An unstable family environment involving violence or alcohol abuse should be considered high-risk for someone at risk for suicide. A family history of suicide or a personal history of sexual abuse are also risk factors for suicide. Other factors such as unemployment and incarceration likewise put one at greater risk. **It is interesting that the prevalence of suicide among minorities is low, and suicide among elderly minorities is rare.** Completed suicide is predominantly carried out by elderly white males in a higher socioeconomic class.

SUGGESTED ADDITIONAL READINGS

Cooper J, Kapur N, Webb R, et al. Suicide after deliberate self-harm: a 4-year cohort study. Am J Psychiatry 2005;162:297–303.

Cooper JB, Lawlor MP, Hiroeh U, et al. Factors that influence emergency department doctors' assessment of suicide risk in deliberate self-harm patients. Eur J Emerg Med 2003;10: 283–287.

Douglas J, Cooper J, Amos T, et al. "Near-fatal" deliberate self-harm: characteristics, prevention and implications for the prevention of suicide. J Affect Disord 2004;79:263–268.

Soomro GM. Deliberate self harm (and attempted suicide). Clin Evid 2005;(13):1200–1211.

III

Patients Presenting with Cardiopulmonary Complaints

Crushing Chest Pain

CC: 54-year-old man with crushing chest pain and difficulty breathing

HPI: C.S. is a 54-year-old man with hypertension who presents
to the ED at 5:00 A.M. with crushing chest pain and difficulty breathing. He awoke at 4:00 A.M. with substernal pressure that he
describes as feeling "as if someone were standing on my chest." He
felt short of breath and began to sweat. His wife called 911, and EMS
arrived 10 minutes later. They put him on 15 liters oxygen by face
mask and gave him four baby aspirins to chew. They started an
18-gauge IV in the right antecubital fossa. His vital signs included a
pulse of 108, blood pressure of 106/64, and oxygen saturation of
96% on oxygen. En route to the hospital he was given a 500-mL
bolus of normal saline. He received sublingual nitroglycerin 0.4 mg
with some relief. He vomited once in the ambulance. On arrival to
the ED, he still complains of chest pressure that radiates to his neck
and jaw. He denies back or abdominal pain. His breathing has
improved with the oxygen and he has mild nausea. He has never
had similar pain and has no history of cardiac disease.

PMHx: Hypertension, hypercholesterolemia

Meds: Amlodipine (Norvasc) 5 mg PO QD, atorvastatin (Lipitor)
40 mg PO QD

ALL: NKDA

SHx: Occasional alcohol use; no cocaine use; smoked 1 ppd for
20 years, quit 10 years ago

FHx: Father died of MI at 58 years of age

VS: Temp 37.2°C (99.0°F), HR 110, BP 96/58, RR 26, Sao$_2$
97% on 15 liters O$_2$

PE: *General:* Pale, diaphoretic, uncomfortable. *HEENT:* Oropharynx moist. *Neck:* Distended neck veins. *CV:* S$_1$, S$_2$; regular; no murmurs; 1+ radial pulses bilaterally. *Chest:* Bibasilar crackles. *Abd:* Soft;

169

nontender; no masses. *Rectal:* Heme-negative brown stool. *Extr:* Trace pedal edema; cool, clammy extremities. *Neuro:* Alert, oriented; grossly intact.

Studies: See Figure 25-1 for EKG.

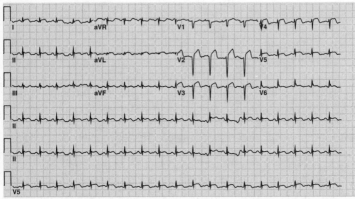

FIGURE 25-1 EKG showing sinus tachycardia with ST-segment elevations in V$_2$ to V$_4$ and poor R wave progression. (*Image courtesy of Massachusetts General Hospital, Boston.*)

THOUGHT QUESTIONS

- Which interventions need to be done immediately?
- What are the five life-threatening causes of acute chest pain, and how do you rule them out?
- What are the three indications for pharmacologic thrombolysis in acute myocardial infarction (AMI)?

Immediate Actions:
Place on oxygen 15 liters by face mask; start second IV; send blood for CBC, chem 7, Ca, Mg, Phos, CPK with isoenzymes, troponin; place on monitor and obtain 12-lead EKG; give aspirin 325 mg to chew; obtain portable chest x-ray.

(Continued)

Discussion:

When a patient presents with chest pain, diagnosis and management occur concurrently and immediately. The most important actions are prompt 12-lead EKG and aspirin administration, regardless of your degree of suspicion for acute coronary syndrome (ACS). Myocardial infarction should top your differential diagnosis. Other causes of life-threatening chest pain include aortic dissection, pulmonary embolism, tension pneumothorax, and pericardial tamponade. Additional common but less urgent causes of chest pain include pneumonia, pleural effusion, myocarditis, esophageal spasm, and reflux disease. It is important to exclude aortic dissection when treating ACS because administration of heparin or thrombolytics to a patient with aortic dissection will result in hemorrhage and death. A portable chest x-ray is obtained to ensure a narrow mediastinum and normal aortic contour, in addition to showing pulmonary edema or other causes of chest pain (e.g., pneumothorax or pneumonia).

Three indications for thrombolytic therapy in patients with onset of chest pain within 12 hours include EKG findings of 1-mm ST-segment elevations in two contiguous limb leads (I and aVL, or II, III, and aVF), 2 mm of ST elevation in two contiguous precordial leads (V_2 to V_6), or new-onset left bundle branch block. Any patient who meets any of these criteria requires immediate coronary revascularization. The first choice is to take the patient to the catheterization lab if a cardiologist and the facilities are available. If this cannot be achieved within 1 hour, the next best option is pharmacologic thrombolysis. There are several different thrombolytics available, including streptokinase (Streptase), alteplase (tPA), and reteplase (Retavase).

   CASE CONTINUED

The patient has large ST elevations in leads V_2 to V_4 consistent with occlusion of the LAD coronary artery with subsequent myocardial infarction (see Table 25-1 for anatomic regions of the EKG). Nitrates and β-blockers are withheld due to hypotension. The patient is given heparin 80 mg/kg IV bolus followed by 18 mg/kg infusion. Cardiology is consulted and the catheterization lab is activated. After 1 liter of normal saline, his blood pressure remains 92/48 mm Hg. Dopamine 5 µg/kg/min is started and titrated to 10 µg/kg/min to maintain systolic blood pressure over 100 mm Hg. Within 30 minutes of arrival, the patient is taken to the cath lab. Angiography reveals a totally occluded mid-LAD. An abciximab (ReoPro) bolus and infusion are given. Angioplasty is performed and a stent is placed, with resultant 100% patency. The patient is transferred to the CCU on heparin, abciximab, and dopamine drips.

TABLE 25-1 Major Cardiac Territories and Their Corresponding Coronary Artery Supply

Location	EKG changes	Coronary Artery
Anterior	V_2-V_4	LAD
Inferior	II, III, aVF	Right coronary, circumflex
Lateral	I, aVL, V_5-V_6	Circumflex, diagonal

QUESTIONS

25-1. A 69-year-old man presents with chest tightness and an EKG showing 3-mm ST elevations in leads II, III, and aVF. Which of the following is an absolute contraindication to thrombolysis?

A. Blood pressure 200/110
B. History of atrial fibrillation on coumadin
C. Ischemic stroke 9 months ago
D. Right total knee replacement 3 weeks ago
E. Hemorrhoids

25-2. A 62-year-old woman presents with substernal chest pain and difficulty breathing. An EKG shows 2-mm ST depressions in leads V_5 and V_6. She receives oxygen, aspirin 325 mg chewed, and three sublingual nitroglycerin tablets separated by 5 minutes. A portable chest x-ray shows no cardiopulmonary disease. Her vital signs are HR 62, BP 126/76, RR 18, and Sao_2 98% on oxygen. Her pain and ST depressions persist. What is the next appropriate action?

A. Start thrombolysis of unstable coronary plaque if no contraindications exist.
B. Start a nitroglycerin drip, start heparin, and consider a IIb/IIIa receptor inhibitor.
C. Start a β-blocker.
D. Await first set of cardiac enzymes before treating for myocardial infarction.
E. Perform an exercise stress test.

25-3. A 42-year-old man who smokes and has hypertension presents with 20 minutes of chest pain while gardening that was relieved with rest. His vital signs, EKG, and chest x-ray are normal. He receives aspirin 325 mg chewed. What is the most appropriate management for this patient?

    A. Discharge home to follow-up with his primary care physician within 1 week for an exercise stress test.

    B. Check cardiac enzymes, repeat EKG in 1 hour, and discharge home.

    C. Administer β-blocker and nitroglycerin paste to maintain SBP less than 120 and HR less than 70, draw cardiac enzymes, and admit the patient for observation and exercise stress test.

    D. Start a nitroglycerin drip, start heparin, and consider a IIb/IIIa receptor inhibitor.

    E. Consult a cardiologist.

25-4. A 70-year-old woman presents with chest heaviness and general weakness for 12 hours. Lab tests are significant for a markedly elevated troponin level. Which of the following is the most common complication of her condition?

    A. Ventricular wall aneurysm

    B. Ventricular arrhythmias

    C. Heart block

    D. Valvular insufficiency

    E. Papillary muscle rupture

ANSWERS

25-1. C. Absolute contraindications to thrombolysis include active internal bleeding, previous hemorrhagic stroke, ischemic stroke within 12 months, and suspected aortic dissection. Relative contraindications include severe, uncontrolled hypertension (BP >180/110), current use of anticoagulants with INR greater than 2.5 or known bleeding disorder, major surgery within 3 weeks, recent internal bleeding within 4 weeks, and pregnancy. If any of these conditions exist, then the risk/benefit ratio must be determined on an individual basis.

25-2. B. The goal for any patient who presents with chest pain, regardless of age, EKG, or suspected etiology, is to alleviate the pain. This is particularly true for patients with possible cardiac etiology, because persistent pain means cardiac myocyte ischemia and death.

All patients receive aspirin and sublingual nitroglycerin if SBP is greater than 90 mm Hg. **Patients with EKG changes suggestive of ischemia (e.g., ST depressions, T-wave flattening or inversion) receive β-blockage, heparin, and consideration of IIb/IIIa receptor inhibition. If pain persists despite this therapy, try morphine 2 to 4 mg IV.** If the suspicion for myocardial ischemia is high, proceed directly to a nitroglycerin drip at 5 μg/min and titrate up until pain-free or SBP is less than 90 mm Hg. Patients with new ST elevations in two contiguous leads should be considered for immediate percutaneous intervention or thrombolysis.

25-3. C. The EKG is only 75% sensitive for detecting myocardial ischemia; therefore, a normal EKG in a patient with risk factors for coronary artery disease is not definitive. Cardiac enzymes and troponin begin to rise 3 to 4 hours after the onset of chest pain, and peak after 12 hours. **Recent studies show that a low-risk patient can safely undergo a cardiac exercise stress test following a brief episode of chest pain if the following criteria apply: no history of coronary disease, no EKG changes, no ongoing chest pain, and two sets of normal cardiac enzymes separated by 6 hours. Emergency department observation units are ideal for patients such as this.** In young patients with no cardiac risk factors and a normal EKG, it may be appropriate to arrange an outpatient stress test and send them home without obtaining cardiac enzymes.

25-4. B. This woman has suffered a myocardial infarction as evidenced by her positive troponin level. Complications of myocardial infarction are lethal. Therefore, it is important to identify patients who are having an acute coronary syndrome and admit them for observation and cardiac monitoring. This is a simple disposition decision for patients who are having an ST-elevation MI. It is more difficult to identify patients who are having a non-ST-elevation MI because these patients will have subtle or no EKG abnormalities, and initial cardiac enzymes may be normal. **Ventricular arrhythmias (VT and VF) are a common complication of acute MI because acute ischemia causes ventricular irritability. These are deadly arrhythmias if they occur at home; however, in a monitored setting, rapid defibrillation of VT results in restoration of normal sinus rhythm in 90% of cases.** Another common complication of acute MI is heart block, which occurs typically with an inferior MI. Cardiac pacing is necessary if the patient is bradycardic with evidence of impaired perfusion (e.g., altered mental status or hypotension). Other complications of myocardial infarction include congestive heart failure, cardiogenic shock, pericarditis, mural thrombosis with possible embolus formation, myocardial wall rupture with possible tamponade, papillary muscle rupture with possible valvular insufficiency, and ventricular aneurysm formation.

 SUGGESTED ADDITIONAL READINGS

Achar SA, Kundu S, Norcross WA. Diagnosis of acute coronary syndrome. Am Fam Physician 2005;72:119–126.

Andersen HR, Nielsen TT, Rasmussen K, et al. A comparison of coronary angioplasty with fibrinolytic therapy in acute myocardial infarction. N Engl J Med 2003;349:733–742.

Antman EM, Anbe DT, Armstrong PW, et al. ACC/AHA guidelines for the management of patients with ST-elevation myocardial infarction-executive summary: a report of the American College of Cardiology/American Heart Association Task Force on Practice Guidelines. Circulation 2004;110:588–636.

Kamineni R, Alpert JS. Acute coronary syndromes: initial evaluation and risk stratification. Prog Cardiovasc Dis 2004;46:379–392.

Tearing Chest and Back Pain

CC: 56-year-old man presents with severe chest pain

HPI: T.P. is a 56-year-old man who presents to the ED with sudden onset of severe anterior chest pain that radiates straight through to the back. The pain started suddenly one hour ago as he was getting out of a chair. He has no shortness of breath, nausea, vomiting, or abdominal pain. He has no history of previous chest pain.

PMHx: Hypertension

Meds: None

ALL: NKDA

SHx: 20 pack-year history of smoking; no alcohol or drug use

VS: Temp 36.9°C (98.4°F), HR 98, BP 196/110, RR 18, Sao$_2$ 100% on RA

PE: *General:* Uncomfortable; diaphoretic; clutching his chest. *HEENT:* Oropharynx moist. *Neck:* No JVD. *CV:* S$_1$, S$_2$; regular; no murmurs; 2+ radial pulses bilaterally. *Chest:* Clear bilaterally. *Abd:* Soft; nontender; no masses. *Rectal:* Heme-negative brown stool. *Extr:* No peripheral edema; well-perfused. *Neuro:* Alert and oriented; CN II to XII intact; 5/5 motor strength all extremities; normal reflexes.

THOUGHT QUESTIONS

- Which immediate actions must be taken?
- What is the differential diagnosis for chest pain radiating to the back?
- How would you control this patient's blood pressure?
- What are the indications for operative intervention for this disease process?

Immediate Actions:
Place on oxygen and cardiac monitor; establish two large-bore IVs; obtain 12-lead EKG; obtain portable chest x-ray; send blood for CBC, chem 7, CK-MB and TnI, PT/PTT, blood-bank sample; order chest CT scan; start esmolol 500 μg/kg bolus followed by 50–150 μg/kg/min drip; start nitroprusside 5–20 μg/kg/min drip.

Discussion:
Acute anterior chest pain radiating to the back can be caused by cardiovascular (e.g., acute MI, aortic dissection), pulmonary (e.g., pneumothorax, PE), or GI (e.g., perforated ulcer, esophageal spasm, Boerhaave's syndrome) pathology. It is important to exclude the diagnosis of aortic dissection before treating a patient with presumed acute coronary syndrome with aspirin, heparin, or thrombolytics, because anticoagulation in the setting of aortic dissection will cause massive retroperitoneal hemorrhage and death. Findings suggestive of aortic dissection on portable chest x-ray are mediastinal widening and blunting of the cardiopulmonary angle, although the chest x-ray is sometimes normal. A STAT chest CT scan should be obtained if there is clinical suspicion for aortic dissection.

Control of the pulse-pressure product (HR × MAP) is essential in aortic dissection. An intimal tear usually occurs at the point in the aorta of maximal hydrodynamic pressure during systole, which is the aortic arch near the ligamentum arteriosum. Blood then tracks between the media and adventitia, which is exacerbated by increased pulse and blood pressure. It is important to first control the heart rate with a β-blocker (e.g., esmolol) and then reduce afterload (e.g., with nitroprusside). Esmolol and nitroprusside are ideal because they are both rapid acting and easy to titrate. Administration of nitroprusside alone will cause a reflex tachycardia and thus an increased pulse-pressure product. IV labetalol can be used as a single agent because it has both α- and β-blocking properties, which will reduce afterload while blunting reflex tachycardia. Surgery is indicated if the dissection involves the aortic arch. Conservative management is indicated for descending aortic dissections.

CASE CONTINUED

The 12-lead EKG shows no ischemic changes, and the portable chest x-ray reveals a widened mediastinum consistent with aortic dissection (Figure 26-1). Esmolol and nitroprusside drips are started to maintain the pulse lower than 70 and systolic blood pressure lower than 120 mm Hg. Surgery is consulted and arranges STAT aortography, which shows an intimal tear beginning in the ascending portion of the aorta, with a dissection and false lumen propagating to the distal portion of the aorta. The patient is taken to the OR, where a thoracotomy is performed and an aortic arch graft that bridges the ascending to descending aorta is placed.

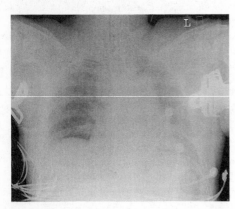

FIGURE 26-1 Portable chest x-ray shows widened mediastinum with indistinct aortic knob, consistent with aortic dissection. (*Image courtesy of Massachusetts General Hospital, Boston.*)

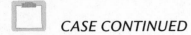 *QUESTIONS*

26-1. A 54-year-old man presents with acute, severe, tearing chest and upper back pain. At triage his HR is 110, BP is 178/110, and oxygen saturation is 98% on room air. The patient is brought to a room immediately, where he is placed on oxygen and a cardiac monitor. A large-bore IV is placed in his right antecubital vein. You suspect aortic dissection and administer labetolol 20 mg IV in order to prevent worsening and potential complications. Which of the following complications of aortic dissection is associated with the highest mortality?

    A. Acute MI

    B. Aortic valve insufficiency

    C. Acute stroke

    D. Horner's syndrome

    E. Aortic rupture

26-2. A 64-year-old man presents with sharp, stabbing anterior chest pain. His vitals are normal and his EKG shows no acute ischemia. Upon further questioning he states that his pain radiates straight through to the back. You are concerned about aortic dissection. Which of the following tests is considered the gold standard for the diagnosis of aortic dissection?

A. Esophageal echocardiogram
B. Aortogram
C. Transthoracic echocardiography
D. Chest MRI
E. Chest CT with IV contrast

26-3. An elderly woman with crushing chest pain radiating to her back, who has a normal EKG, undergoes a chest CT scan that shows an aortic dissection originating distal to the take-off of the left subclavian artery and extending down to the bifurcation of the aorta. How is this dissection classified?

A. Stanford type A
B. Stanford type B
C. DeBakey type I
D. DeBakey type II
E. DeBakey type A

26-4. A 62-year-old woman with a history of CAD presents with crushing chest pain that radiates to the midscapular area. Her pulse is 92 and her blood pressure is 178/92. She has a midsternal II/VI diastolic murmur. Her EKG shows 2-mm ST elevations in II/III/aVF. Her portable chest x-ray is normal. What is the best next step in this patient's management?

A. Consult a cardiologist for coronary catheterization.
B. Administer aspirin and heparin for treatment of acute MI.
C. Obtain a STAT echocardiogram.
D. Obtain a STAT chest CT scan.
E. Administer thrombolytic therapy.

ANSWERS

26-1. E. Acute aortic dissection has numerous grave complications, with the worst being rupture and massive hemorrhage. A dissection will often propagate proximally and occlude the right coronary artery, resulting in acute MI. Aortic valve involvement and regurgitation is also common. If the dissection progresses into the pericardial space, cardiac tamponade will result. As a dissection propagates distally, it can occlude the arteries that branch from the aortic arch, including the left common carotid artery, resulting in acute ischemic stroke. Occlusion of the left subclavian artery can result in decreased pulse and blood pressure in the left arm, although this is observed in fewer than 40% of aortic arch dissections. Horner's syndrome (unilateral miosis, ptosis, and anhydrosis) can result as the false lumen of blood expands in the posterior mediastinum and compresses the superior sympathetic ganglion.

26-2. B. Aortogram, which is fluoroscopy during the injection of IV contrast, is still considered the gold standard for the diagnosis of aortic dissection. This modality can detect the location of the intimal tear, the presence of aortic regurgitation, and involvement of major branch arteries. Newer modalities include echocardiography, spiral CT scan, and MRI. Echocardiography is not as sensitive as other modalities, but it has the advantage of being performed at the bedside, which is preferable in a patient who is unstable. Chest CT is often used for diagnosis in the ED because of its wide availability and increasing sensitivity given new-generation, spiral CT technology. The disadvantage of CT scan is that it cannot detect aortic regurgitation. In practice, a CT diagnosis of aortic dissection is often followed by aortogram or echocardiography in order to plan for surgery. MRI is often used to follow the progression of a chronic descending aortic dissection.

26-3. B. There are two widely used classification systems for aortic dissection. The older system is DeBakey: Type I is a dissection involving both ascending and descending aorta, type II involves only the ascending aorta, and type III involves only the descending aorta. Both type I and type II require surgery. **Stanford developed a simplified system: Type A is any dissection involving the ascending arch (DeBakey type I or type II) and thus requiring surgery, whereas type B is any dissection not involving the ascending arch (DeBakey type III).** Dissections involving only the descending aorta (DeBakey type III and Stanford type B) do not require surgery. DeBakey type A (choice E) does not exist.

26-4. D. An aortic dissection commonly dissects retrograde, occluding the right coronary artery and resulting in an acute inferior MI with ST elevations resembling thrombotic coronary artery occlusion. If aspirin, heparin, or thrombolytics are administered to an acute aortic dissection, retroperitoneal rupture and massive hemorrhage can result. If you suspect aortic dissection (e.g., tearing chest pain radiating to the back, aortic regurgitation murmur, decreased pulse or blood pressure in the left arm compared with the right, neurologic deficits) and the patient is stable, chest CT

with IV contrast is the best test to quickly make the diagnosis. If the patient is unstable with evidence of pericardial tamponade or loud aortic regurgitation murmur, then a STAT echocardiogram or immediate OR thoracotomy is indicated.

SUGGESTED ADDITIONAL READINGS

Borioni R, Garofalo M, De Paulis R, et al. Abdominal aortic dissections: anatomic and clinical features and therapeutic options. Tex Heart Inst J 2005;32:70–73.

Hagan PG, Nienaber CA, Isselbacher EM, et al. The international registry of acute aortic dissection (IRAD): new insights into an old disease. JAMA 2000;283:897–903.

Mariani MA, D'Alfonso A, Nardi C, et al. Aortic dissection: diagnosis, state-of-the-art of imaging and new management acquisitions. Ital Heart J 2004;5:648–655.

Mukherjee D, Eagle KA. Aortic dissection—an update. Curr Probl Cardiol 2005;30:287–325.

Syncope

CC: 77-year-old man with syncopal episode

HPI: S.E. is a 77-year-old man who underwent a CABG 1 year ago and who has been feeling weak for 3 days, followed today by an episode of syncope as he was getting up to open the door. He was caught by his wife; he had no head trauma, though did have loss of consciousness for approximately 2 minutes. He does not remember falling and denies vertigo or focal weakness, but does remember feeling palpitations and lightheadedness just before he fell. Afterward, he complained of chest discomfort and shortness of breath, both of which resolved before arrival to the ED. He denies nausea, vomiting, headache, abdominal pain, back pain, or any other symptoms. He has not had any recent illnesses or previous syncopal episodes.

PMHx: CAD s/p MI 12 years ago, s/p four-vessel CABG 1 year ago; paroxysmal AF; claudication; hypercholesterolemia

Meds: Triamterene/HCTZ (Maxzide) 25 mg PO QD; amiodarone 200 mg PO QD; warfarin (Coumadin) 2 mg PO QD; metoprolol (Lopressor) 25 mg PO QD; simvastatin (Zocor) 20 mg PO QD

ALL: NKDA

SHx: Lives with wife; past tobacco use; occasional alcohol; no drugs

VS: Temp 36.8°C (98.2°F), HR 52, BP 116/55, RR 16, Sao_2 99% on RA

PE: *General:* Healthy-appearing older gentleman; alert and responsive; no apparent distress. *HEENT:* Atraumatic; moist mucous membranes. *Neck:* No JVD; no bruits. *CV:* S_1, S_2; irregular; brady-cardic; II/VI SEM right upper sternal border; 2+ radial and DP pulses. *Chest:* Lung sounds clear bilaterally; median sternotomy scar well-healed. *Abd:* Soft; nontender; nondistended; bowel sounds present; no organomegaly or masses. *GU:* Guaiac-negative; nontender; mildly decreased tone. *Extr:* Warm; no edema; s/p left SVG harvest. *Neuro:*

Alert, oriented; CN II to XII intact; 5/5 motor strength in all extremities; normal sensation and reflexes throughout; normal finger-to-nose test; normal gait.

THOUGHT QUESTIONS

- What is the initial management for this patient?
- What is the differential diagnosis for syncope?
- Which patients with syncope should be admitted to the hospital?

Immediate Actions:
Place on cardiac monitor and oxygen 2 liters by nasal cannula; obtain 12-lead EKG; establish IV access; send for CBC, chem 7, Ca, Mg, phosphate, CK and TnI; obtain portable chest x-ray.

Discussion:
Syncope is defined as an abrupt decrease in cerebral perfusion producing a temporary loss of consciousness and postural tone, with subsequent spontaneous recovery. It is best thought of as a transient cessation of blood flow to the brainstem, either caused by hypovolemia (e.g., profound dehydration), hemorrhage (e.g., ruptured aortic aneurysm, ectopic pregnancy, GI bleeding), cardiac pump failure (e.g., tachy- or bradydysrhythmia, AMI), mechanical flow obstruction (e.g., massive PE, aortic stenosis, pericardial tamponade, aortic dissection), or loss of vascular tone or neuroautonomic reflex (e.g., vasovagal response, micturition or defecation, hypoadrenalism, carotid sinus sensitivity). Central CNS events (e.g., stroke) do not typically cause syncope, with the exception of spontaneous subarachnoid or subdural hemorrhage. Seizures and hypoglycemia should also be considered in the differential diagnosis for syncope.

The workup for syncope varies depending on the age of the patient, risk factors for serious disease, and the findings on history and exam. The latter is critical in excluding life-threatening etiologies, and a detailed inquiry should include questions regarding severe headache (SAH), neck pain (vertebrobasilar

(Continued)

dissection), chest or back pain (AMI, aortic dissection), difficulty breathing (PE), and abdominal pain (AAA). Tachycardia or hypotension is evidence for hypovolemia, hemorrhage, or cardiac pump failure. Pearls for the physical exam include listening for carotid bruits (carotid artery stenosis) and cardiac murmurs (aortic regurgitation or stenosis), doing a rectal exam to exclude massive GI bleeding, and doing a thorough neurologic exam to exclude central CNS processes. Essential lab tests include hematocrit, potassium, and glucose, as well as other electrolytes and cardiac enzymes in those at risk for cardiac ischemia. Urine hCG is critical in women to screen for possible ectopic pregnancy. Syncope is also more common during pregnancy in general. An EKG (AMI, arrhythmias, heart block, hyperkalemia) and chest x-ray (aortic dissection, PE) should also be done on all patients presenting with syncope. Depending on the patient's complaints or physical exam, a CT scan may be indicated in diagnosing SAH or SDH, aortic dissection, or AAA. A V/Q scan or CT angiography may be indicated if PE is suspected. An echocardiogram may be indicated if pericardial tamponade or valvular disease is suspected.

If no clear source for syncope is found, hospital admission depends on the age of the patient and his or her underlying risk factors. Most patients younger than 40 years can be safely discharged home given a normal ED evaluation, especially if evidence points toward a benign etiology such as vasovagal syncope, viral illness and dehydration, or micturition syncope. After 40 years of age, cardiac ischemia and malignant cardiac arrhythmias become significantly more prevalent. Therefore, unless there is clearly a benign etiology, these patients should be admitted for observation and further work-up.

CASE CONTINUED

The patient is mildly orthostatic and has equal BP measurements in both arms. EKG shows atrial flutter with variable block in the 50s without evidence of ischemia. CBC is within normal limits; chemistries are significant for BUN 38 mg/dL, Cr 1.9 mg/dL, both up from the patient's baseline (24 mg/dL and 1.4 mg/dL, respectively). Cardiac enzymes are normal. Chest x-ray reveals mild cardiomegaly but no acute pulmonary process. IV normal saline is started, and the patient is admitted for further work-up. During admission, MI is ruled out, and the patient is found to have episodes of bradycardia to the 30s at night. His syncope is thought to be due to bradycardia caused by his antihypertensives. His Lopressor is discontinued with resolution of his episodic bradycardia. His Cr improves with hydration, and he is discharged home.

QUESTIONS

27-1. A 62-year-old man with history of colon cancer status post resection, COPD, MI status post CABG, hypertension, hypercholesterolemia, and recent pneumonia presents to the ED after a syncopal episode. Which of his medications, if any, is most likely to have caused his syncope?

A. Atorvastatin (Lipitor)
B. Levofloxacin
C. Aspirin
D. Hydrochlorothiazide
E. Albuterol

27-2. A 59-year-old man presents after a syncopal episode. Which of the following symptoms on review of systems would make you most concerned about pulmonary embolism, aortic stenosis, acute MI, pericardial tamponade, and aortic dissection as possibilities in the differential diagnosis?

A. Dizziness
B. Back pain
C. Chest pain
D. Abdominal pain
E. Leg swelling

27-3. A third-year medical student presents after a syncopal event. She states that it was her first day on the surgical rotation; she had gotten up very early that morning, had not had time for breakfast, and had been standing for several hours in the OR observing a case. She had been watching a particularly bloody part of the surgery just prior to fainting. Which of the following signs or symptoms would be expected in her case?

A. Elevated blood pressure
B. Tachycardia
C. Blurring of vision
D. Flushing
E. Hot, dry skin

27-4. A 74-year-old woman with history of hypertension, high cholesterol, and diabetes, presents after a syncopal event. She says the only thing she remembers was feeling unwell for a couple seconds before she fainted. Which of the following is most likely to cause syncope with a prodrome lasting less than 3 seconds?

A. Aortic stenosis
B. Aortic dissection
C. Acute MI
D. Dysrhythmia
E. Pulmonary embolism

ANSWERS

27-1. D. Antipsychotics, antidepressants, antihypertensives, and antiparkinsonian drugs are commonly implicated in syncope, with antihypertensives and antidepressants leading the list. Additional medications that may cause syncope include β-blockers, cardiac glycosides, diuretics, antidysrhythmics, phenothiazines, nitrates, alcohol, and cocaine.

27-2. C. Chest pain in the setting of syncope is an ominous symptom, and a specific diagnosis should be aggressively pursued. An EKG will quickly give an answer as to whether acute cardiac ischemia exists. In the absence of ischemia, other etiologies to consider include aortic dissection, pericardial tamponade, and pulmonary embolism. Aortic stenosis can cause syncope because it poses a mechanical obstruction to cardiac output. This is especially true during times of exertion when the basal oxygen demand increases but the heart can only supply a fixed maximum flow rate due to the mechanical obstruction. This results in myocardial ischemia and chest pain, as well as cerebral hypoperfusion.

27-3. C. The patient described likely had vasovagal (or reflex-mediated) syncope. Nausea, dizziness, blurring of vision, pallor (not flushing), and diaphoresis are common prodromal symptoms of vasovagal syncope. Vasovagal syncope occurs when the normal sympathetic outflow in response to a physical or emotional stress is inappropriately absent, withdrawn, or replaced with vagal tone. This leads to decreased heart rate, decreased blood pressure, decreased cerebral perfusion, and finally syncope. Vasovagal syncope usually has a benign etiology and the patient will typically give a history of previous syncopal events, usually in the setting of fear, surprise, or extreme stress. Extreme caution should be taken in making this diagnosis in someone who has not previously had syncope, or in patients older than 40 years who are at risk for cardiac arrhythmias.

27-4. D. All of the choices listed are causes of cardiac syncope. **Dysrhythmias, including both bradydysrhythmias and tachydysrhythmias, are the most likely cause of syncope with an extremely brief prodrome (less than 3 seconds).** Bradydysrhythmias include sinus node disease, pacemaker malfunction, and first- or third-degree heart block. Tachydysrhythmias include narrow-complex (e.g., atrial fibrillation, atrial flutter, PSVT) and wide-complex (e.g., VT, torsades de pointes) tachycardias. Structural cardiopulmonary lesions are also a major etiology for cardiac syncope, with aortic stenosis being the most common. Other types of structural lesions include PE, mitral or tricuspid stenosis, pulmonary hypertension, and aortic dissection. Myocardial ischemia and infarction are also causes of cardiac syncope.

 SUGGESTED ADDITIONAL READINGS

Goldschlager N, Epstein AE, Grubb BP, et al. Etiologic considerations in the patient with syncope and an apparently normal heart. Arch Intern Med 2003;163:151–162.

Grubb BP. Neurocardiogenic syncope. N Engl J Med 2005;352: 1004–1010.

Strieper MJ. Distinguishing benign syncope from life-threatening cardiac causes of syncope. Semin Pediatr Neurol 2005;12:32–38.

Vincent GM. The long QT and Brugada syndromes: causes of unexpected syncope and sudden cardiac death in children and young adults. Semin Pediatr Neurol 2005;12:15–24.

Palpitations and Lightheadedness

CC: 58-year-old woman with palpitations and lightheadedness

HPI: P.L. is a 58-year-old healthy woman who one hour ago started feeling palpitations as if her heart were racing. She also started feeling lightheaded at the same time. She denies chest pain or diaphoresis but feels like she cannot take in a deep breath. She has no headache, vision changes, fevers, chills, nausea, vomiting, abdominal pain, dysuria, or diarrhea. She has had no recent illnesses, and she has never had a similar sensation.

PMHx: Abdominal hysterectomy

Meds: None

ALL: NKDA

SHx: No tobacco or drugs; occasional alcohol

FHx: No heart disease

VS: Temp 37.2°C (99.0°F), HR 140, BP 102/58, RR 16, Sao_2 100% on RA

PE: *General:* Healthy-appearing; mildly anxious; mild pallor. *HEENT:* Conjunctiva clear; oropharynx moist. *Neck:* Supple; no JVD. *CV:* S_1, S_2; tachycardic; no murmurs; 1+ radial pulses. *Chest:* Clear bilaterally. *Abd:* Soft; nontender; no masses. *Extr:* Well-perfused; no edema. *Neuro:* Alert and oriented; grossly intact.

Studies: See Figure 28-1 for the EKG.

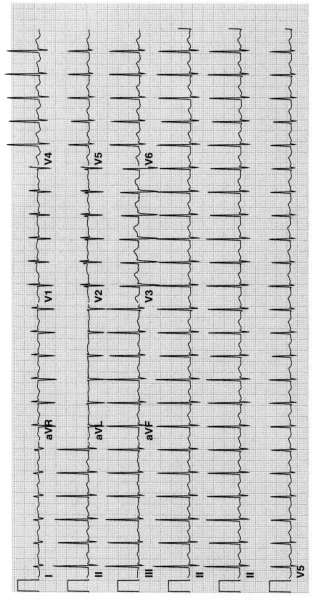

FIGURE 28-1 EKG demonstrates narrow-complex tachycardia at a rate of about 140/min with retrograde P waves (best seen in lead II as a small downward deflection following the QRS complex), characteristic of AV nodal reentrant tachycardia. (*Image courtesy of Massachusetts General Hospital, Boston.*)

THOUGHT QUESTIONS

- What is the initial management for this patient?
- What are the possible etiologies for this woman's tachycardia?
- Which medication can be both diagnostic and therapeutic for this patient?
- What further workup does this woman require?

Immediate Actions:
Place on oxygen 2 liters by nasal cannula; place on cardiac monitor; obtain 12-lead EKG; place large-bore antecubital IV; send blood for CBC, chem 7, Ca, Mg, phosphate; obtain portable chest x-ray; attempt carotid massage; administer adenosine 6 mg fast IV push.

Discussion:
Tachycardias can have many etiologies, but it is useful to break them down into three major groups: sinus tachycardia, narrow-complex tachycardia (i.e., supraventricular tachycardia [SVT]), and wide-complex tachycardia. Sinus tachycardia is a normal response to a systemic stress and therefore is not considered an arrhythmia. Narrow-complex tachycardias consist of multifocal atrial tachycardia, atrial fibrillation, atrial flutter, paroxysmal supraventricular tachycardia (PSVT), and junctional tachycardia. Wide-complex tachycardias are usually ventricular tachycardia, but can also be any one of the SVTs with aberrant conduction (e.g., bundle branch block or WPW syndrome).

It is often difficult to make a specific diagnosis for SVT because of the rapid rate; therefore, vagal maneuvers (e.g., carotid massage) and adenosine are used to slow conduction through the AV node in order to reveal the native rhythm. If the rhythm is irregular (e.g., atrial fibrillation) or the rate is exactly 150/min (i.e., implying atrial flutter with a 2:1 AV block), then longer-acting nodal blocking agents (e.g., β-blocker, calcium channel

(Continued)

blocker, digoxin) are used to control the ventricular rate. If the rate is 200/min or greater, the rhythm is likely PSVT, although PSVT is also common at rates less than 200/min. PSVT is a reentrant tachycardia at the AV node, and adenosine will act to break the circuit movement of the electrical impulse and reset the sinus mechanism. It is common to see a retrograde P wave (negative deflection) just after each QRS complex as the electrical impulse from the AV node travels backward up into the atrium. Any patient with narrow- or wide-complex tachycardia and signs of myocardial ischemia (e.g., chest pain) or pump failure (e.g., hypotension) requires immediate cardioversion. Patients with PSVT that breaks with adenosine and without evidence of cardiac ischemia need no further immediate workup and can be discharged home.

CASE CONTINUED

The rhythm strip shows a narrow-complex tachycardia at a regular rate of 140/min with retrograde P waves best seen in lead II, consistent with AV node reentrant tachycardia, a specific variety of PSVT. There is no response to carotid massage or Valsalva maneuvers. Adenosine 6 mg IV is pushed rapidly without response. Several minutes later adenosine 12 mg is pushed rapidly and a 3-second pause is displayed on the rhythm strip, followed by a sinus rhythm at 72/min (Figure 28-2). Her electrolyte panel is normal. She is told to avoid coffee and other stimulants and to see her doctor in one week for follow-up and a cardiac stress test.

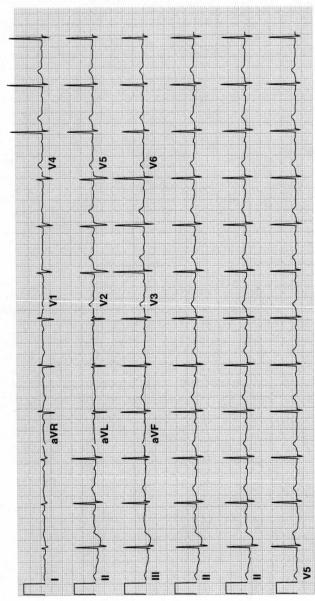

FIGURE 28-2 Normal EKG with a sinus rhythm at a rate of about 70/min after administration of adenosine. (*Image courtesy of Massachusetts General Hospital, Boston.*)

QUESTIONS

28-1. A 56-year-old woman with a previous episode of AF presents with palpitations and difficulty breathing. On the monitor her heart rate is 158 and irregular. There are no identifiable P-waves. Her blood pressure is 134/88. You consider using a pharmacologic agent to convert her to sinus rhythm. Which one of the following agents used to facilitate conversion from AF back to normal sinus rhythm is associated with polymorphic VT?

    A. Amiodarone
    B. Ibutilide
    C. Procainamide
    D. Sotalol
    E. Flecainide

28-2. An elderly woman presents to the ED with a chief complaint of weakness. She is very vague about her past medical history but can tell you that she takes a special medicine for a "funny heart beat." On EKG you notice a corrected QT interval of 550 ms. Which of the following agents *decreases* the QT interval (and thus would not be her "special" medicine?

    A. Procainamide
    B. Quinidine
    C. Lidocaine
    D. Sotalol
    E. Amiodarone

28-3. A 52-year-old man presents to the ED with palpitations about an hour before arrival. He takes no medications and has never had heart problems. You notice his heart rate on the monitor is 140 and irregular. What is the preferred initial agent to treat AF with RVR in this patient?

    A. Amiodarone
    B. Metoprolol
    C. Procainamide
    D. Sotalol
    E. Digoxin

28-4. A 64-year-old man with a history of CAD and coronary stents presents to the ED with lightheadedness, chest pain, difficulty breathing, and nausea. The cardiac monitor shows him to be in a wide-complex tachycardia at a rate of 164. His blood pressure is 92/46. He looks pale and mildly diaphoretic. What is the appropriate treatment for this patient?

    A. Amiodarone
    B. Lidocaine
    C. Synchronized cardioversion
    D. Procainamide
    E. Metoprolol

ANSWERS

28-1. B. All of the following agents have been used to facilitate the termination of AF and thereafter to maintain normal sinus rhythm: procainamide, propafenone, flecainide, amiodarone, ibutilide, and sotalol. **Ibutilide is a short-acting agent that has relatively high success in converting AF of relatively short duration. However, ibutilide has been shown to cause polymorphic VT in 2% to 5% of patients; therefore, a 4- to 6-hour observation period is required after its use.** Amiodarone and sotalol are both class III antiarrhythmics and thus have wide utility in both atrial and ventricular dysrhythmias. Procainamide is a class Ia agent, while flecainide and propafenone are class Ic agents; these all act to block sodium current and therefore slow conduction velocity in both atrial and ventricular myocardium.

28-2. C. The QT interval reflects the length of the ventricular action potential (AP). Class Ia agents (e.g., quinidine, procainamide) act to prolong the AP and thus the QT interval. Class III agents (e.g., sotalol, amiodarone, bretylium) block potassium efflux from activated myocardium, which prolongs the plateau of the AP, thus also prolonging the QT interval. Prolongation of the AP results in a prolonged effective refractory period. This inhibits repeated rapid ventricular activation, the hallmark of SVT. Both class Ia and class III agents act on atrial and ventricular myocardium. **Class Ib agents (e.g., lidocaine, mexiletine) act only on ventricular myocardium and *decrease* AP duration.**

28-3. B. The first priority for this patient is to control his ventricular rate. **As long as he has an otherwise healthy heart with a good EF, the first-line agents are β-blockers (e.g., metoprolol),**

calcium channel blockers (e.g., verapamil, diltiazem), and digoxin. Since digoxin will take several hours to take effect, metoprolol would be the best drug initially to control his rate. Digoxin can then be added for long-term rate control. For those with a known low EF, the recommended agents for rate control are diltiazem, amiodarone, or digoxin. If the patient has been in AF for more than 48 hours or if the duration is unclear, then anticoagulation and delayed cardioversion are indicated.

28-4. C. Wide-complex tachycardia should be presumed to be VT unless the patient is stable and has a known history of preexcitation syndrome (e.g., Wolff-Parkinson-White) or bundle branch block. The latter conditions may masquerade as VT during episodes of SVT. **Regardless of the etiology of a wide-complex tachycardia, if the patient is unstable (e.g., chest pain, difficulty breathing, hypotension), then cardioversion is indicated.** The following agents may be useful in monomorphic VT in stable patients: procainamide, sotalol, amiodarone, and lidocaine.

SUGGESTED ADDITIONAL READINGS

Chen-Scarabelli C. Supraventricular arrhythmias: an electrophysiology primer. Prog Cardiovasc Nurs 2005;20:24–31.

Hebber AK, Hueston WJ. Management of common arrhythmias: Part I. Supraventricular arrhythmias. Am Fam Physician 2002;65:2479–2486.

Sarkozy A, Dorian P. Advances in the acute pharmacologic management of cardiac arrhythmias. Curr Cardiol Rep 2003;5:387–394.

Van der Merwe DM, Van der Merwe PL. Supraventricular tachycardia in children. Cardiovasc J S Afr 2004;15:64–69.

Sudden Collapse in a Dialysis Patient

CC: 62-year-old woman with abdominal pain and diarrhea

HPI: S.C. is a 62-year-old woman who presents to the ED with one day of abdominal pain and diarrhea. She usually receives hemodialysis every Monday, Wednesday, and Friday. On Sunday evening she developed crampy abdominal pain and watery, non-bloody diarrhea. Overnight she had about 10 episodes of diarrhea. She missed her Monday morning dialysis and presents to the ED in the afternoon for persistent diarrhea. She denies fevers, chills, or vomiting. Two days prior, she took care of her 2-year-old grandson, who has had gastroenteritis. In the waiting room, she collapses and becomes unresponsive; she is taken quickly to the resuscitation room.

PMHx: Long-standing hypertension, end-stage renal disease, stable angina

Meds: Aspirin 325 mg PO QD, lisinopril (Zestril) 20 mg PO QD, atenolol (Tenormin) 100 mg PO QD, amlodipine (Norvasc) 5 mg PO QD, Nephrocaps one tablet PO QD, isosorbide mononitrate (Imdur) 60 mg PO QD

ALL: NKDA

SHx: No tobacco, alcohol, or drug use

VS: Vitals: Unable to obtain vital signs

PE: *General:* Unresponsive; warm. *Primary survey:* No spontaneous respirations; no femoral or carotid pulses. *Cardiac monitor:* See Figure 29-1.

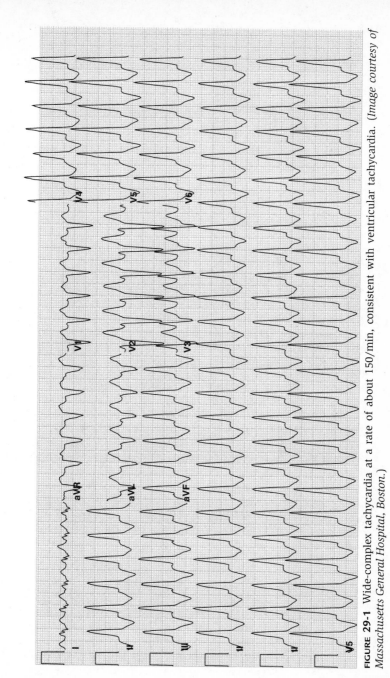

FIGURE 29-1 Wide-complex tachycardia at a rate of about 150/min, consistent with ventricular tachycardia. (*Image courtesy of Massachusetts General Hospital, Boston.*)

THOUGHT QUESTIONS

- Which immediate actions must be taken?
- What are the most likely etiologies for this patient's arrhythmia?
- Which medications should this patient receive to correct the underlying metabolic abnormality?

Immediate Actions:
Defibrillate with 200 J, 300 J, and then 360 J; perform orotracheal intubation via laryngoscopy without medication; start CPR; place a femoral triple-lumen catheter; send blood for CBC, chem 7, Ca, Mg, Phos, CK-MB and TnI; send venous blood gas; administer amiodarone (150 mg IV over 10 min, then 1 mg/min) and vasopressin 40 U IV.

Discussion:
Wide-complex tachycardia in elderly patients usually represents ventricular tachycardia secondary to cardiac ischemia. Other etiologies can include metabolic abnormalities (e.g., hyperkalemia, hypomagnesemia, hypocalcemia), hypoxia, and drug toxicity (e.g., tricyclic antidepressants, cocaine, antiarrhythmics). Wide-complex tachycardia in a dialysis-dependent patient should be treated as hyperkalemia before a potassium level is obtained. All patients who present with a wide-complex tachycardia without a pulse must receive immediate electrical defibrillation before all else. This is the only therapy shown effective for VT. The next priority is orotracheal intubation and mechanical ventilation, IV access, and initiation of chest compressions. Only after these life-saving interventions are performed should medications be considered, such as vasopressin, amiodarone, epinephrine, or lidocaine.

Treatment for life-threatening hyperkalemia begins with calcium chloride, which immediately stabilizes the myocardial cell membrane and lowers the depolarization threshold. Insulin followed by glucose IV push acts to drive potassium into peripheral tissues. Bicarbonate IV acts to alkalinize the serum and drive potassium into cells via hydrogen-potassium exchange.

(Continued)

> Sodium polystyrene sulfonate (Kayexalate) is an oral agent that causes sodium–potassium exchange in the colon and thus excretion of potassium. The most effective means of lowering serum potassium is by hemodialysis.

 ## CASE CONTINUED

The patient is administered electrical defibrillation at 200 J, which results in a sinus rhythm with a markedly prolonged QRS to 130 ms. A weak carotid pulse is obtained. She is intubated with a 7.5 ETT. Vitals include a pulse of 130 and a blood pressure of 78/42. She is given calcium chloride 5 mL of 5% solution IV, regular insulin 10 U IV, dextrose 25 g in 50 mL IV (D50W), and bicarbonate one ampule (44 mEq) IV. Her QRS interval narrows and her blood pressure rises. Her potassium level subsequently comes back at 7.5 mEq/L. She is taken immediately for dialysis and has a successful recovery.

 ## QUESTIONS

29-1. A previously healthy 17-year-old boy presents to the ED after 5 days of profuse watery diarrhea. Which primary acid–base abnormality would you expect him to have?
   A. Metabolic alkalosis
   B. Anion gap metabolic acidosis
   C. Non-anion-gap metabolic acidosis
   D. Respiratory acidosis
   E. Respiratory alkalosis

29-2. A 77-year-old patient in the ED complains of episodes of palpitations and lightheadedness. She is triaged to a room, seen by the nurse, placed on oxygen and cardiac monitor, and is undergoing IV placement when she suddenly becomes unresponsive. The monitor shows a wide QRS complex that is regular at roughly 150-200 bpm. You are unable to feel a femoral or carotid pulse. Which of the following is the first-line intervention?
   A. Epinephrine
   B. Lidocaine
   C. Electrical defibrillation
   D. Atropine
   E. Amiodarone

29-3. A 44-year-old dialysis patient is found to have a potassium level of 6.0 mEq/L on routine bloodwork. Which of the following EKG findings is seen earliest in his condition?

A. Flattened T waves
B. Sine waves
C. Widened QRS interval
D. Peaked P waves
E. Shortened QT interval

29-4. A 56-year-old man complains of weakness and abdominal cramping. Electrolytes reveal a potassium level of 2.5 mEq/L. Which of the following may have led to his hypokalemia?

A. Lactic acidosis
B. Massive blood transfusion
C. Hyperaldosteronism
D. NSAID use
E. Sepsis

ANSWERS

29-1. C. Diarrhea causes an excessive loss of bicarbonate, which leads to a metabolic acidosis. A primary loss of bicarbonate, whether via the GI tract or the kidneys (e.g., proximal or distal renal tubular acidosis, acetazolamide therapy), is followed by a compensatory elevation of chloride, which results in a hyperchloremic non-anion-gap metabolic acidosis. Anion gap metabolic acidosis is caused by the introduction of acidic anions and secondary consumption of serum bicarbonate. Common causes for anion gap metabolic acidosis (mnemonic: MUDPILES) include methanol, uremia, diabetic ketoacidosis, paraldehyde, infection/intoxication (alcohol, iron, isoniazid), lactic acidosis (e.g., from hypoxia or sepsis), ethylene glycol, and salicylates. Primary respiratory acidosis is due to inadequate ventilation (i.e., elimination of carbon dioxide) combined with inadequate diffusion of oxygen across the pulmonary capillary beds. This acid–base disorder is seen with respiratory failure, ARDS, massive PE, and severe COPD.

29-2. C. The first priority in pulseless ventricular tachycardia is electrical defibrillation, which is the only intervention shown to improve outcome. Second priority is orotracheal intubation, mechanical ventilation, and initiation of CPR. If these measures fail to restore spontaneous circulation, then Code medications should be administered. Epinephrine and vasopressin are both potent vasopressors that act to increase peripheral vasoconstriction and increase cerebral perfusion. Approved antiarrhythmic agents include lidocaine, amiodarone, procainamide, and bretylium. These act to stabilize cardiac cell membranes and decrease automaticity. Atropine blocks muscarinic parasympathetic receptors and increases cardiac automaticity, which in theory perpetuates ventricular tachycardia. Atropine is indicated for symptomatic bradycardia and asystole, not tachyarrhythmias.

29-3. E. Early hyperkalemia is characterized by peaked T waves and QT shortening. As hyperkalemia progresses, the PR and QRS intervals widen, and the P-wave amplitude decreases. Eventually, P waves disappear and the QRS widens to the point at which the tracing resembles a sine wave. Following that, the rhythm will degenerate into ventricular fibrillation and then asystole.

29-4. C. Aldosterone acts at the kidneys to absorb sodium at the distal renal tubule in exchange for potassium excretion. Therefore, hyperaldosteronism would result in sodium retention and potassium wasting. Symptoms of hypokalemia may include palpitations, muscle weakness or cramping, nausea, vomiting, constipation, abdominal cramping, polyuria/polydipsia, psychosis, or depression. Causes of *hyperkalemia,* on the other hand, are divided into extrarenal, renal, and lab error. The most common extrarenal cause is acidosis of any etiology, but especially mesenteric ischemia, crush and burn injuries, and sepsis. Other extrarenal causes include potassium supplements, β-blocker administration, massive blood transfusions, and tumor lysis syndrome. Renal causes include any condition leading to worsening renal failure, which results in impaired ability to excrete potassium. Many drugs can affect kidney function and result in hyperkalemia, including NSAIDs, ACE inhibitors, and potassium-sparing diuretics.

 SUGGESTED ADDITIONAL READINGS

Mahoney BA, Smith WA, Lo DS, et al. Emergency interventions for hyperkalemia. Cochrane Database Syst Rev 2005;2:CD003235.

Saxon LA. Sudden cardiac death: epidemiology and temporal trends. Rev Cardiovasc Med 2005;6 Suppl 2:S12–20.

Schaefer TJ, Wolford RW. Disorders of potassium. Emerg Med Clin North Am 2005;23:723–747.

Wenzel V, Krismer AC, Arntz HR, et al. A comparison of vasopressin and epinephrine for out-of-hospital cardiopulmonary resuscitation. N Engl J Med 2004;350:105–113.

Shortness of Breath and Fatigue

CC: 76-year-old woman with shortness of breath and fatigue

HPI: D.F. is a 76-year-old woman with COPD, CHF, AF, and hypertension; she is on home O_2. She has been feeling fatigued for the past several days, and has required 4 liters O_2 instead of her usual 3 liters. She denies fevers, chills, chest pain, nausea, vomiting, diarrhea, or abdominal pain, and has been tolerating liquids but has a decreased appetite. She has not skipped any medications, though has been to several family gatherings recently for holiday meals.

PMHx: Hypertension, atrial fibrillation, CHF, COPD, s/p three-vessel CABG; s/p right inguinal hernia repair at age 61

Meds: Warfarin (Coumadin) 6 mg PO QD, furosemide (Lasix) 40 mg PO QD, captopril 12.5 mg PO TID, digoxin 0.125 mg PO QD, metoprolol (Lopressor) 50 mg PO BID, esomeprazole (Nexium) 20 mg PO QD, fluticasone (Flovent) 2 puffs BID, albuterol 1.25 mg inh Q4–6 hr PRN, ipratropium inh PRN

ALL: Penicillin

FHx: Brother with CAD and CHF; sister with NIDDM

SHx: Lives with husband; no tobacco, alcohol, or drug use

VS: Temp 36.4°C (97.5°F), HR 96, BP 186/105, RR 24, Sao_2 82% to 90% on RA, 93% on 4 liters NC

PE: *General:* Well-developed elderly woman, alert and appropriate, in mild respiratory distress. *HEENT:* Moist mucous membranes. *Neck:* Elevated JVP. *CV:* S_1, S_2; irregularly irregular rhythm; no murmurs or gallops; 2+ radial and DP pulses. *Chest:* Rales audible bilaterally throughout lung fields. *Abd:* Soft; nontender; nondistended; no hepatomegaly; bowel sounds present. *GU:* Heme-negative stool. *Extr:* 2+ pedal edema to distal calves bilaterally; no lesions. *Neuro:* Nonfocal.

THOUGHT QUESTIONS

- What is the initial management for this patient?
- What is the differential diagnosis for this patient?
- Which diagnostic tests, if any, should be performed?
- What is the approach to treatment?

Immediate Actions:
Place on 100% oxygen by face mask; obtain 12-lead EKG; establish IV and send CBC, chem 7, cardiac enzymes, digoxin level; place Foley catheter and send urinalysis; get portable chest x-ray; administer aspirin 325 mg PO, Lasix 60 mg IV, and nitroglycerin paste 2 inches to her chest wall.

Discussion:
This patient's symptoms are most consistent with acute pulmonary edema (acute CHF), although one must also consider COPD flare, pulmonary embolism, and acute pneumonia. Common precipitants for CHF include acute MI, valvular abnormalities, poorly controlled hypertension, dietary indiscretion, medication noncompliance, or underlying infection. An EKG is important to evaluate for cardiac ischemia, and a chest x-ray will confirm the suspicion of pulmonary edema. ABG may be helpful to evaluate the extent of respiratory acidosis and to follow the effectiveness of treatment. However, the decision to intubate or provide noninvasive positive-pressure ventilation should be based on the clinical appearance of the patient.

Treatment for acute CHF involves oxygenation and ventilation (including positive-pressure ventilation via mask or ETT if the patient is in extremis), diuretics (e.g., Lasix), and preload reduction via vasodilatation (e.g., nitrates). Patients with acute CHF are typically hypertensive and tolerate aggressive diuresis and preload reduction; however, if the patient is hypotensive, inotropic agents (e.g., dopamine) may be required in order to increase cardiac output and reverse pulmonary congestion.

CASE CONTINUED

The patient is placed on 100% O_2 by face mask. Her EKG shows AF at 96 bpm without evidence of ischemia. Portable chest x-ray reveals moderate to marked pulmonary edema (Figure 30-1). Her labs show Hct 31.1% (same as patient's baseline Hct), normal cardiac enzymes, and digoxin 0.3 ng/mL (therapeutic 0.6–1.2 ng/mL). The patient is given Lasix 60 mg IV and 2 inches of nitroglycerin paste, resulting in greater than 2 liters of urine output and rapid improvement in her symptoms; her O_2 saturation improves to 98%. She is admitted for further treatment of her acute CHF exacerbation, fine-tuning of her cardiac medications, and work-up of her mild anemia.

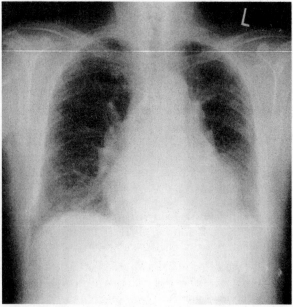

FIGURE **30-1** Upright chest x-ray shows bilateral interstitial edema characterized by diffuse hazy appearance, indistinct vascular borders, peribronchial cuffing, and Kerley B lines seen peripherally. There is also mild cardiomegaly and a small left pleural effusion. (*Image courtesy of Massachusetts General Hospital, Boston.*)

QUESTIONS

30-1. An elderly woman presents with chest pain; you do a chart review and notice that she has a history of right-sided heart failure. Which of the following would be consistent with right-sided heart failure?
A. Orthopnea
B. Paroxysmal nocturnal dyspnea
C. Peripheral edema
D. S_3 gallop
E. Pulmonary rales

30-2. A woman presents to the ED with general malaise, weakness, and shortness of breath. She has a history of a low ejection fraction due to ischemic cardiomyopathy. Her blood pressure typically runs low, but today it is lower than usual, at 86/62 mm Hg. On exam, she has bilateral rales. After a discussion with the attending physician, the conclusion is that she likely has impaired stroke volume (the volume of blood expelled from the left ventricle into the aorta with each heart beat) and acute CHF. In order to maximize her cardiac output, which of the following do you want to reduce?
A. Contractility
B. Heart rate
C. Preload
D. Oxygenation
E. Stroke volume

30-3. A patient presents to the clinic with a history of chronic CHF; she has been off her medications for the past two months and is starting to have symptoms of exertional dyspnea, peripheral edema, orthopnea, and weight gain. Which of the following would exacerbate her symptoms?
A. Reduction of cardiac work
B. Enhancement of myocardial contractility
C. Reduction of fluid retention
D. Symptomatic relief
E. Increased peripheral vascular resistance

30-4. A 56-year-old man with a history of CHF presents with a sudden onset of difficulty breathing, wheezing, and chest tightness. On arrival by EMS, he is sitting bolt upright and taking rapid, shallow breaths. His skin is cool and clammy. His vitals are HR 124, BP 88/46, RR 36, and oxygen saturation 88% on room air. He has elevated neck veins, an S_3 murmur, and bilateral crackles half way up his lungs. Which of the following should be avoided until his blood pressure has improved?
A. Oxygen
B. Dobutamine
C. Furosemide
D. Nitroglycerin
E. Continuous positive airway pressure (CPAP)

ANSWERS

30-1. C. Peripheral edema is a sign of right-sided heart failure. The other options listed (orthopnea, paroxysmal nocturnal dyspnea, and S_3 gallop) are found in left-sided heart failure. Additional signs and symptoms of left-sided failure include dyspnea, fatigue, mental status changes, pulmonary rales or wheezes, tachycardia, tachypnea, S_4, nocturia, and diaphoresis. **Additional signs and symptoms of right-sided failure include JVD, hepatomegaly and RUQ pain, nausea, anorexia, dependent edema, and hepatojugular reflux.**

30-2. C. Stroke volume and heart rate together determine cardiac output (CO = HR × SV). Heart rate is not a factor in determining ventricular stroke volume. Stroke volume depends on contractility of the myocytes, preload (the amount of myocardial stretch, or end-diastolic ventricular volume), and afterload (effective resistance to ventricular outflow). The Frank-Starling curve relates preload (measured as left ventricular end-diastolic volume or pressure) to ventricular stroke volume or cardiac output. **The greater the filling of the ventricle during diastole (i.e., greater preload), the more the ventricular myocytes stretch and the greater the resultant contractility and cardiac output. However, excessive preload and myocardial stretch (as seen with fluid overload and CHF) causes a decrease in cardiac output. Therefore, preload reduction is the goal for acute CHF in order to optimize myocardial stretch and cardiac output.**

30-3. E. This patient has an exacerbation of her chronic CHF. Enhancement of myocardial contractility (e.g., digoxin), reduction of cardiac work (e.g., afterload reduction with ACE inhibitors and other antihypertensive agents), and decreasing fluid retention (e.g., diuretics) are all important factors in treatment for chronic CHF. Correction of any underlying cause of the CHF (e.g., ongoing cardiac ischemia, aortic stenosis, mitral insufficiency, anemia, or thyrotoxicosis), if present, should be pursued. If the cause of CHF is not correctable, treatment is aimed at symptomatic relief. **Increased peripheral vascular resistance, in effect increasing afterload, would increase the workload placed on the heart and therefore exacerbate CHF.**

30-4. D. This patient has acute cardiogenic CHF. **Oxygen, dobutamine (or other inotropic agents), morphine, CPAP, furosemide (and/or other diuretics), and nitroglycerin (or other venodilators) can all be useful in treatment of acute cardiogenic CHF. In this particular patient with a low blood pressure, however, morphine and nitroglycerin should be avoided until his blood pressure has normalized.** CPAP is the application of positive airway pressure via a tight-fitting mask attached to a pressure source, referred to as noninvasive positive-pressure ventilation. This acts to reopen (or recruit) alveoli that have collapsed because of the interstitial edema and alveolar exudates. This increases the delivery of oxygen and improves alveolar gas exchange.

 SUGGESTED ADDITIONAL READINGS

Diamond JA, Phillips RA. Hypertensive heart disease. Hypertens Res 2005;28:191–202.

Gallagher MJ, McCullough PA. The emerging role of natriuretic peptides in the diagnosis and treatment of decompensated heart failure. Curr Heart Fail Rep 2004;1:129–135.

Izzo JL Jr, Gradman AH. Mechanisms and management of hypertensive heart disease: from left ventricular hypertrophy to heart failure. Med Clin North Am 2004;88:1257–1271.

Mitchell J, Taylor A. Congestive heart failure in women. J Fam Pract 2005;Suppl:6–7.

Shortness of Breath and Chest Pain

CC: 36-year-old woman with shortness of breath and chest pain

HPI: S.B. is a 36-year-old woman with sudden onset last night of left-sided chest pain and mild shortness of breath. She was able to get to sleep but woke up this morning with persistent pain. The pain is worse when she takes a deep breath. She walked up the stairs at home and became very short of breath, which made her come to the ED. She has no fevers, chills, back or abdominal pain, or recent illnesses. One week ago she took a 14-hour flight from Australia, and since then has had soreness in her right calf.

PMHx: None

Meds: OCPs

ALL: NKDA

FHx: Parents with CAD; grandfathers died of CVA

SHx: 16 pack-year smoker, no alcohol or drug use

VS: Temp 37.4°C (99.3°F), HR 108, BP 146/76, RR 26, Sao$_2$ 94% on RA

PE: *General:* Healthy-appearing woman; mild dyspnea. *HEENT:* Oropharynx clear; membranes moist. *Neck:* No JVD; no adenopathy. *CV:* S$_1$, S$_2$; regular rhythm; no murmurs or gallops; 2+ radial and DP pulses. *Chest:* Clear bilaterally; chest wall nontender. *Abd:* Soft; non-tender. *Extr:* No edema; right calf mildly tender and swollen. *Neuro:* Alert and oriented.

THOUGHT QUESTIONS

- What is the initial management for this patient?
- What is the differential diagnosis?
- Which diagnostic tests need to be done in the ED?
- What is the long-term treatment for this disease?

Immediate Actions:
Place on oxygen by nasal cannula; obtain 12-lead EKG; establish IV and send CBC, chem 7, and PT/PTT; obtain chest x-ray.

Discussion:
The differential diagnosis for pleuritic chest pain and dyspnea includes cardiac (e.g., acute MI, pericarditis), pulmonary (e.g., pulmonary embolism, spontaneous pneumothorax, pneumonia, pleurisy), and musculoskeletal (e.g., intercostal muscle strain, costochondritis) pathology. Pulmonary embolism is the most concerning diagnosis because untreated it may lead to progressive clot formation, pulmonary ischemia, cardiovascular collapse, and death. Most PEs result from propagation of a clot from a lower-extremity DVT. Therefore, patients who have a DVT and new dyspnea can be given the presumptive diagnosis of PE. In this patient it would be reasonable to stop the workup if she has a lower-extremity ultrasound that shows a venous clot. In patients with no clinical evidence of lower-extremity clot, a V/Q scan or CT angiography can be done. A V/Q scan can show areas of lung tissue that have adequate ventilation but decreased perfusion, which would be suspicious for a pulmonary embolus. A V/Q scan is not 100% sensitive; therefore, if the clinical suspicion for PE is high and the V/Q scan indeterminate, then a pulmonary arteriogram is the gold standard for diagnosis. Spiral CT scan technology has developed to the point where CT angiography is now being used to diagnose PE as well.

Treatment for pulmonary embolism or deep venous thrombosis includes initial anticoagulation with unfractionated heparin followed by 6 months of warfarin (Coumadin) therapy. Recurrent PEs or DVTs require permanent anticoagulation or placement of an inferior vena cava filter.

CASE CONTINUED

A lower-extremity ultrasound shows a popliteal DVT. She is started on heparin and admitted to the hospital with a presumptive diagnosis of PE. She undergoes chest CT angiography to characterize the extent of the clot. She is screened for protein C, protein S, and antithrombin III deficiency (which would lead to a hypercoagulable state). She is started on Coumadin on hospital day 2, and is discharged from the hospital on day 5 when her INR is therapeutic at greater than 2.0. She is advised to quit smoking and stop taking oral contraceptives (both risk factors for DVT, especially in combination).

QUESTIONS

31-1. A 54-year-old woman who had right total hip replacement one week earlier complains of sudden-onset chest pain and shortness of breath that woke her from sleep. Her pain is worse with deep inspiration. She has no history of coronary artery disease. On exam, her oxygen saturation is 92% on room air and her right leg is markedly swollen compared with the left leg; she is also tender to palpation behind the right knee. What is the most common EKG finding in her condition?
A. Tachycardia or nonspecific ST or T-wave changes
B. $S_1Q_3T_3$ syndrome
C. P-pulmonale
D. Right axis deviation
E. Atrial fibrillation

31-2. A 21-year-old man with no past medical history presents to the ED with a complaint of left leg swelling for 5 days and acute onset of severe shortness of breath one hour prior to presentation. He says he has left-sided chest pain when trying to breathe. He denies any other recent illnesses and denies alcohol or drug use, other than being a 2-pack-per-day smoker. He recently took a 2-week cross-country road trip with his girlfriend from Massachusetts to California and back. He is afebrile and denies cough. Which of the following chest x-ray findings is most likely?
A. Elevated hemidiaphragm
B. Hampton's hump
C. Westermark's sign
D. Pleural effusion
E. Clear lungs

31-3. A 56-year-old woman with a history of ovarian cancer presents to the ED with acute onset of right-sided chest pain and dyspnea. Her pulse is 106, blood pressure 126/84, and oxygen saturation 94% on room air. EKG and chest x-ray are normal. What is the appropriate next management step?

    A. Start heparin therapy

    B. Administer thrombolytic therapy

    C. Obtain V/Q scan

    D. Obtain bedside echocardiography

    E. Obtain chest CT

31-4. A 58-year-old woman with a history of breast cancer presents to the ED with acute onset of right-sided chest pain and shortness of breath. Her pain is worse on inspiration. Her pulse is 126, blood pressure 74/42, and oxygen saturation 82% on room air. Her EKG shows a right bundle branch block, and a portable chest x-ray is normal. In addition to orotracheal intubation, what is the appropriate next management step?

    A. Start heparin therapy

    B. Administer thrombolytic therapy

    C. Obtain V/Q scan

    D. Obtain bedside echocardiography

    E. Obtain chest CT

ANSWERS

31-1. A. This patient likely has a pulmonary embolus, with venous stasis due to immobilization after surgery as a risk factor. **EKG abnormalities should not be expected in the presence of PE. The most common abnormalities are sinus tachycardia and nonspecific ST or T-wave changes.** A larger pulmonary embolus will result in elevated pulmonary artery pressure and right heart strain. EKG changes consistent with right heart strain include P-pulmonale (large P waves), right axis deviation, right bundle branch block, atrial fibrillation, and $S_1Q_3T_3$ syndrome. The last consists of a deep S wave in lead I, a Q wave in lead III, and an inverted T wave in lead III. $S_1Q_3T_3$ syndrome is considered the classic EKG finding with PE but is only present in fewer than 10% of cases.

31-2. E. This patient likely has a DVT and PE. Chest x-ray has low sensitivity and specificity for PE. Over 30% of patients with PE have a totally normal chest x-ray. Approximately 30% will have an infiltrate that resembles pneumonia. Other common findings include an elevated hemidiaphragm, focal atelectasis, and pleural effusion. Hampton's hump is a triangular infiltrate with its rounded base abutting the pleura and its apex pointing toward the hilum. Westermark's sign is dilatation of the pulmonary vessels proximal to a large clot, with a sharp cutoff and distal vessel collapse. The last two findings are rare.

31-3. A. In this patient with a history of cancer and a classic presentation for PE, initiation of heparin therapy should not be delayed. This is especially true because the patient may need to leave the ED in order to obtain a V/Q scan or CT angiography, where immediate resuscitative help may not be available if her clot burden progresses. After heparin is started, the best next step in this stable patient is to obtain a V/Q scan to confirm the diagnosis. If the V/Q scan is entirely normal, then the heparin can always be stopped. If the V/Q scan is low probability (i.e., probably negative, but cannot entirely exclude PE), it would not be unreasonable to obtain pulmonary arteriography given that this patient is at high risk because of her malignancy. An intermediate- or high-probability V/Q scan would be enough to make the diagnosis.

31-4. B. Immediate thrombolytic therapy is indicated in this patient, who gives a classic history for PE, has a right bundle branch block on EKG, and is hypoxic with unstable vital signs. This woman will die without immediate therapy. Thrombolytics are indicated in patients with unstable vital signs and severe right heart strain. If the diagnosis is in doubt in a patient who presents with unstable vital signs, bedside echocardiography can be done to look for evidence of right heart strain.

 ## SUGGESTED ADDITIONAL READINGS

Dunn KL, Wolf JP, Dorfman DM, et al. Normal d-dimer levels in emergency department patients suspected of acute pulmonary embolism. J Am Coll Cardiol 2002;40:1475–1478.

Fedullo PF, Tapson VF. The evaluation of suspected pulmonary embolism. N Engl J Med 2003;349:1247–1256.

Laack TA, Goyal DG. Pulmonary embolism: an unsuspected killer. Emerg Med Clin North Am 2004;22:961–983.

Chest Pain and Fever

CC: 54-year-old woman with chest pain and fever

HPI: C.P. is a 54-year-old woman who developed right-sided chest pain somewhat suddenly 2 days prior to presentation, with mild nausea, occasional shortness of breath, and some pain in the right back. She has spent the past 2 days in bed with general malaise and anorexia. She has also had a fever (unmeasured) and a mild, dry cough. Her pain is worse with deep inspiration and movement. She has no recent history of air or car travel, no history of clotting disorders, and no leg pain or swelling. The patient has no known cardiac history or prior lung disease.

PMHx: Hysterectomy

Meds: Ibuprofen (Motrin) PRN, tramadol (Ultram) PRN

ALL: Penicillin, codeine, doxycycline

FHx: Noncontributory

SHx: Past tobacco use; occasional alcohol; no illicit drugs

VS: Temp 37.7°C (99.9°F), HR 106, BP 116/68, RR 16, SaO$_2$ 96% on RA

PE: *General:* Alert, middle-aged woman in mild discomfort. *HEENT:* No pharyngeal erythema; dry mucous membranes; no conjunctival injection. *CV:* S$_1$, S$_2$; mildly tachycardic; regular rhythm; no murmurs. *Chest:* Rales audible throughout right chest; left chest has clear sounds. *Back:* Mild tenderness to palpation over right back overlying base of scapula. *Abd:* Soft; nontender; obese; nondistended; bowel sounds present. *Extr:* No palpable cords; no leg tenderness; no edema; intact pulses. *Neuro:* Alert and oriented.

THOUGHT QUESTIONS

- What is the initial management for this patient?
- What is the differential diagnosis for this patient?
- Which diagnostic tests, if any, should be performed?
- Does this woman require hospitalization?

Immediate Actions:

Place O_2 by nasal cannula; obtain 12-lead EKG and PA and lateral chest x-ray; hang a liter of NS; send blood for CBC with differential and basic electrolytes.

Discussion:

The broad differential diagnosis for this patient includes pneumonia, bronchitis, viral upper respiratory infection, pulmonary embolus, and (less likely) cardiac ischemia. Pneumonia types can include pneumococcal, staphylococcal, other bacterial (e.g., *Klebsiella, Haemophilus influenzae, Moraxella*), and atypical (e.g., *Mycoplasma, Chlamydia, Legionella*). EKG is quick and easy, and thus should be done on any patient who has a remote chance of cardiac cause of symptoms. A chest x-ray should be obtained. For patients with productive sputum, Gram's stain and culture of the sputum should be sent. Blood cultures are low yield, but are indicated if the patient appears very ill or has rigors or other evidence of bacteremia. Occasionally a pulmonary embolus can present with fever and an infiltrate on chest x-ray; therefore, risk factors for PE (e.g., smoking, oral contraceptives, recent immobilization, history of PE or DVT) should be elicited. This diagnosis should be considered if a previously diagnosed pneumonia is not responding to antibiotics. The majority of patients with community-acquired pneumonia are able to go home with oral antibiotics; patients who require hospital admission include those with respiratory distress or hypoxemia, inability to keep down food or liquid, evidence of severe dehydration, or hypotension. Elderly patients and those with significant comorbidities (e.g., coronary disease, diabetes, renal disease) can decompensate rapidly and usually require admission.

CASE CONTINUED

EKG is normal. Pertinent labs include WBC 13.8 k/mm^3 with 90% polys. Chest x-ray reveals a right upper lobe opacity, consistent with lobar pneumonia (Figure 32-1). The patient is admitted to the observation unit for IV hydration, IV cefuroxime 1.5 g IV Q8 hr, azithromycin (Zithromax) 500 mg PO, and pain control. She feels improvement of her symptoms by morning and is discharged home with a 5-day course of azithromycin; she plans to see her primary care physician within 1 week for follow-up of her community-acquired pneumonia. Given that she had an upper lobe pneumonia, reactivation tuberculosis is considered. However, she has no risk factors (previous exposure, previous positive PPD, imprisonment or impoverished living conditions, or overseas travel).

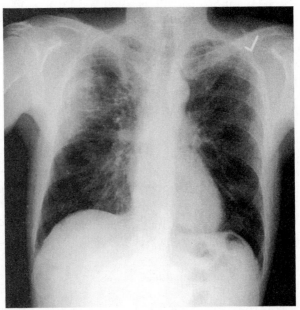

FIGURE 32-1 Chest x-ray shows right upper lobe airspace disease consistent with lobar pneumonia. (*Image courtesy of Massachusetts General Hospital, Boston.*)

QUESTIONS

32-1. A 54-year-old man with a history of renal failure, alcohol abuse, diabetes, and COPD presents to the ED with hematemesis. His vital signs are normal other than tachycardia to 108 bpm. An NG tube is placed with return of coffee-ground contents. His porta-cath is accessed for labwork and shows a hematocrit of 39%. He is admitted to the hospital for an upper GI bleed and endoscopy in the morning. Which of the following places this patient at risk for developing pneumonia due to increased risk of bacteremia?

   A. Portacath
   B. Alcoholism
   C. COPD
   D. Diabetes
   E. Nasogastric tube

32-2. A 24-year-old man presents to the ED with a dry cough and low-grade fever. He has had several days of malaise. A chest x-ray shows diffuse, hazy, interstitial infiltrates. Which of the following antibiotics provides poor coverage for the likely pathogen in his condition?

   A. Azithromycin
   B. Cefuroxime
   C. Doxycycline
   D. Levofloxacin
   E. Clarithromycin

32-3. An HIV-positive patient with CD4 count of 90 cells/μL has had several weeks of increasing cough and dyspnea. His chest x-ray reveals bilateral alveolar and interstitial infiltrates (resembling ground glass). What is the most likely pneumonia this patient has?

   A. Pneumococcus
   B. *Pneumocystis carinii*
   C. *Cryptococcus neoformans*
   D. *Coccidioides immitis*
   E. *Histoplasma capsulatum*

32-4. A 74-year-old man with a history of CAD, hypertension, and a prior stroke presents to the ED with 2 days of fever and a dry cough. Which of the following statements about pneumonia in the elderly is accurate?

A. Pneumonia is the second most common infection in the elderly, after urinary tract infection.

B. Elderly patients with pneumonia may present with weakness, GI symptoms, or confusion instead of respiratory symptoms.

C. *Mycoplasma* is the most common atypical agent of pneumonia in the elderly.

D. The chest x-rays of elderly patients with bacterial pneumonia do not show a classic lobar opacity.

E. Atypical agents are uncommon in the elderly.

ANSWERS

32-1. A. All of the options listed are risk factors for pneumonia, but the portacath specifically increases this patient's risk of bacteremia. Pneumonia risk factors include presence of chronic diseases (e.g., diabetes, CHF, renal failure), pulmonary disorders (e.g., COPD, viral lung infections, chest wall disorders), aspiration risk (e.g., esophageal motility disorder, stroke, NGT), bacteremia risk (e.g., intrathoracic or indwelling vascular devices), and debilitation (e.g., immunosuppression, alcoholism, age >70 years).

32-2. B. Atypical pathogens for pneumonia (e.g., *Mycoplasma*, *Legionella*, *Chlamydia*) lack a cell wall and therefore do not respond to β-lactam antibiotics; hence, they are not covered by second-generation cephalosporins (e.g., cefuroxime). Recommended antibiotics for atypical coverage include tetracyclines (e.g., doxycycline), macrolides (e.g., azithromycin or erythromycin), or a newer fluoroquinolone (e.g., levofloxacin).

32-3. B. Although all of the choices listed are possible infections in HIV-positive patients, *Pneumocystis carinii* pneumonia (PCP) is the most likely ailment of the patient presented. PCP is usually characterized as causing weeks of cough and dyspnea with rapid worsening. There is an increased risk of PCP once the CD4 count falls below 200 cells/μL. The characteristic chest x-ray in PCP shows "ground glass opacities" throughout the lungs, representing alveolar and interstitial infiltrates. Pneumococcus is the most common cause of pneumonia in the general population, although atypical and opportunistic agents are becoming increasingly more common. Pneumococcal pneumonia usually presents with sudden onset of symptoms, including fever, sputum, chest pain, and rigors; chest x-ray classically reveals a lobar infiltrate. *Cryptococcus neoformans* is the most common fungal cause of life-threatening infection among immunocompromised HIV patients, usually causing meningitis but also causing pneumonia. *Coccidioides immitis* is a fungus endemic in the southwestern United States that can cause granulomatous and pyogranulomatous pneumonia. *Histoplasma capsulatum* is another fungus, endemic in the Ohio, Missouri, and Mississippi River valleys; it can cause a granulomatous pneumonia.

32-4. B. Elderly patients with pneumonia may present with weakness, GI symptoms, or confusion instead of respiratory symptoms. *Legionella*, not *Mycoplasma*, is the most common cause of atypical pneumonia in the elderly and accounts for approximately 10% of community-acquired pneumonias among the elderly; atypical agents of pneumonia are becoming more common in the elderly. Pneumonia, not urinary tract infection, is the most common infection in the elderly. The chest x-ray of elderly patients with bacterial pneumonia may show a bronchial pattern rather than a classic lobar opacity.

 SUGGESTED ADDITIONAL READINGS

Loeb M. Community acquired pneumonia. Clin Evid 2005;(13): 1862–1875.

Marik PE. Aspiration pneumonitis and aspiration pneumonia. N Engl J Med 2001;344:665–671.

Segreti J, House HR, Siegel RE. Principles of antibiotic treatment of community-acquired pneumonia in the outpatient setting. Am J Med 2005;118(Suppl 7A):21S–28S.

Weiss K, Tillotson GS. The controversy of combination vs monotherapy in the treatment of hospitalized community-acquired pneumonia. Chest 2005;128:940–946.

Shortness of Breath and Wheezing

CC: 24-year-old woman with shortness of breath

HPI: W.H. is a 24-year-old woman with a history of asthma who presents to the ED with chest tightness, wheezing, and shortness of breath. Her triggers include fir trees, dust, cats, pollen, and cold air. She had been asymptomatic earlier today. She is visiting from out of town, is staying with a friend who owns three cats, and went with the friend today to buy a Christmas tree. By evening she had begun feeling progressively worse, with chest tightness and difficulty breathing that did not improve with several puffs of her albuterol MDI.

PMHx: Asthma, Crohn's disease

Meds: Albuterol MDI two puffs Q4–6 hr PRN

ALL: Demerol

FHx: No family history of rhinitis, urticaria, or eczema

SHx: Past tobacco history, quit 1 year ago; occasional alcohol; occasional marijuana and ecstasy

VS: Temp 35.6°C (96.1°F), HR 100, BP 116/80, RR 22, Sao$_2$ 95% on RA

PE: *General:* Young woman, healthy-appearing, though in mild to moderate respiratory distress. *HEENT:* No pharyngeal erythema; no rhinitis or rhinorrhea; no conjunctivitis. *CV:* S$_1$, S$_2$; mildly tachycardic; regular rhythm; no murmurs; good pulses. *Chest:* Tachypneic; wheezes bilaterally with expiration, prolonged expiratory phase; decreased air movement; use of accessory muscles with suprasternal retractions. *Abd:* Soft; nontender; nondistended. *Extr:* Warm; no rashes. *Neuro:* Alert and oriented.

THOUGHT QUESTIONS

- What is the initial management for this patient?
- What is the mainstay of treatment for patients with an acute asthma exacerbation?
- Which diagnostic tests, if any, should be performed?
- Which risk factors predict increased morbidity and mortality in an asthma exacerbation?
- Which preventive measures can be taken to avoid future exacerbations?

Immediate Actions:
Place on O_2 by nasal cannula; use continuous pulse oximetry; obtain bedside spirometry; administer albuterol (Ventolin) 3 mL and ipratropium (Atrovent) 500 µg mixed with 3 mL NS by nebulizer; give prednisone 60 mg PO.

Discussion:
Treatment for acute asthma exacerbation includes β-adrenergic agonists (e.g., albuterol), anticholinergics (e.g., ipratropium), and glucocorticoids. Albuterol and ipratropium by nebulizer can be given every 20 minutes or continuously as needed in the first hour. If these methods fail to relieve bronchospasm, subcutaneous epinephrine or terbutaline, IV magnesium, and inhaled heliox have been shown to be effective. In the ED, glucocorticoids can be given orally (40–60 mg of prednisone) or intravenously if unable to tolerate PO (125 mg, or 2 mg/kg of methylprednisolone); this can be followed by a nontapered steroid burst of 40 to 60 mg prednisone per day for 4 to 5 days. Serial bedside spirometry measurement of peak expiratory flow rate (PEFR) is a useful measure to follow the effectiveness of treatment. Pulse oximetry is helpful, but does not always correlate with adequate response to therapy. Indeed, a young, healthy asthmatic patient may maintain adequate oxygenation until the point when respiratory failure occurs. Chest x-ray, ABG, and routine labs are not usually indicated unless there is a clinical suspicion for an underlying pneumonia or other pulmonary process.

(Continued)

Various risk factors have been associated with poor outcome in asthma, such as recent hospitalization for asthma, recent systemic steroid use for asthma, recent ED visits for asthma, poor ability to recognize the severity of one's own air-flow obstruction, history of intubation for asthma, and history of ICU admission for asthma (Table 33-1).

Preventive measures for asthma include use of mast cell stabilizers (e.g., cromolyn sodium), use of leukotriene inhibitors [e.g., montelukast (Singulair), zafirlukast (Accolate), zileuton (Zyflo)] or long-acting inhaled steroids [e.g., triamcinolone acetonide (Azmacort), fluticasone (Flovent), beclomethasone dipropionate (Vanceril)], avoidance of known triggers, and early use of home MDIs and home peak flow monitoring.

TABLE 33-1 Risk Factors for Poor Outcome in Asthma

History of prior intubation or ICU admission for asthma
History of sudden severe exacerbation of asthma
Recent or current systemic steroid use for asthma
≥3 ED visits for asthma in the last 12 months
≥2 hospital admissions for asthma in the last 12 months
ED visit or hospitalization for asthma in the last month
Poor ability to recognize the severity of one's own airflow obstruction
Use of >2 albuterol MDI canisters per month
Significant comorbidities and/or significant psychiatric disease
Illicit drug use (especially inhaled cocaine and heroin)

CASE CONTINUED

The patient's initial peak flow measurement is 100 L/min, 29% of her usual 350 L/min. She is given nebulized albuterol/ipratropium doses every 20 minutes, with improvements in PEFR to 150 L/min, 230 L/min, and 290 L/min, respectively. By the end of her third neb-ulized treatment, her PEFR is at 83% of her personal best, and her oxygen saturation improves to 98% on room air; she feels much better, her lungs sound clearer, and her expiratory phase has nor-malized. She is monitored for an additional hour, continues to do well, and is discharged home with instructions to take prednisone

40 mg PO QD for 4 days and albuterol MDI two puffs every 4 to 6 hours as needed, with follow-up in her primary care physician's clinic within 1 week.

 QUESTIONS

33-1. A 19-year-old man with history of asthma presents to the ED with moderate respiratory distress after jogging in cold air. On exam, he has bilateral wheezing and increased expiratory phase. Which of the following would you also expect?

A. Diaphragmatic flattening on chest x-ray
B. Increased PEFR on bedside spirometry
C. Decreased lung volumes
D. Decreased airway resistance
E. Bronchial dilation

33-2. A 32-year-old woman with long-standing asthma history presents to the ED with 2 days of worsening shortness of breath, typical of her usual asthma flares. In the room next to hers, a 67-year-old man with history of CHF presents with 2 days of worsening shortness of breath and lower extremity edema, typical of his usual CHF exacerbations. Which of the following do these two patients likely have in common?

A. Kerley B lines on chest x-ray
B. Air trapping
C. Wheezing
D. Improvement with administration of furosemide (Lasix)
E. Increased airway resistance

33-3. A 33-year-old man with history of asthma presents to the ED with severe respiratory distress, unable to speak in full sentences. His wife says that he had been feeling short of breath since last night when they walked past a building construction site. She further says that he was up intermittently overnight using his albuterol inhaler without noticeable improvement. Which of the following is a risk factor for death from asthma?

A. Low sensitivity for perceiving airflow obstruction
B. No prior intubation for asthma
C. Past use of systemic corticosteroids
D. Alcohol use
E. Hospitalization for asthma one year ago and an ED visit for asthma 6 months ago

33-4. A 52-year-old woman with long history of asthma presents to the ED with moderate-severe respiratory distress, using accessory muscles and audibly wheezing. She has trouble speaking more than a couple words at a time. After appropriate treatments in the ED, which of the following would indicate that she can be admitted to the regular hospital floor instead of the intensive care unit?

A. Mild confusion

B. $Paco_2$ less than 35 mm Hg after initial ED treatments

C. PEFR less than 50% after initial ED treatments

D. Respiratory arrest

E. Respiratory fatigue with good oxygenation (Sao_2 98% on room air after nebulized treatments)

ANSWERS

33-1. A. The patient described is suffering from an asthma attack. Increased lung volumes are typical during an asthma exacerbation; therefore, a chest x-ray typically shows hyperexpansion and diaphragmatic flattening. Asthma is characterized by bronchiolar constriction and inflammation, resulting in narrowing of the bronchi and bronchioles, increased airway resistance, and decreased PEFR. Because expiration is usually a passive process, it is difficult to expel air through this resistance, and air trapping occurs. As ventilation worsens, the patient becomes hypercarbic (increased $Paco_2$), followed by hypoxia and respiratory failure.

33-2. C. CHF, as well as other conditions such as bronchogenic carcinoma, vocal cord dysfunction, aspiration of gastric acid, and upper airway obstruction, can present similarly to asthma with shortness of breath, wheezing, and chest tightness. Aspiration of a foreign body, metastatic carcinoma, and sarcoidosis (with endobronchial obstruction) can also present with similar symptoms; all of these should be considered in the differential diagnosis when evaluating a patient who presents with chest discomfort, trouble breathing, and wheezing. Kerley B lines may be seen on chest x-ray in CHF, but are not typical in asthma. Air trapping and increased airway resistance are descriptive of asthma. Improvement of symptoms after furosemide (Lasix) administration is typical of CHF.

33-3. A. Low sensitivity for perceiving airflow obstruction or its severity is a risk factor for death from asthma. Other risk factors include prior intubation for asthma, current use of corticosteroids, illicit drug use, past admission to an ICU for asthma, two or more hospitalizations or three or more ED visits for asthma in the past year, hospitalization or ED visit for asthma within the last month, past history of sudden severe asthma exacerbation, comorbidity, and serious psychiatric illness or psychosocial problem (see Table 33-1).

33-4. B. After initial treatment in the ED with O_2, albuterol and ipratropium nebulizers, and corticosteroids, a patient who still has a PEFR less than 50% of expected, who appears drowsy or confused, or who continues to have severe symptoms should be admitted to the ICU. Any patient with worsening respiratory fatigue should be intubated, administered continuous nebulized medication, and admitted to the ICU. Arterial blood gas can be helpful to follow the trend of $Paco_2$ **Asthmatic patients who are ventilating properly should develop a respiratory alkalosis (i.e., they will have a $Paco_2$ less than 40 mm Hg).** Values greater than 40 mm Hg indicate that the patient is tiring and requires more aggressive treatment. However, the decision to intubate should be based on the overall appearance of the patient and not on the results of a blood gas test.

 SUGGESTED ADDITIONAL READINGS

Ram FS, Wellington S, Rowe B, et al. Non-invasive positive pressure ventilation for treatment of respiratory failure due to severe acute exacerbations of asthma. Cochrane Database Syst Rev 2005;(3):CD004360.

Rodrigo GJ, Rodrigo C, Hall JB. Acute asthma in adults: a review. Chest 2004;125:1081–1102.

Roy SR, Milgrom H. Management of the acute exacerbation of asthma. J Asthma 2003;40:593–604.

Wood-Baker RR, Gibson PG, Hannay M, et al. Systemic corticosteroids for acute exacerbations of chronic obstructive pulmonary disease. Cochrane Database Syst Rev 2005; (1):CD001288.

Difficulty Breathing after an Insect Sting

 CC: 22-year-old woman presents with difficulty breathing after an insect sting

HPI: I.B. is a 22-year-old healthy woman who presents to the ED 15 minutes after being stung by a bee. She was at a picnic playing softball when a bee stung her in the back of the arm. She had been stung by a bee once before but recalls having had only a rash near the sting site. Within 5 minutes of today's sting, she began to feel lightheaded, nauseated, and "uneasy." She then had difficulty taking a deep breath and felt as if her throat were closing shut. Her friends put her in the car and took her to the hospital.

PMH: Seasonal allergies

Meds: None

ALL: NKDA

VS: Temp 37.0°C (98.6°F), HR 110, BP 80/40, RR 20, SaO_2 91% on RA

PE: *General:* Appears very anxious, diaphoretic, taking gasping shallow breaths. *HEENT:* Oropharynx without obvious swelling. *Neck:* Supple; no stridor. *CV:* S_1, S_2; tachycardic; no murmurs; weak thready pulses. *Chest:* Bilateral inspiratory and expiratory wheezes; supraclavicular retractions. *Abd:* Soft; nontender. *Extr:* Small welt on posterior aspect of left arm; no peripheral cyanosis. *Skin:* Warm and diffusely flushed. *Neuro:* Fully alert and oriented; grossly intact.

THOUGHT QUESTIONS

- Which interventions need to be done immediately?
- How is epinephrine dosed in the treatment of anaphylaxis?

- Which type of hypersensitivity reaction is insect-sting anaphylaxis?
- What are the four types of intravenous medications administered during anaphylaxis?

Immediate Actions:
Place a nonrebreather face mask with 15 liters O_2; rapidly obtain peripheral IV access while someone retrieves epinephrine; give 0.5 mL of 1:1000 epinephrine subcutaneously in the deltoid region; hang normal saline wide open; *remove* the stinger if present; give albuterol nebulizer 0.5 mL in 2.5 mL of normal saline, diphenhydramine (Benadryl) 50 mg IV, methylprednisolone (Solu-Medrol) 125 mg IV, and ranitidine (Zantac) 50 mg IV.

Discussion:
Anaphylaxis is a truly frightening experience for both patient and physician. If rapid and appropriate action is not taken, the patient will die. Every emergency physician must memorize the dose for epinephrine used in treating anaphylaxis: 0.5 mL of 1:1000 strength epinephrine subcutaneously in adults (for kids it's 0.01 mL/kg of 1:1000 epinephrine). Subcutaneous epinephrine should take effect within 2 minutes and, in addition to the other medications mentioned, will result in rapid improvement in the majority of patients. If the patient's condition continues to deteriorate, epinephrine 0.1 mL of 1:1000 mixed in 10 mL of normal saline (1:100,000 strength) administered IV over 10 minutes is required.

Bee sting anaphylaxis is considered a type I hypersensitivity reaction. This requires prior sensitization to a foreign protein; reexposure results in activation of IgE receptors on the surface of mast cells, with release of preformed mediators. The most important mediators include histamine, eosinophil and neutrophil chemotactic factors, and platelet activating factor. Arachidonic acid is also metabolized into leukotrienes, which play a major role as well. These substances result in increased vascular permeability (urticaria, angioedema, laryngeal swelling, pulmonary edema),

(*Continued*)

vasodilation (flushing, hypotension, syncope), contraction of smooth muscle (bronchospasm, abdominal cramping), and coronary vasoconstriction leading to decreased myocardial contractile force. Epinephrine acts to increase myocardial contraction via β-adrenergic agonism and to increase peripheral vascular resistance via α-adrenergic agonism. Diphenhydramine and ranitidine antagonize histamine at the H_1 and H_2 receptors, respectively. Methylprednisolone inhibits the breakdown of membrane phospholipids to arachidonic acid, thus preventing synthesis of leukotrienes, which are responsible for the delayed phase of anaphylaxis.

CASE CONTINUED

Within 15 minutes of initial treatment, the patient begins to feel better. Repeat blood pressure is 110/68, with an SaO_2 of 98% on a nonrebreather mask. Her bilateral inspiratory and expiratory wheezes diminish to a mild wheeze upon expiration, and supra-clavicular retractions have ceased. Her skin has cleared. Two addi-tional albuterol nebulizer treatments are given. She is admitted to the hospital for 24-hour observation in a monitored bed. She receives prednisone PO 60 mg every 6 hours and Benadryl 50 mg PO every 4 hours to prevent relapse of symptoms. She is discharged home 22 hours after admission.

QUESTIONS

34-1. A 24-year-old woman presents to the ED with a sudden onset of diffuse hives, throat and tongue swelling, and stridor. Her vital signs are HR 118, BP 86/40, RR 32, and oxygen saturation 92% on room air. She is promptly administered epinephrine subcu-taneously while preparations are made for intubation. What is the most common cause of fatal anaphylaxis?

    A. Food ingestion, including shellfish, nuts, and eggs

    B. Insect sting

    C. Penicillin

    D. Aspirin

    E. Contrast dye

34-2. A young man presents to the ED after having eaten Chinese food with crushed peanuts, to which he has had severe anaphylactic reactions. Involvement of which system in severe anaphylaxis is both common and deadly?

A. Cardiovascular
B. Respiratory
C. Dermal
D. Gastrointestinal
E. Neurologic

34-3. A 32-year-old man started penicillin for an infected tooth. He presents to the ED with hives and wheezing. On exam he has posterior pharyngeal edema but no stridor. He has bilateral wheezes. His symptoms improve significantly after administration of subcutaneous epinephrine. Which of the following is important to prescribe when he is discharged in order to prevent relapse of late-phase reactants of his condition?

A. Prednisone 60 mg daily for 5 days
B. Benadryl 25 to 50 mg every 4 to 6 hours
C. Epi-Pen
D. Cimetidine 300 mg every 6 hours
E. Albuterol inhaler two puffs every 4 hours

34-4. Which of the following is highest in your differential diagnosis along with anaphylactic reaction after an anxious patient receives a painful IM antibiotic injection and begins to have symptoms of difficulty breathing?

A. Acute stroke
B. Seizure
C. Status asthmaticus
D. Foreign body airway obstruction
E. Vasovagal reaction

ANSWERS

34-1. C. Penicillin accounts for 90% of cases (up to 500 cases annually in the United States) of fatal anaphylaxis, and most of these follow parenteral administration. Hymenoptera insects (yellow jackets, honeybees, wasps, hornets) account for approximately 50 deaths annually. Allergic reactions to various foods are common, especially in children, in whom the incidence is about 5%; however, fatal anaphylaxis is extremely rare. Reactions to aspirin and other NSAIDs constitute anaphylactoid reactions, which are independent of IgE antibodies. These substances inhibit synthesis of prostaglandins from arachidonic acid via the cyclooxygenase pathway. Thus, arachidonic acid is preferentially converted to leukotrienes via the lipoxygenase pathway. In sensitized individuals, this alternative pathway is accentuated.

34-2. B. In contrast to a simple allergic reaction, anaphylaxis is characterized by acute systemic involvement of multiple organ systems in response to IgE-mediated immunologic reaction in previously sensitized individuals. Respiratory and dermal manifestations are most common in anaphylaxis. These include airway edema and swelling, bronchospasm, histamine-mediated cutaneous flushing, and urticaria. Respiratory and cardiac compromise predominate in fatal cases of anaphylaxis. **Therefore, respiratory compromise is both common and deadly in anaphylaxis. For this reason, intubation and mechanical ventilation should be undertaken at the first sign of respiratory difficulty, because a delay may result in airway edema to such an extent that intubation is impossible.**

34-3. A. All of these medications except albuterol inhaler could be useful in preventing a relapse and should thus be prescribed when a patient is ready to go home following treatment for anaphylaxis. Oral Benadryl and cimetidine should be the first-line treatment for recurrent mild wheezing. However, if not improved, the patient should return immediately to the ED. It is essential to prescribe an Epi-Pen to anyone who presents to the emergency department with a severe allergic reaction that involves respiratory or cardiovascular compromise. The Epi-Pen allows self-administration of 0.3 mL of 1:1000 epinephrine subcutaneously via a spring-loaded system. **A short course of prednisone is important to prevent relapse of late-phase reactants such as leukotrienes that are liberated from arachidonic acid via the lipoxygenase pathway.**

34-4. E. There are many conditions included in the differential diagnosis of anaphylaxis, including seizure, status asthmaticus, foreign body airway obstruction, and vasovagal reaction. The differential diagnosis further includes arrhythmias, drug reactions, epiglottitis, and hereditary angioedema. **Vasovagal syncope is not uncommon with administration of IV medication due to pain and anxiety, and this may be misinterpreted as anaphylaxis.** Tachycardia, hypotension, altered mental status, respiratory distress, stridor, cutaneous hives, pallor, and diaphoresis will differentiate anaphylaxis from vasovagal syncope.

SUGGESTED ADDITIONAL READINGS

Borchers AT, Naguwa SM, Keen CL, et al. The diagnosis and management of anaphylaxis. Compr Ther 2004;30:111–120.

Chiu AM, Kelly KJ. Anaphylaxis: drug allergy, insect stings, and latex. Immunol Allergy Clin North Am 2005;25:389–405, viii.

Sheikh A, Walker S. Anaphylaxis. BMJ 2005;331:330.

Wiener ES, Bajaj L. Diagnosis and emergent management of anaphylaxis in children. Adv Pediatr 2005;52:195–206.

IV

Patients Presenting with Eye, ENT, Upper Respiratory, or Febrile Illnesses

Acute Vision Loss

CC: 36-year-old woman with acute vision loss

HPI: V.L. is a 36-year-old woman who presents to the ED with complaint of blurred, fogged vision in the left eye for 4 days. She has pain when she looks from side to side, and she has a constant headache centered behind her eye. She denies tearing, itching, discharge, flashes, floaters, or trauma. She gives no history of extremity weakness, bowel or bladder incontinence, or recent URIs or vaccines. She also denies any history of similar symptoms or migraines in the past.

PMHx: None

Meds: None

ALL: NKDA

SHx: 1/2 ppd tobacco; denies alcohol and drugs

VS: Temp 37.2°C (99.0°F), HR 81, BP 156/72, RR 14, SaO$_2$ 100% on RA

PE: *General:* Very anxious, mildly overweight woman. *HEENT:* Pupils 3 mm to greater than 2 mm OU; afferent pupillary defect present OS; acuity 20/20 OD, counting fingers at 6 inches OS; EOM full OU; confrontation visual fields full OU. *Slit lamp exam:* Lids, lashes, conjunctiva, cornea, anterior chamber, iris, and lens normal OU. *Dilated retinal exam:* Normal OD, with minimal/mild swelling of optic disk and normal peripheral retina OS. Tonometry 12 mm Hg OD, 11 mm Hg OS (normal range 10–20 mm Hg). *CV:* RRR; no murmurs. *Chest:* Clear bilaterally. *Abd:* Soft, nontender, nondistended; bowel sounds present. *Extr:* Normal pulses; no edema or rashes. *Neuro:* Alert, oriented; CN III to XII intact, CN II as above; 5/5 motor all extremities; sensation to pinprick intact throughout; normal finger-to-nose test; normal gait.

THOUGHT QUESTIONS

- What is the immediate intervention for patients with acute vision loss or reduction?
- What is the differential diagnosis for acute vision loss or acute vision reduction that is painful?
- What is the differential diagnosis for acute vision loss or acute vision reduction that is painless?
- Are there any diagnostic tests that should be performed?

Immediate Actions:
Send blood sample for CBC, basic chemistries, and ESR; order MRI of brain; consult ophthalmology.

Discussion:
History and eye examination must quickly establish the likely cause of vision loss. If acute angle-closure glaucoma is suspected (severe pain and vision loss, steamy appearance of cornea, conjunctival injection, mid-positioned sluggish pupil), intraocular pressure (IOP) should be checked and reduction should be initiated immediately with topical β-blockers [timolol (Timoptic) 0.5%], α_2-adrenergic agonists [apraclonidine (Iopidine) 0.1%], oral or IV carbonic anhydrase inhibitors [acetazolamide (Diamox)], IV mannitol 1 to 2 g/kg, and topical steroids [prednisolone (Pred Forte) 1%]; after IOP is less than 40 mm Hg, pilocarpine 1% to 2% should be started. The first three agents act to decrease production of aqueous humor; the last agent causes pupillary constriction in order to maintain patency of the angle between the cornea and iris; keep in mind that topical β-blockers can be absorbed systemically.

If central retinal artery occlusion (CRAO) is suspected (painless vision loss with blanching of the retina and a "cherry-red spot" over the fovea), ophthalmology must be immediately consulted and ocular massage administered along with IOP-lowering medications and vasodilation techniques; ophthalmology may consider performing an anterior chamber paracentesis to further lower IOP.

(Continued)

The differential diagnosis for painful acute vision loss or vision reduction includes acute angle-closure glaucoma and optic neuritis. The differential diagnosis for painless acute vision loss or vision reduction includes CRAO, central retinal vein occlusion (CRVO), retinal detachment, vitreous hemorrhage, and temporal arteritis (giant-cell arteritis). Timely and thorough history and examination are very important and can be vision-sparing in the cases of acute angle-closure glaucoma, CRAO, and temporal arteritis. IOP should be measured in all patients with vision loss. ESR and CRP can help suggest the diagnosis of temporal arteritis, but temporal artery biopsy is the confirmational test. Optic neuritis is characterized by focal demyelination of the optic nerve; it is often the first manifestation of multiple sclerosis (30% incidence at 5 years), but more often optic neuritis is idiopathic and self-limited. It causes monocular vision loss, swelling of the optic disc, and pain with extraocular movements; optic neuritis is always associated with an afferent pupillary defect (the bad eye's pupil dilates when a flashlight is swung from the good eye to the bad eye). Its natural history is spontaneous improvement in 2 to 3 weeks; a 3-day course of IV steroids may accelerate improvement. An MRI is indicated to look for evidence of multiple sclerosis.

CASE CONTINUED

Ophthalmology is consulted in the ED. An MRI is obtained and shows markedly high T2 signal abnormality in the posterior segment of the left optic nerve, consistent with left (retrobulbar) optic neuritis. The patient is admitted for high-dose IV methylprednisolone. She slowly regains her vision over the next month and has no long-term sequelae.

QUESTIONS

35-1. A 60-year-old woman with history of polymyalgia rheumatica presents with headache, jaw claudication, and painless left eye vision loss. Which diagnosis is most likely?

A. CRAO
B. Retinal detachment
C. Temporal arteritis
D. Acute angle-closure glaucoma
E. Vitreous hemorrhage

35-2. A 66-year-old woman presents with new-onset monocular painful vision loss and has a mid-dilated and nonreactive pupil on the affected side. She reports that she had been fine at lunchtime, but developed symptoms while watching a movie at the theater with her husband. She denies any history of trauma to the eyes or any prior eye problems. Which diagnosis is most likely?

    A. CRAO

    B. CRVO

    C. Retinal detachment

    D. Acute angle-closure glaucoma

    E. Primary open-angle glaucoma

35-3. A 61-year-old man with history of hypertension, diabetes, and coronary artery disease presents to the ED with complaint of trouble seeing from his left eye. He hadn't noticed any problems with his vision yesterday, but has had blurring since awakening this morning. Funduscopic examination on the left is shown in Figure 35-1. What is his likely diagnosis?

    A. CRAO

    B. CRVO

    C. Conjunctivitis

    D. Vitreous hemorrhage

    E. Orbital cellulites

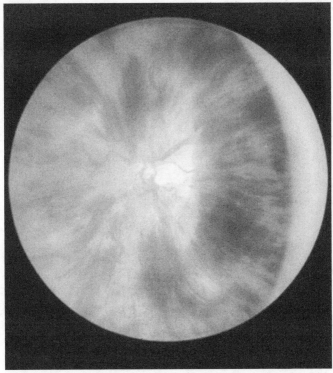

FIGURE 35-1 Fundoscopic examination for the patient in Question 35-3. (*Image reprinted with permission from Harwood-Nuss A, Wolfson AB, et al. The Clinical Practice of Emergency Medicine, 3rd Ed. Philadelphia: Lippincott Williams & Wilkins, 2001.*)

35-4. A 41-year-old man with sickle-cell anemia presents to the ED with complaint of pain in his back and legs, similar to his usual sickle-cell crises, but also trouble seeing out of his right eye, which has never happened before. His back and leg pain started last night, and his vision problem was evident from the time he woke up this morning. Funduscopic examination is shown in Figure 35-2. Other than sickle cell crisis, what is his likely diagnosis?

    A. Primary open-angle glaucoma
    B. Retinal detachment
    C. CRAO
    D. CRVO
    E. Optic neuritis

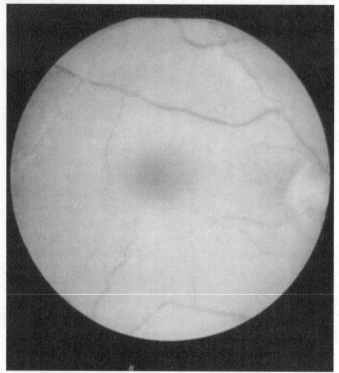

FIGURE 35-2 Fundoscopic examination for the patient in Question 35-4. (*Image reprinted with permission from Harwood-Nuss A, Wolfson AB, et al. The Clinical Practice of Emergency Medicine, 3rd Ed. Philadelphia: Lippincott Williams & Wilkins, 2001.*)

ANSWERS

35-1. C. Temporal arteritis is more common in women than men and generally affects patients older than 50 years. Symptoms include painless vision loss, headache, pain over the temporal artery, jaw claudication, fatigue, myalgias, fever, and anorexia. Patients usually have markedly elevated ESR and CRP. The contralateral eye can also become involved with subsequent contralateral eye vision loss, hence the need for immediate initiation of IV steroids in any patient highly suspected of having temporal arteritis, even before biopsy results are established.

35-2. D. A mid-dilated, nonreactive pupil with sudden painful vision loss or vision reduction is classic for acute angle-closure glaucoma. This generally occurs in patients without any previous history of glaucoma. These patients present also with headache or eye pain, cloudy vision, nausea, and vomiting. Patients typically have narrow anterior chamber angles to begin with; acute closure of the angle can occur with the iris touching the lens, obstructing normal aqueous humor flow from the posterior chamber to the anterior chamber where it is normally filtered out of the eye. Continued production of aqueous humor in the setting of obstructed outflow causes increased IOP, which leads to corneal edema and clouding (the normal corneal pump mechanism can no longer function correctly in the setting of high IOP). Primary open-angle glaucoma is the most common form of glaucoma and the leading cause of blindness in the United States. Its onset is more insidious, often bilateral, and painless. Significant optic nerve damage has already occurred before significant vision loss is realized. These patients benefit from surgery to open the trabecular meshwork.

35-3. B. CRVO occurs when there is thrombosis of the central retinal vein. This leads to venous stasis, edema, and hemorrhage diffusely, causing the classic "blood and thunder" appearance of the retina on funduscopic examination, as shown in Figure 35-1. These patients often have a history of hypertension. There is no specific treatment; daily aspirin is sometimes started.

35-4. C. CRAO occurs when embolus, thrombus, arteritis, vasculitis, trauma, or sickle-cell disease causes occlusion of the central retinal artery, a branch of the ophthalmic artery. Central retinal artery occlusion leads to retinal infarction; this causes the retina to become pale, edematous, and less transparent. The underlying choroidal circulation at the macula, however, remains visible because the macular portion of the retina is thinnest. The "cherry-red spot" thus refers to the normal-appearing, red-colored macula ("spot") in a sea of surrounding infarcted, pale retina, as shown in Figure 35-2. Digital massage is performed in an attempt to dislodge a clot. Intraocular pressure should be reduced with topical agents and acetazolamide to improve the perfusion gradient.

 SUGGESTED ADDITIONAL READINGS

Gariano RF, Kim CH. Evaluation and management of suspected retinal detachment. Am Fam Physician 2004;69:1691–1698.

Manolopoulos J. Emergency primary eye care. Tips for diagnosis and acute management. Aust Fam Physician 2002;31:233–237.

Purvin V, Kawasaki A. Neuro-ophthalmic emergencies for the neurologist. Neurologist 2005;11:195–233.

CASE 36

Red Eye

CC: 29-year-old woman presents with both eyes red and irritated

HPI: R.E. is a 29-year-old woman who presents to the ED complaining of bilateral red eyes for several days. She reports that she had gotten sunscreen in her eyes 4 days earlier while on a beach in Mexico. Although she had rinsed her eyes, they became red. The redness improved somewhat until yesterday, when she had spent the entire day near seawater. Now both eyes feel "sensitive" with some itching and tearing. She denies eye pain, photophobia, vision change, coughing, sneezing, runny nose, fevers, or chills. She has not had any recent illnesses, sick contacts, or history of trauma to the eyes. She wears corrective lenses but does not wear contact lenses.

PMHx: None

Meds: Oral contraceptive pills

ALL: None

VS: Temp 35.9°C (96.6°F), HR 75, BP 129/83, RR 16, SaO₂ 98% on RA

PE: *General:* Pleasant, healthy-appearing young woman in no distress. *Ocular exam:* Visual acuity 20/20 bilaterally with glasses, diffuse conjunctival injection bilaterally; minimal clear discharge without pus or eyelash matting; no periorbital edema or lid lesions; pupils 4 mm and reactive bilaterally; extraocular movements intact without pain. *Confrontation exam:* Vision normal in all four quadrants bilaterally. *Funduscopic exam:* Optic disc margins sharp; normal vessels; no retinal hemorrhages or exudates bilaterally. *Slit-lamp exam:* Conjunctivae injected and chemotic bilaterally; no corneal abrasions, dendrites, or perforations seen with fluorescein staining; small papillae on palpebral conjunctivae. *Neck:* No preauricular lymph nodes. *Skin:* Intact; warm; no rashes. *Neuro:* Alert and oriented.

THOUGHT QUESTIONS

- What is the most emergent disorder that causes red eye?
- What is the differential diagnosis of red eye?
- How can you narrow the differential diagnosis?
- Does contact lens use make any difference in management?

Discussion:

Acute angle-closure glaucoma is the most concerning potential cause for red eye. Glaucoma results from closure of the canals of Schlemm that drain aqueous humor from the anterior chamber. This results in an increase in the intraocular pressure and ultimately retinal ischemia and permanent vision loss. Glaucoma is unilateral and is associated with significant eye pain; the patient typically has nausea and vomiting as well. Risk factors for glaucoma include family history of glaucoma, African ancestry, diabetes, severe nearsightedness, previous eye injury, old age, and steroid use. More common causes of red eye include viral, bacterial, or allergic conjunctivitis, conjunctival or corneal abrasion and foreign bodies, subconjunctival hemorrhage, corneal ulcer, herpes zoster ophthalmicus, and HSV. Periorbital cellulitis, as well as lid pathology, can also cause red eye.

History and examination are key in making a diagnosis in red eye. Viral or bacterial conjunctivitis is more likely than allergic conjunctivitis in this patient because she has not had previous episodes of red eye and she has no other allergic symptoms. Viral conjunctivitis is the most common cause of conjunctivitis and is associated with intense itching, irritation, and preauricular adenopathy, usually lasting 1 to 2 weeks. Pus or eyelid matting is consistent with bacterial conjunctivitis, which usually lasts up to 1 week with appropriate antimicrobial therapy. Corneal and conjunctival abrasion, ulceration, or foreign body is usually obvious on slit-lamp exam with fluorescein staining because the stain deposits

(Continued)

in the area of the defect. Subconjunctival hemorrhage has a distinct appearance of a confluent, raised, deep red patch on the conjunctiva and typically follows eye trauma or bouts of forceful coughing. HSV infection is characterized by dendritic lesions on the cornea by fluorescein exam. Herpes zoster ophthalmicus is usually associated with vesicular cutaneous lesions within the trigeminal nerve V_1 distribution. Contact lens wearers, especially those with extended-wear lenses, are predisposed to developing corneal abrasions and ulcers, which have a high incidence of *Pseudomonas* superinfection. Therefore, contact lens wearers with bacterial conjunctivitis should be treated with a fluoroquinolone or aminoglycoside to cover for *Pseudomonas* in addition to the more common pathogens, *Staphylococcus aureus* and *Streptococcus pneumoniae*. These patients should not wear contact lenses until they have fully recovered from their ophthalmic condition.

CASE CONTINUED

The patient is diagnosed with viral conjunctivitis. She is discharged with erythromycin ointment 0.5% to both eyes four times per day for 7 days to prevent bacterial superinfection, and ketorolac (Acular) 0.5% drops to both eyes four times a day for pain relief. She is also instructed to use cool compresses four times per day, with follow-up in the ophthalmology clinic within 7 days.

QUESTIONS

36-1. A 36-year-old man presents to the ED with pain, redness, and tearing in his left eye. He works with metal tools and has had eye pain since leaving work yesterday. Slit-lamp examination shows a small, superficial corneal foreign body with associated rust ring. Which of the following is appropriate management?

   A. Use topical anesthetic in both eyes prior to attempting foreign body removal.
   B. Remove the foreign body under slit-lamp magnification using a 14-gauge needle.
   C. Remove rust ring with an ophthalmic burr; be certain to remove all traces of rust.
   D. If the patient still has a foreign body sensation after removal, evert the eyelid to ascertain presence of any additional foreign bodies.
   E. Remove a full-thickness foreign body as long as ophthalmology follow-up is within 24 hours.

36-2. A factory worker is repairing machinery when he is sprayed in the face with an unknown chemical. He is brought to a decontamination area where his face and eyes are irrigated with water. He presents to the ED with tearing, red eyes, and blurriness. Which of the following statements regarding chemical injury to the eye is accurate?

   A. Acid burns are usually more severe than alkali burns.
   B. Alkali burns are usually more severe than acid burns.
   C. Acid and alkali burns are usually of equal severity.
   D. The physiologic pH of tear fluid is acidic.
   E. The physiologic pH of tear fluid is alkaline.

36-3. A new mother brings her 3-day-old home-birthed neonate to the ED because of red eye. Of the following choices, which is the most likely cause of this baby's condition?

   A. *Chlamydia*
   B. *Neisseria gonorrhoeae*
   C. *Staphylococcus aureus*
   D. *Haemophilus*
   E. *Streptococcus pneumoniae*

36-4. A 64-year-old man presents to the ED with painful erythema and vesicles in a V_1 facial nerve distribution on his left forehead. Given this distribution, you are concerned about herpes zoster involving the eye as well. Which of the following is atypical of herpes zoster ophthalmicus?

A. Hutchinson sign
B. Iritis
C. Corneal dendrites
D. Photophobia
E. Pain

 ANSWERS

36-1. A. The use of topical anesthetic in both eyes is to suppress the blink reflex during foreign body removal and to alleviate pain. A 25-gauge or 30-gauge needle can be used to remove a superficial foreign body if an ophthalmic burr is not available; removal should be done under adequate magnification, such as that afforded by the slit lamp. Full-thickness foreign bodies should be removed by an ophthalmologist. Superficial rust that is not located over the pupil can be removed in the ED; additional burring is usually necessary the following day, so it is not necessary to remove all traces of rust on the first day in the ED. The patient's resulting corneal abrasion (due to foreign body removal) should be treated with a topical cycloplegic and erythromycin ointment. The patient should be seen by an ophthalmologist within 24 hours for follow-up. All patients should have the eyelid everted to search for any additional foreign bodies (not just those with persistent foreign body sensation, as in choice D).

36-2. B. Alkali burns are worse than acid burns because alkali causes liquefactive necrosis that penetrates and dissolves tissue until the alkali is removed. Acid burns cause protein coagulation, which limits the depth of acid penetration. Chemical injury to the eye is a true ocular emergency. In a patient with chemical injury to the eye, copious irrigation with at least 2 liters of sterile saline should be done prior to a full examination. Irrigation should continue until the pH of the tears is between 7 and 8. The physiologic pH of tear fluid is neutral.

36-3. B. Neonatal conjunctivitis within the first 3 days of life is usually caused by chemical irritation caused by the silver nitrate drops they receive at birth to prevent gonorrheal conjunctivitis; this baby, born at home, may not have received silver nitrate drops, and thus choice B is the best answer of the options listed.

Although uncommon, pathogens that cause conjunctivitis in the first few days of life include *Neisseria gonorrhoeae* and HSV-2 (HSV-2 can manifest any time within the first 2 weeks). At 5 to 10 days of life, *Staphylococcus aureus*, *Streptococcus pneumoniae*, *Chlamydia*, and *Haemophilus* are common pathogens. Diagnosis is made by Gram's stain and culture of exudates or viral culture from conjunctival scrapings. Treatment for chlamydial conjunctivitis is oral erythromycin for 14 to 21 days; neisserial conjunctivitis treatment is IV ceftriaxone for 7 days, while HSV-2 treatment is IV acyclovir for 10 days. Appropriate treatment is crucial to prevent permanent vision loss and systemic neisserial, chlamydial, or HSV infection.

36-4. C. All of the features listed except corneal dendrites characterize herpes zoster ophthalmicus. While HSV is associated with true dendrites (corneal epithelial defect resembling a fern), zoster is associated with "pseudodendrites," which are poorly staining mucous plaques on the cornea without epithelial erosion. The Hutchinson sign refers to vesicular lesions on the tip of the nose characteristic of cutaneous herpes zoster. Iritis can occur in zoster, causing photophobia and pain. Treatment for herpes zoster ophthalmicus includes cycloplegic pain reduction, erythromycin ophthalmic ointment to prevent bacterial superinfection, oral narcotics as necessary, prednisolone (Pred Forte) for iritis, and possible admission to the hospital for IV acyclovir.

 SUGGESTED ADDITIONAL READINGS

Bal SK, Hollingworth GR. Red eye. BMJ 2005;331:438.

Greenberg MF, Pollard ZF. The red eye in childhood. Pediatr Clin North Am 2003;50:105–124.

Kuckelkorn R, Schrage N, Keller G, et al. Emergency treatment of chemical and thermal eye burns. Acta Ophthalmol Scand 2002;80:4–10.

Nosebleed

CC: 25-year-old man presents with nosebleed

HPI: N.B. is a 25-year-old man with history of one prior nose-bleed 4 months earlier who now presents to the ED complaining of nosebleed today. He had been at work driving a bus when his nose started bleeding after having sneezed. He has been holding pressure to his nose for 1 hour but the blood continues to dribble down the back of his throat. He felt dizzy, nauseated, and vomited once before arriving to the ED. He denies any history of melena or hematemesis, recent trauma, or cocaine use. He has had a head cold for one week and has been blowing his nose frequently. He denies history of head or neck tumor or surgery, and does not use NSAIDs, aspirin, or anticoagulants.

PMHx: None

Meds: None

ALL: None

FHx: No known bleeding or clotting disorders

VS: Temp 37.0°C (98.6°F), HR 88, BP 114/74, RR 18, SaO$_2$ 99% on RA

PE: *General:* Sitting upright, holding pressure to nose. *HEENT:* A gush of blood comes out of the left nostril as he releases pressure; pressure is quickly reapplied; some blood is present in the oropharynx but he is easily maintaining his airway. *CV:* S$_1$, S$_2$; regular rate and rhythm; no murmurs, rubs, or gallops; pulses normal. *Chest:* Lungs clear to auscultation bilaterally; no respiratory distress. *Abd:* Soft, nontender, nondistended; bowel sounds present. *Skin:* Intact, warm; no rashes.

THOUGHT QUESTIONS

- What is the initial management for this patient?
- Into what two broad categories are nosebleeds (epistaxis) divided?
- What are common etiologies of epistaxis?
- How is epistaxis treated?

Immediate Actions:
Put on gown and face mask before examining the patient; have the patient blow his nose into a towel to clear any clots; have patient snort oxymetazoline (Afrin) two sprays; apply cotton swabs doused in 4% cocaine (a potent topical vasoconstrictor) with McGill forceps and reapply pressure for 10 minutes; remove cotton and reexamine nostril now that vasoconstriction has been achieved; cauterize bleeding source with silver nitrate if visualized; insert anterior nasal packing.

Discussion:
Nosebleeds are categorized according to origin of bleeding into either anterior or posterior epistaxis. Anterior epistaxis is more common in young people and represents 90% of nosebleeds. These include nosebleeds due to nose-picking and dry mucosa; the site of bleeding can usually be visualized. Posterior epistaxis is more common in the elderly and represents only 5% of patients with nosebleeds presenting to the ED. Posterior nosebleeds often occur posterior to the inferior turbinate; their origins usually cannot be seen. Common etiologies of epistaxis include trauma (e.g., nose-picking, foreign body, and local irritants such as nasal cocaine, dry nasal mucosa, and OTC nasal sprays) and infection (e.g., rhinitis, nasopharyngitis, sinusitis). Allergic or atrophic rhinitis can also cause epistaxis. Hypertension and arteriosclerosis are common cofactors in posterior epistaxis among the elderly.

Treatment of epistaxis includes direct pressure (useful for anterior epistaxis only), vasoconstrictive agents (e.g., epinephrine, phenylephrine, oxymetazoline), nasal packing, and cautery

(Continued)

(with silver nitrate or electrocautery). Patients with nasal packs should be given antistaphylococcal prophylaxis and should see an otolaryngologist in 2 to 3 days for pack removal. Patients with posterior epistaxis should be admitted to the hospital because of the nasopulmonary reflex, which can cause decreased respiratory drive, bradycardia, and hypoxia. If posterior bleeding persists, intra-arterial embolization or ligation by an otolaryngologist or interventional radiologist may be required.

CASE CONTINUED

With the anterior packing, the patient's nosebleed does not recur after 30 minutes of observation in the ED. Because of his complaint of dizziness, a hematocrit is checked and found to be 40.5%. The patient is sent home with cephalexin (Keflex) 500 mg four times daily. He follows up with otolaryngology in 3 days and the packing is removed, at which time the irritated mucosa has healed. He is sent home with instructions to use saline spray in both nares several times daily and apply Vaseline around the inlet of both nares to keep the mucosa moist.

QUESTIONS

37-1. A 41-year-old man presents to the ED complaining of fever, nausea, vomiting, and lightheadedness. He had been seen in the ED for a nosebleed 4 days earlier but has no other medical problems and takes no medications. Vital signs are significant for a temperature of 39°C (102.2°F), heart rate of 110 bpm, and blood pressure of 89/55 mm Hg. On examination, he has anterior nasal packing in place in the right nostril, without any visible acute bleeding. His oropharynx is unremarkable. Which of the following is his likely diagnosis?

    A. Dislodgment of the pack
    B. Sinusitis
    C. Toxic shock syndrome
    D. Septal necrosis
    E. Persistent bleeding

37-2. A 74-year-old male on warfarin (Coumadin) for atrial fibrillation presents to the ED with left-sided anterior epistaxis. Direct pressure for 15 minutes fails to provide hemostasis. Epinephrine 4% nasal spray also fails to provide hemostasis. What should be done next?

A. Electrocautery in the ED
B. Anterior nasal packing
C. Cautery with silver nitrate
D. Posterior nasal packing
E. Direct pressure for another 30 minutes

37-3. A 25-year-old man returns to the ED 2 days after being seen for anterior epistaxis that had been controlled with a nasal pack; he is now complaining of severe left-sided headache and facial pain extending from the top of his head down to his jaw. What has happened?

A. Nasal mucosa trauma
B. Sinusitis
C. Septal perforation
D. Dislodgment of pack
E. Toxic shock syndrome

37-4. A 30-year-old woman is brought to the ED with blood all over her shirt and a washcloth held in front of her nostrils. She says she has no past medical history but has been suffering from an upper respiratory infection for the past several days, with sinus congestion alternating with rhinorrhea. An hour prior to arrival, she had been blowing her nose when suddenly bright red blood was "gushing out." What is the likely source of her nosebleed?

A. Kiesselbach's plexus
B. Lateral nasal branch of sphenopalatine artery
C. Lingual branch of external carotid artery
D. Maxillary artery
E. Temporal artery

ANSWERS

37-1. C. All of the choices listed, including dislodgment of the pack, sinusitis, toxic shock syndrome, persistent bleeding, and septal necrosis, are possible complications of anterior nasal packing. **In a patient returning with fever, nausea, vomiting, or rash, however, one should suspect toxic shock syndrome. This is a rare but possible complication of anterior nasal packing, caused by *Staphylococcus aureus* infection with exotoxin release.** The toxic shock exotoxin has severe systemic effects, including fever, rash with desquamation, multiorgan system failure (ARDS, renal failure, coagulopathy, myocardial depression), and hypotension. Because complications of anterior nasal packing can occur, it is important that patients are given follow-up with an otolaryngologist. Patients being discharged with anterior nasal packing in place should also be started on antistaphylococcal antibiotics.

37-2. B. Anterior nasal packing is the next step. Silver nitrate cautery can only be used when the bleeding has already stopped and the bleeding site is well visualized. Electrocautery should usually be performed by an otolaryngologist because of the potential for significant trauma to surrounding tissues. **Posterior nasal packing is not yet indicated in this patient, whose bleeding source has been localized as anterior. However, it is difficult sometimes to locate the source of bleeding, and if several attempts at anterior packing fail, then posterior packing may be required.** Direct pressure for 15 minutes has already been attempted and has failed to provide hemostasis, so it would not be the appropriate next step.

37-3. B. The patient derives incomplete yet significant symptom relief from removal of his anterior nasal packing. He has no further epistaxis following pack removal. Sinus CT shows acute sinusitis throughout the paranasal sinuses, a complication of his nasal packing. He is discharged home on amoxicillin-clavulanate (Augmentin) 875 mg PO BID for 10 days and oxymetazoline two sprays BID for 3 days. A complication of overzealous use of cautery (electrical or silver nitrate) is septal perforation. Complications of electrocautery further include trauma to the nasal mucosa and to the skin surrounding the nares.

37-4. A. The majority of nosebleeds are anterior nosebleeds, and the majority of anterior nosebleeds originate from an area called Kiesselbach's plexus at the nasal septum. The majority of posterior nosebleeds originate from the lateral nasal branch of the sphenopalatine artery.

   SUGGESTED ADDITIONAL READINGS

Leong SC, Roe RJ, Karkanevatos A. No frills management of epistaxis. Emerg Med J 2005;22:470–472.
Pope LE, Hobbs CG. Epistaxis: an update on current management. Postgrad Med J 2005;81:309–314.

Fever and Sore Throat

CC: 34-year-old woman with fever and sore throat

HPI: S.T. is a 34-year-old woman who presents to the ED complaining of fever to 38.9°C (102°F) and sore throat for 3 days. Today she has difficulty swallowing because of the pain. She has a mild cough but denies rhinorrhea, congestion, nausea, vomiting, diarrhea, dysphagia, drooling, SOB, or urinary symptoms.

PMHx: None

Meds: None

ALL: NKDA

FHx: Noncontributory

SHx: Denies tobacco, alcohol, or drug use

VS: Temp 38.8°C (101.8°F), HR 105, BP 120/70, RR 18, SaO$_2$ 99% on RA

PE: *General:* Healthy-appearing woman sitting on bed in no apparent distress. *HEENT:* Tonsils erythematous with moderate whitish-yellow exudate bilaterally; erythematous pharynx; mild uvular edema; no petechiae noted; nostrils clear bilaterally; TM normal bilaterally; no conjunctival injection; mucous membranes mildly dry. *Neck:* Mildly enlarged, tender anterior cervical lymph nodes; no stridor. *CV:* S$_1$, S$_2$; tachycardic; no murmurs, rubs, or gallops; 2+ radial and 2+ DP pulses. *Chest:* Clear bilaterally. *Abd:* Soft, nontender, nondistended; bowel sounds present. *Extr:* No edema; well-perfused.

THOUGHT QUESTIONS

- What is the initial management for this patient?
- What is the differential diagnosis?

- Which diagnostic tests, if any, should be performed?
- Which patients should get antibiotics?

Immediate Actions:
Ensure adequate airway patency; obtain pharyngeal swab for rapid strep test.

Discussion:
The differential diagnosis for sore throat includes pharyngitis, epiglottitis, and peritonsillar or retropharyngeal abscess. Causes for pharyngitis include viruses, bacteria, fungi, and parasites. The most common viral causes of pharyngitis are adenovirus and rhinovirus; the most common bacterial causes are *Streptococcus pyogenes, Mycoplasma, Chlamydia, Neisseria,* and *Corynebacterium.* Infection with *S. pyogenes,* or group A β-hemolytic streptococcus (GABHS), can lead to development of acute rheumatic fever (ARF). Antibiotics, therefore, are given to those thought to have GABHS to prevent ARF. The incidence of ARF following GABHS pharyngitis is less than 1%, and it can be prevented if antibiotics are started within 10 days of the onset of infection. Throat culture and/or rapid strep test (antigen detection test on throat swab) can be performed to assess for GABHS, but neither is 100% sensitive, and cultures require at least a couple of days to obtain results. Some physicians therefore prefer to treat presumptively without testing. Patients with GABHS pharyngitis are typically young, have a high fever, tonsillar exudates, tender anterior cervical lymph nodes, and lack a cough or rhinorrhea. Any patient with confirmed or suspected GABHS pharyngitis should be given 10 days of an antibiotic such as penicillin (erythromycin or first- or second-generation cephalosporin for patients allergic to penicillin). EBV infection or mononucleosis should be considered in patients who have a prolonged course of pharyngitis not responsive to antibiotics. These patients classically develop a diffuse macular rash to ampicillin or amoxicillin.

CASE CONTINUED

The rapid strep comes back positive for streptococcal pharyngitis. She is given water and juice to drink, which she tolerates well. A repeat heart rate is 80. She is discharged with a 10-day course of penicillin 500 mg PO BID, Tylenol for fever, and instructions to gargle with warm saltwater, get plenty of rest, and drink warm liquids. She recovers uneventfully.

QUESTIONS

38-1. An 18-year-old man presents to the ED with 2 days of sore throat, fever to 38.9°C (102°F), and malaise. A pharyngeal swab is sent for a rapid-strep antigen test, which returns positive. Left untreated, which of the following is a nonsuppurative complication of pharyngitis?
- A. Peritonsillar abscess
- B. Sinusitis
- C. Otitis media
- D. Acute rheumatic fever
- E. Retropharyngeal abscess

38-2. A mother brings her daughter to the ED for a sore throat and refusal to swallow solids. Which of the following choices correlates with peak occurrence of pharyngitis in children?
- A. Age younger than 3 years and fall season
- B. Age younger than 3 years and winter season
- C. Age 4 to 7 years and fall season
- D. Age 4 to 7 years and winter season
- E. Age 8 to 11 years and fall season

38-3. A father brings his 6-year-old son to the ED for sore throat, hoarse voice, and fever to 39.2°C (102.6°F). The boy appears ill and he refuses to talk. You consider epiglottitis based on the history. Which of the following is characteristic of epiglottitis?
- A. Dry mucous membranes
- B. Tongue protrusion
- C. Expiratory stridor
- D. Neck flexed with head toward chest
- E. Lying supine

38-4. A 5-year-old girl presents to the ED with a fever, hoarse voice, and drooling. Her temperature is 39.3°C (102.8°F) and she appears ill. She is sitting upright with her head jutting forward and her neck extended. A lateral x-ray in the bay shows the "thumb sign." She is taken to the OR for intubation and IV placement. In considering appropriate antibiotics, what has historically been the most common cause of her condition?

A. *Streptococcus pyogenes* (GAS)
B. *Haemophilus influenzae* type b
C. *Moraxella catarrhalis*
D. Respiratory syncytial virus
E. Adenovirus

ANSWERS

38-1. D. Suppurative complications of pharyngitis include peritonsillar abscess, sinusitis, otitis media, cervical lymphadenitis, and retropharyngeal abscess. These can result from all types of pharyngitis. **Nonsuppurative complications of GABHS pharyngitis include acute rheumatic fever and poststreptococcal glomerulonephritis.** GABHS is also associated with scarlet fever, which is characterized by a sandpaper erythematous rash that subsequently desquamates.

38-2. D. Pharyngitis peaks in the age range of 4 to 7 years and has a higher incidence in the winter. Pharyngitis is uncommon in infants younger than 2 years. GABHS accounts for only 15% of pharyngitis in patients older than 15 years.

38-3. B. Patients with epiglottitis usually appear uncomfortable or apprehensive, prefer to sit upright leaning forward with head extended, and have difficulty lying supine. **These patients are often drooling and panting with mouth open and tongue protruding.** They frequently have inspiratory, not expiratory, stridor. Children with epiglottitis are a respiratory emergency and require endotracheal intubation in the OR, where a surgical airway can be quickly achieved if all else fails. Until they can be taken to the OR, they require IV steroids and nebulized racemic epinephrine. A tongue blade should not be used to look at the throat of a child with suspected epiglottitis because this could cause laryngospasm and respiratory arrest.

38-4. B. Epiglottitis in children was previously caused almost exclusively by *Haemophilus influenzae* B (HIB), although its occurrence today is relatively rare. Epiglottitis can also be caused by other bacteria, viruses, or fungi. Other bacterial causes include *Streptococcus* species, *Staphylococcus* species, *Moraxella catarrhalis*, *Klebsiella pneumoniae*, and *Mycobacterium tuberculosis*. Viral causes include RSV, adenovirus, and herpesvirus. Fungal causes include *Candida* species. Since the advent of the HIB vaccine, epiglottitis occurs much less frequently in younger children, and GABHS is emerging as a more predominant organism. While epiglottitis is not uncommon in older children and adults, it does not result in airway compromise as it does in small children.

 SUGGESTED ADDITIONAL READINGS

Gerber MA. Diagnosis and treatment of pharyngitis in children. Pediatr Clin North Am 2005;52:729–747, vi.

McIsaac WJ, Kellner JD, Aufricht P, et al. Empirical validation of guidelines for the management of pharyngitis in children and adults. JAMA 2004;291:1587–1595.

Tewfik TL, Al Garni M. Tonsillopharyngitis: clinical highlights. J Otolaryngol 2005;34 Suppl 1:S45–49.

Wei JL, Kasperbauer JL, Weaver AL, et al. Efficacy of single-dose dexamethasone as adjuvant therapy for acute pharyngitis. Laryngoscope 2002;112:87–93.

Fever and Back Pain

CC: 26-year-old intravenous drug user with fever and malaise

HPI: D.U. is a 26-year-old woman who has used intravenous heroin for 4 years. She began feeling ill 2 weeks ago with malaise, decreased appetite, and muscle soreness. She has been having fevers up to 39.4°C (103°F) and night sweats. She has also had mild headaches, neck stiffness, and low back pain. She has no sore throat, cough, chest or abdominal pain, dysuria, or diarrhea. Her back pain has been worsening over the past day with some radiation into her buttocks bilaterally. She has bilateral thigh numbness and numbness around her anus and vagina. She has not been incontinent of urine or stool.

PMHx: Hepatitis C

Meds: None

ALL: Penicillin

SHx: 1 ppd smoker; uses IV heroin

VS: Temp 39.0°C (102.2°F), HR 116, BP 112/64, RR 18, Sao$_2$ 100% on room air

PE: *General:* Cachectic, chronically ill-appearing. *HEENT:* Conjunctiva pink, no scleral icterus; PERRL, EOMI, oropharynx clear, no exudates; sinuses nontender. *Neck:* Supple; no adenopathy; full ROM. *CV:* S$_1$, S$_2$; tachycardic; soft systolic ejection murmur just to the right of the sternum. *Chest:* Normal breath sounds. *Abd:* Soft, nondistended; normal bowel sounds. *Back:* Tender over the lumbar spine. *Rectal:* Perianal numbness, decreased rectal tone. *Extr:* Nontender; no edema or swelling. *Skin:* Warm, dry; no petechiae or rashes. Pulses: Strong radial and pedal pulses. *Neuro:* Alert and oriented; CN II-XII intact; 5/5 motor in upper extremities; 4/5 ankle dorsiflexion bilaterally; decreased sensation lateral legs and feet bilaterally; decreased patellar reflexes bilaterally.

THOUGHT QUESTIONS

- Which high-risk infections should be considered in IV drug abusers?
- What are the signs of cauda equina syndrome?
- Which test is a priority for this patient?
- What is the treatment for this disease process?

Immediate Actions:
IV placement; send blood for CBC with manual differential, electrolytes, LFTs, and two sets of blood cultures; send urinalysis and culture; obtain STAT MRI of the spine; consult neurosurgery.

Discussion:
It is important to ask about IV drug use when evaluating a patient with fever. IV drug users are at high-risk for bacteremia and seeding of bacteria, usually *Staphylococcus,* in any organ system. They are particularly at high risk for endocarditis, usually involving the tricuspid valve. Abscesses secondary to IV drug abuse can form in the brain, lungs, liver, and kidneys. IV drug abusers are also at higher risk for sepsis, osteomyelitis, septic joint, and soft-tissue infections. Spinal epidural abscess should always be considered in IV drug abusers with fever and back pain. An epidural abscess is a collection of pus between the epidural space and the posterior wall of the spinal canal, and it will often span longitudinally along the canal. It is often insidious and causes no neurologic symptoms but can cause cord compression once large enough. Epidural abscess is usually a result of hematogenous seeding of bacteria but can also result from direct extension from vertebral osteomyelitis, especially in IV drug abusers. A spinal epidural abscess requires surgical drainage and a 4- to 6-week course of IV antibiotics.

Cauda equina syndrome is a complication of epidural abscess, and it refers to compression of the nerve roots within the spinal canal below the level of the L1 vertebra at the termination of the spinal

---

(*Continued*)

cord. Below this level the nerve roots course through the canal and exit the vertebral foramina from L1-S5. Compression of the cauda equina in the canal results in lower extremity neurologic deficit including numbness, weakness, decreased reflexes, and difficulty walking. Sacral nerve root dysfunction will cause "saddle anesthesia," referring to loss of perianal and perineal sensation, decreased or absent rectal tone, and incontinence of urine or stool. Loss of perianal sensation is usually the first finding, and therefore a rectal exam is essential. Cauda equina syndrome is a neurosurgical emergency that requires surgery for decompression. If suspected, an MRI is required immediately to confirm the diagnosis and identify an etiology.

 CASE CONTINUED

The patient has signs of cauda equina syndrome on exam. She is taken immediately for an MRI of her spine, which shows a large epidural abscess spanning from T10 to L3. Neurosurgery is consulted and arrangements are made for emergent surgery. IV nafcillin 2 g and vancomycin 1 g are administered in the meantime. She undergoes a laminectomy with drainage of the abscess and she is admitted to the ICU. The next day she has regained full lower extremity motor strength but has residual leg numbness.

 QUESTIONS

39-1. An IV drug abuser has had 3 weeks of intermittent fever, chills, and night sweats. His physical exam is only remarkable for a soft systolic murmur at the right sternal border. An echocardiogram shows a vegetation on the tricuspid valve. What is the most likely etiologic agent?

    A. *Staphylococcus aureus*
    B. *Streptococcus pneumoniae*
    C. *Streptococcus viridans*
    D. *Escherichia coli*
    E. *Pseudomonas*

39-2. A 75-year-old man with a history of prostate cancer and metastases to the spine presents with sudden-onset low back pain and leg numbness. He is unable to get out of a chair. He has weakness with both ankle dorsiflexion and extension. He has right lateral leg numbness. He has decreased perianal sensation and decreased rectal tone. What is the most immediate step necessary in this patient's management?
- A. Immediate surgery for decompression
- B. Angiogram to rule out aortic thrombus
- C. MRI of spine to elucidate etiology of cauda equina syndrome
- D. CT scan to characterize extent of bone metastases
- E. High-dose steroids for likely cord compression

39-3. A 32-year-old woman is working in the yard and develops sudden low back pain with bending. The pain radiates to her left buttock and she is having difficulty walking. She has no medical history, does not take medications, and does not use IV drugs. On exam she has no midline back tenderness; she does have pain in the left posterior leg with passive leg raising, normal distal strength, and normal pedal pulses. She has mildly decreased sensation over the lateral aspect of her left lower leg. What is the most appropriate management for this patient in the ED?
- A. Analgesia, ambulation, and follow-up with primary doctor for re-examination
- B. Lumbar x-ray to evaluate for compression fracture
- C. Neurosurgical evaluation for likely sciatica
- D. CT scan to evaluate for compression fracture
- E. MRI to evaluate for lumbar disc herniation

39-4. A 65-year-old man is referred to your ED to rule out spinal cord compression because your hospital has an MRI scanner and a neurosurgeon. The patient has a history of coronary bypass and takes aspirin, atenolol, and isosorbide. He also has a history of colon cancer that was resected 5 years ago. Today he had a sudden onset of lower back pain and bilateral leg weakness. On exam he is diffusely weak in his lower extremities and has diffuse leg tenderness. His legs also seem cool and you have a difficult time finding his pulses in both legs. Which test is necessary to make the diagnosis?
- A. MRI of the spine
- B. Doppler ultrasound of the legs
- C. CT of the abdomen without contrast
- D. CT of the abdomen and pelvis with IV contrast
- E. Lumbar puncture

ANSWERS

39-1. A. IV drug abusers are at extremely high risk for developing bacterial endocarditis. The most common pathogen is *S. aureus* in 75% of cases, with many of these being methicillin-resistant. The second most common pathogen in IV drug abusers is *S. pneumoniae* in about 20%. Gram-negative organisms and *Pseudomonas* must also be considered in these patients. *S. viridans* is the most common etiologic agent in subacute bacterial endocarditis in those who do not use IV drugs. This pathogen usually attaches to left-sided valves (i.e., mitral and aortic) that are calcified or previously damaged from rheumatic fever, in contrast to IV drug abusers who often have an infected tricuspid valve. If endocarditis is suspected, three sets of blood cultures should be obtained from different veins and the patient should be admitted for IV antibiotics and echocardiography.

39-2. C. This patient has signs of cauda equina syndrome, which include lower extremity numbness and weakness, decreased perianal and perineal sensation, decreased rectal tone, and incontinence. This is a neurosurgical emergency that requires prompt surgical intervention, but first an MRI is required to identify the level of compression and the etiology. Acute aortic thrombus or dissection must also be considered in the setting of acute low back pain and lower extremity weakness. It is essential to do a thorough pulse exam when assessing lower extremity weakness. Absent pulses should prompt an angiogram to find the level of arterial occlusion.

39-3. A. Low back pain is a common presenting complaint in the ED. Although we are trained to think of the worst possible etiology, most back pain is benign. A thorough exam must be done to rule out cauda equina syndrome and aortic pathology, including an abdominal and back exam, neurologic exam, and rectal exam. Thereafter, most patients can be treated conservatively. X-rays would be considered to evaluate for compression fracture if there was a history of trauma or significant axial loading, or if the patient's pain is refractory to narcotic analgesia. An MRI should be considered if there is a suspicion for cauda equina syndrome or for focal leg weakness. **This patient has evidence of sciatica, which is irritation of the sciatic nerve either via compression, stretching, or inflammation. Initial treatment should be with analgesia, assurance that the patient is able to ambulate, and follow-up with a primary care physician for re-examination.**

39-4. D. It is important to remember that extremity weakness does not necessarily mean a primary neurologic process. **Acute arterial occlusion must always be considered and cannot be excluded by a normal-appearing extremity. In the case of bilateral leg weakness and absence of pulses, an arterial occlusion at the level of the aorta must be present.** An aortic dissection would typically result in unilateral arterial occlusion. **An aortic thrombus must be considered if both femoral artery pulses are absent. The diagnosis is made by angiography, which today can be accomplished with CT of the abdomen and pelvis with IV contrast.** Modern multi-detector CT scanners can reformat images to obtain a three-dimensional arteriogram. Treatment of arterial occlusion is emergent thombectomy, which entails surgical removal of the thombus.

 ## SUGGESTED ADDITIONAL READINGS

Bluman EM, Palumbo MA, Lucas PR. Spinal epidural abscess in adults. J Am Acad Orthop Surg 2004;12:155–163.

Bremer AA, Darouiche RO. Spinal epidural abscess presenting as intra-abdominal pathology: a case report and literature review. J Emerg Med 2004;26:51–56.

Calder KK, Severyn FA. Surgical emergencies in the intravenous drug user. Emerg Med Clin North Am 2003;21:1089–1116.

Rapidly Spreading Skin Redness

CC: 46-year-old diabetic with leg redness

HPI: E.G. is a 46-year-old man with 3 days of left lower leg redness that started with a superficial shin abrasion 2 days ago. He presents to the ED with spreading redness, a fever to 39.1°C (102.4°F), chills, leg pain, and dizziness. He has not seen his doctor and has not taken antibiotics. His initial triage blood pressure is 112/60. After sitting in the waiting room for an hour, he vomits and the triage nurse brings him to a treatment room. He states the redness has progressed significantly over the past 2 hours.

PMHx: IDDM

Meds: Insulin

ALL: None

SHx: No tobacco or alcohol

VS: Temp 39.0°C (102.2°F), HR 106, BP 88/64, RR 24, Sao_2 94% on room air

PE: *General:* Mild pallor, ill-appearing. *HEENT:* Conjunctiva pink; oropharynx clear, no exudates. *Neck:* Supple; no adenopathy; full ROM. *CV:* S_1, S_2; tachycardic; no murmur. *Chest:* Scattered bilateral rhonchi. *Abd:* Soft, nondistended; normal bowel sounds. *GU:* Normal genitals. *Extr:* Erythema and warmth over medial aspect of left lower leg with streaking up medial thigh. *Pulses:* Weak radial and pedal pulses. *Neuro:* Alert and oriented; CN II-XII intact; 5/5 motor in all extremities; pain in left lower leg with range of motion of ankle; normal sensation in all dermatomes of legs.

THOUGHT QUESTIONS

- What is the most worrisome potential soft-tissue infection in this patient?
- What are worrisome symptoms and signs to watch for?
- What is the notorious "flesh-eating" bacterium?
- What is the key to management of a critically ill patient with a skin infection?

Immediate Actions:
Place two large-bore IVs; send blood for CBC with manual differential, electrolytes, LFTs, coagulation panel, and two sets of blood cultures; send urinalysis and culture; administer 2 L normal saline over 30 minutes; administer nafcillin 2 g IV, gentamicin 80 mg IV, and metronidazole 500 mg IV; if persistent hypotension after 2 L normal saline, place central venous catheter and measure central venous pressure (CVP); if CVP <8 mm Hg continue fluid boluses, otherwise start norepinephrine 2 to 10 μg/kg/min and titrate to mean arterial pressure (MAP) >70 mm Hg; obtain portable x-ray of leg to look for subcutaneous air; consult surgery for potential necrotizing fasciitis.

Discussion:
Necrotizing fasciitis should be the first consideration in patients with rapidly spreading skin infections who are critically ill. Necrotizing fasciitis is defined as infection of subcutaneous tissue and fascia, with relative sparing of muscle, which rapidly leads to systemic toxicity, sepsis, and death. The deceiving aspect of this disease is that in its early stages, external manifestations may be minimal. It may present as a focal skin infection or cellulitis and rapidly progress with nondistinct, spreading erythema. A concerning sign is localized pain out of proportion to external appearance. Subcutaneous tissue gas, supposedly a hallmark of the disease and apparent on x-ray, is present in less than half of cases. *Streptococcus* is the most-often implicated organism, followed by *Staphylococcus;* however, most

(Continued)

cases are polymicrobial with no specific predominant organism isolated. Group A β-hemolytic strep (GABHS) has been associated with necrotizing fasciitis, despite being isolated in only about 15% of cases, because it can result in a "toxic shock"-type syndrome with profound discoloration and sloughing of skin. This has led to the term "flesh-eating" bacteria.

If necrotizing fasciitis is considered, the key to management is aggressive treatment of sepsis and early surgical intervention. These patients can deteriorate very quickly despite an initial benign appearance of their soft-tissue infection. Early goal-directed therapy for sepsis should be initiated, including rapid crystalloid bolus and broad-spectrum antibiotics, followed by central venous access and vasopressors if necessary. Antibiotic therapy should be aimed at gram-positive cocci, gram-negative rods, and anaerobes. A good initial choice would be nafcillin, gentamicin, and metronidazole or clindamycin. The key to management of necrotizing fasciitis is early surgical debridement once the disease is considered. A bedside tissue biopsy can be performed, but this results in many false-negatives. Patients who are critically ill should be taken to the operating room for extensive tissue debridement down to viable tissue. Repeat operation is required within 24 to 48 hours to assure that necrosis has not progressed. Despite the best efforts, mortality of necrotizing fasciitis is about 25% to 50% depending on the time of presentation.

CASE CONTINUED

The patient remains hypotensive after 2 liters of crystalloid and antibiotics, and he requires central venous access and a norepinephrine drip. He becomes hypoxic and requires intubation, all consistent with severe sepsis and adult respiratory distress syndrome (ARDS). His left medial thigh develops a deep-purple hue, and he is taken to the OR for soft-tissue debridement. He continues to require full-dose norepinephrine and dopamine 4 hours postop, but thereafter slowly begins to improve. The next day he is taken to the OR again and is found to have no progression of necrosis. He recovers over the next 2 weeks and later requires skin grafting over the large wound in his left leg.

QUESTIONS

40-1. It is mid-August in Mississippi during a hot, humid heat wave. An 8-year-old boy is bitten numerous times on the legs by mosquitos. Two days later he develops several small papules over his anterior shin that rapidly progress to small vesicles and pustules that rupture over the next 24 hours. In the ED, there is a large patch on his lower leg of thick, amber-colored, crusty exudates on an erythematous base. He has no fever and his leg is minimally tender. What is the appropriate treatment?

    A. Broad-spectrum IV antibiotics and admission
    B. Oral prednisone and topical neomycin
    C. Iodine scrub and saline gauze dressings
    D. Oral penicillin, erythromycin, cephalexin, or clindamycin
    E. No treatment required

40-2. An 83-year-old man with a history of diabetes, hypertension, and dementia presents to the ED with a fever to 39.2°C (102.6°F), chills, and a blood pressure of 84/46. He complains of low abdominal pain. He appears ill and is disoriented. He has mild low abdominal tenderness. His testicles are tender and he has bilateral inguinal adenopathy. You notice significant perineal edema, bogginess, and tenderness. What is an appropriate step in his management?

    A. Open fasciotomy and perineal tissue debridement
    B. Bedside incision and drainage of perineal abscess
    C. Antibiotic coverage for gram-positive organisms
    D. Testicular ultrasound to identify scrotal abscess
    E. CT abdomen to rule out incarcerated scrotal hernia

40-3. A 42-year-old man is struck by a car at moderate speed, resulting in a comminuted midshaft femur fracture that requires surgery. On the second post-op day he develops increased thigh pain and a fever to 38.7°C (101.6°F). Over the next 2 hours, the thigh swells and a brownish, sweet-smelling exudate is present. There are several purplish blebs around the wound and crepitus is palpated. What is the most likely responsible organism?

    A. *Staphylococcus aureus*
    B. *Bacteroides fragilis*
    C. Group A β-hemolytic streptococcus (GABHS)
    D. *Escherichia coli*
    E. *Clostridium perfringens*

40-4. A 56-year-old woman went to a clinic for epistaxis that was not controlled with direct pressure and ice. She required nasal packing with an absorptive tampon to stop the bleeding. She was sent home with the packing in place and told to follow-up in 5 to 7 days. Four days later, she develops high fever, vomiting, and a diffuse, erythematous, macular rash over the chest, back, and arms with areas of desquamation. Upon arrival to the ED, her pulse is 134 and blood pressure is 78/43; she appears very ill. What is the most likely etiology of the rash?

- A. Viral exanthem
- B. Febrile reaction
- C. Necrotizing fasciitis
- D. Bacterial endotoxin
- E. Drug reaction

ANSWERS

40-1. D. This is a classic presentation for impetigo contagiosa, a very common skin infection in children, especially in summer months in warm, humid climates. It usually starts in the area of insect bites or abrasions, typically legs more than upper extremities or trunk. The inciting organism is usually group A β-hemolytic streptococcus (GABHS), but also coagulase-positive *Staphylococcus aureus* as well. Lesions start as small papules that progress to vesicles and pustules, which rupture, coalesce, and form a thick, yellowish crust. The patient is typically not ill. **Washes, steroids, or topical antibiotics can be of some benefit, but oral antibiotics are the most effective treatment. Coverage is similar to that for simple cellulitis, including penicillin or erythromycin, first-generation cephalosporins, or clindamycin.**

40-2. A. This presentation is consistent with Fournier's gangrene, a necrotizing subcutaneous infection in older men affecting the perineum, scrotum, and penis. It is more common in chronically ill, immunocompromised, or diabetic patients with mild local trauma to or skin breakdown of the perineum. Organisms are usually colonic, most commonly *Bacteroides fragilis* and *Escherichia coli*. With local edema and inflammation within a limited space, infection can progress rapidly to subcutaneous tissue necrosis. Antibiotic coverage should be broad, covering gram-positive, gram-negative, and anaerobic organisms. **Early operative fasciotomy is required to debride necrotic tissue and prevent further spread.**

40-3. E. Clostridial myonecrosis, or gas gangrene, is a gas-forming infection of deep muscle and usually follows trauma or surgery. *Clostridium* is an anaerobic gram-positive bacillus, ubiquitous in the soil and in the human colon. Clostridia produce a toxin that results in myonecrosis and a local anaerobic environment, thus promoting its own growth. Skin manifestations are usually minimal but can include blebs. **Clostridial myonecrosis classically produces a sickly sweet smelling, brownish exudate.**

40-4. D. Toxic shock syndrome (TSS), the result of *S. aureus* infection, was publicized in the early 1980s in association with high-absorbency vaginal tampons. This disease is now known to be the result of either locally invasive *Staphylococcus* or *Streptococcus* infections, not particularly related to tampon use. **TSS is characterized by a sepsis-like syndrome and a diffuse "sunburn" or "sandpaper" rash that may desquamate. However, the rash is the result of a circulating bacterial endotoxin as opposed to direct bacterial invasion. Endotoxin production results in the wide proliferation of T-cells and subsequent release of cytokines TNF-α, IL-1, and IL-6. These circulating cytokines result in the clinical picture of multi-organ failure, including the desquamating rash.**

 SUGGESTED ADDITIONAL READINGS

Falagas ME, Vergidis PI. Narrative review: diseases that masquerade as infectious cellulitis. Ann Intern Med 2005;142:47–55.

Hasham S, Matteucci P, Stanley PR, et al. Necrotising fasciitis. BMJ 2005;330:830–833.

McGee EJ. Necrotizing fasciitis: review of pathophysiology, diagnosis, and treatment. Crit Care Nurs Q 2005;28:80–84.

Wong CH, Wang YS. The diagnosis of necrotizing fasciitis. Curr Opin Infect Dis 2005;18:101–106.

Painful Head and Neck Rash with a Fever

CC: 35-year-old man with headache, neck pain, rash, and fever

HPI: H.N. is a 35-year-old man who presents with 5 to 6 days of right-sided neck pain, thought by his PCP 4 days ago to be inflamed lymph nodes and neck spasm. He has been taking Vicodin and ibuprofen without improvement. Two days ago, he developed a frontal headache, fevers, chills, nausea, and a rash on his head. He says it hurts the right side of his neck when he moves it. He denies photophobia, sore throat, cough, joint pains, sick contacts, or any other symptoms. He does not recall any specific insect bites, but was camping on Cape Cod a few days prior to the onset of his symptoms.

PMHx: Seborrheic dermatitis, mononucleosis at age 18, anxiety

Meds: Escitalopram (Lexapro) 10 mg PO QD, Vicodin (hydrocodone + acetaminophen) 5 mg/500 mg PO Q 4-6 hr PRN, ibuprofen 600 mg PO Q6 hr PRN

ALL: NKDA

SHx: Lives with wife, no tobacco or drugs, occasional alcohol

VS: Temp 37.3°C (99.1°F), HR 72, BP 163/90, RR 16, SaO$_2$ 98% on room air

PE: *General:* Well-developed, well-nourished, in mild discomfort. *HEENT:* Nonicteric sclerae; pupils 3 mm and reactive bilaterally; no retinal hemorrhages or papilledema; oropharynx moist without exudates; no hemotympanum. *Neck:* Supple; no discomfort to passive flexion; moderate tenderness of right anterior cervical lymphadenopathy. *CV:* S$_1$, S$_2$; regular; no murmurs; 2+ radial and DP pulses bilaterally. Chest: Clear bilaterally. *Abd:* Soft; nontender. *Skin:* Right-sided parietal scalp erythematous macules and papules, almost confluent, extending only to midline of head with a few small, grouped clear vesicles; right anterior neck with a few small areas of similar erythema and vesicles; no other rashes. *Neuro:* Alert and oriented; cranial nerves II to XII intact; normal speech; 5/5 motor strength in major muscle groups in upper and lower extremities; normal sensation to light touch and sharp object in all extremities; no pronator drift.

THOUGHT QUESTIONS

- How do you protect yourself when evaluating patients with headache and fever?
- What are the different types of isolation precautions to consider in ED patients?
- What are some insect-borne illnesses that might present with headache and fever?
- Which disease presents with a rash found in a dermatomal distribution?

Immediate Actions:
Wear a mask while evaluating any patient with complaint of headache and fever in case of bacterial (e.g., meningococcal) meningitis; no further immediate action is required after history and physical exam.

Discussion:
Universal or standard precautions, contact precautions, droplet precautions, and airborne precautions should be kept in mind when working in the ED. Universal precautions entail handwashing after patient contact and wearing gloves, masks, or eyewear when anticipating potential contact with body secretions. Contact precautions entail gloves and gowns for preventing transmission of organisms such as MRSA and *C. difficile.* Droplet precautions require a mask to prevent transmission of diseases such as pertussis and *Neisseria meningitidis* via droplets of greater than 5 microns, which can result from talking, coughing, or sneezing. Airborne precautions

(Continued)

are to prevent infections such as TB via droplets of 5 microns or less, which can be widely dispersed in a room through coughing. This mandates the use of an "N95" mask and placement of the patient in a negative-pressure room.

Important insect-borne illnesses to consider in the differential of a patient presenting with headache and fever include tick- and mosquito-borne illnesses. Tick-borne bacterial illnesses include Lyme disease, tularemia, and relapsing fever (tularemia, however, is not generally associated with a headache). Tick-borne rickettsial illnesses include Rocky Mountain spotted fever (RMSF), Eastern spotted fever, Q fever, and ehrlichiosis. Colorado tick fever and tick-borne encephalitis (viral illnesses), as well as babesiosis (a protozoal illness), are also transmitted by infected ticks. Lyme disease is often seen in conjunction with the characteristic erythema migrans rash, which expands gradually and then may have central clearing. RMSF is often seen with a rash that characteristically starts as maculopapular on the palms and soles, then spreads centripetally and becomes petechial. Babesiosis and Q fever are not generally associated with a rash. Antibiotics are the mainstay of treatment in all of these diseases except for Colorado tick fever and tick-borne encephalitis. Some mosquito-borne illnesses to consider in the United States include West Nile virus, St. Louis encephalitis, eastern equine encephalitis (EEE), Western equine encephalitis (WEE), and Venezuelan equine encephalitis (VEE). Treatment is supportive in these illnesses. Of note, West Nile virus had not been seen in the United States prior to 1999, the year in which 62 cases were reported; during January 1 to December 1, 2005, 2,744 cases were reported in the United States. Most patients who get West Nile virus are asymptomatic; treatment is supportive for those with symptoms, which can range from a mild febrile illness to meningoencephalitis.

Rashes that are found in a dermatomal distribution are classically due to herpes zoster (shingles), which is caused by reactivation of the latent varicella-zoster virus that resides in dorsal root ganglion cells. Zoster is characterized by pain located in a dermatomal distribution and general flu-like malaise symptoms followed in 1 to 10 days by the characteristic rash of grouped vesicles on an erythematous base involving one or more dermatomes. Treatment is generally supportive, although antivirals such as acyclovir or valacyclovir, if started within 72 hours of rash onset, decrease symptom severity and postherpetic neuralgia. Use of

(Continued)

corticosteroids with antivirals is controversial, but tricyclic antidepressants and anticonvulsants have been found helpful for postherpetic neuralgic pain. When zoster involves cranial nerve V_1, care must be taken to assess for eye involvement, which can cause permanent vision damage; prompt use of antivirals and ophthalmology referral are vital.

CASE CONTINUED

This patient's rash is located in a C_1-C_2 dermatome distribution involving the anterior portion of the right neck and right parietal scalp. The rash is characteristic of herpes zoster with painful vesicles on an erythematous base. Because his rash has only been present for 2 days, he is prescribed valacyclovir 1,000 mg PO TID for 7 days. He is also given amitryptylline 25 mg PO QHS for neuropathic pain and to help him sleep. Until the lesions have crusted over, he is advised to avoid anyone who has not been immunized or who has not had chickenpox as a child, anyone who is immunocompromised (e.g., cancer patients, patients with AIDS), pregnant women, and infants.

QUESTIONS

41-1. A healthy 27-year-old woman who is at 20 weeks gestation is found to have an erythematous rash with prominent central clearing located on her leg. She does not recall any tick bites, although she did go to Martha's Vineyard and Cape Cod a week earlier. She is otherwise asymptomatic. Which of the following is the best treatment for her?

A. Supportive; start antibiotics for any development of other symptoms
B. Doxycycline 200 mg PO single-dose therapy
C. Doxycycline 100 mg PO BID for 21 days
D. Amoxicillin 500 mg PO TID for 7 days
E. Amoxicillin 500 mg PO TID for 21 days

41-2. A previously healthy 30-year-old male patient presents with severe headache, fever of 39°C (102.2°F), and neck stiffness. Which of the following is most appropriate to protect yourself and the staff?
   A. Airborne precautions
   B. Droplet precautions
   C. Contact precautions
   D. Universal precautions
   E. No special precautions are necessary in an immunocompetent patient

41-3. A 72-year-old man complains of severe headache for the past week. On your examination of the patient, you find grouped vesicles and erythema on the left side of his forehead. Which of the following is required?
   A. Cardiac monitoring for potential cardiac involvement with heart block
   B. Antibiotics before lumbar puncture
   C. Prompt surgical referral
   D. Prompt ophthalmologic referral
   E. Contact precautions for care providers who have never had chickenpox or the varicella vaccine

41-4. A 64-year-old woman with a history significant only for high cholesterol presents with complaints of headache, nausea, malaise, and fever for the past 5 days. She denies any rashes or sick contacts but does walk in the woods near her New Jersey home a couple times per week during the summer months. Which of the following results is most likely from her lumbar puncture?
   A. Normal pressure, normal glucose, mildly high protein, WBC 55/mm^3 with mostly lymphocytes
   B. Normal pressure, high glucose, high protein, WBC 125/mm^3 with mostly lymphocytes
   C. Normal pressure, high glucose, mildly low protein, WBC 1100/mm^3 with mostly neutrophils
   D. Normal pressure, low glucose, low protein, WBC 350/mm^3 with mostly neutrophils
   E. Elevated pressure, normal glucose, normal protein, WBC 1/mm^3

ANSWERS

41-1. E. This patient's rash is characteristic of erythema migrans, the rash seen in Lyme disease. Erythema migrans can also be seen in other conditions, but given the patient's travel to an endemic area (Cape Cod and the Islands of Martha's Vineyard and Nantucket in Massachusetts), it is safer to presume that she has Lyme disease. Many patients do not recall a specific tick bite because the nymph stage of the *Ixodes* tick is only a bit larger than a speck of pepper. **A full course of antibiotics (21 days) is recommended for pregnant patients with possible Lyme disease to prevent transplacental transmission. Amoxicillin is safe during pregnancy, whereas doxycycline is not recommended.** Single-dose doxycycline may be effective in preventing Lyme disease if given within 72 hours of a tick bite. Treatment of uncomplicated Lyme disease in a patient who is not pregnant is doxycycline 100 mg PO BID for 14 to 21 days.

41-2. B. The patient described has symptoms concerning for potential bacterial meningitis. Droplet precautions are thus warranted while evaluation is being undertaken. Droplets—for example, due to talking, coughing, or sneezing—do not typically travel more than 3 feet or remain suspended in the air; thus health care workers should wear masks when going within 3 feet of the patient.

41-3. D. This patient's rash is concerning for herpes zoster affecting the first division of the trigeminal nerve, and therefore potentially involving the ipsilateral eye as well. Rash involvement on the tip of the nose is referred to as Hutchinson's sign and signifies that the nasociliary branch of the ophthalmic nerve is affected. Examples of ocular complications include conjunctivitis, iritis, corneal ulcers, anterior uveitis, and secondary glaucoma. Prompt referral to ophthalmology is thus critical. Heart block is a potential complication of advanced Lyme disease. Health care workers who are not immune to varicella should avoid patients with suspected chickenpox or zoster; airborne precautions (rather than droplet or contact) are needed to effectively reduce spread of varicella virus because the pathogen is smaller than 5 microns. Antibiotics should be given as soon as possible, without delay for lumbar puncture, in cases of suspected bacterial meningitis.

41-4. A. This patient likely has a mild case of aseptic meningitis (nonbacterial meningitis), given that her symptoms have already lasted for 5 days, though one would not be able to rule out bacterial meningitis until seeing results of a Gram's stain and culture. The fact that she lives near woods in New Jersey suggests that she was either bitten by mosquitos or ticks and may have West Nile virus, Lyme disease, or one of the other insect-borne illnesses; she does not have a rash, however, which is commonly seen in many of the tick-borne diseases. **In aseptic meningitis, the CSF usually has**

normal opening pressure, normal glucose, normal to mildly elevated protein, and a slight pleocytosis (WBC < 100–500/mm³), with a lymphocytic predominance. In the case of bacterial meningitis, CSF usually has a normal opening pressure, decreased glucose, elevated protein, and a pleocytosis (WBC > 500–1,000/mm³) with a predominance of polymorphonuclear leukocytes (see Table 14-1 for further details). Although history alone is not sufficient to rule out bacterial meningitis in this patient, none of the answer choices provides the correct CSF findings for bacterial meningitis. Choice E is consistent with benign intracranial hypertension, but those patients generally are not febrile.

 SUGGESTED ADDITIONAL READINGS

Centers for Disease Control and Prevention (CDC). West Nile Virus activity—United States, January 1–December 1, 2005. MMWR Morb Mortal Wkly Rep 2005;54:1253–1256.

Hengge UR, Tannapfel A, Tyring SK, et al. Lyme borreliosis. Lancet Infect Dis 2003;3:489–500.

Petersen LR, Marfin AA, Gubler DJ. West Nile Virus. JAMA 2003; 290:524–528.

Sandy MC. Herpes zoster: medical and nursing management. Clin J Oncol Nurs 2005;9:443–446.

Tabamo RE, Donahue JE. Eastern equine encephalitis: case report and literature review. Med Health RI 1999;82:23–26.

CASE **42**

Fever in an Infant

CC: 3-month-old girl with fever

HPI: I.F. is a 3-month-old healthy girl who is brought to the ED by her parents for fever. She was fussy yesterday; this morning she had a temperature of 38.3°C (101°F) at 10 A.M. Her parents gave her one-half teaspoon of ibuprofen but she was still irritable and crying, with decreased PO intake. She has not had vomiting, diarrhea, cough, or rhinorrhea, and has not been noted to pull at her ears. She continued to have damp diapers today. She was full-term at birth and has otherwise been doing well since birth.

PMHx: Full-term vaginal delivery to GBS-negative mother without complication

Meds: Ibuprofen elixir today

ALL: NKDA

DevHx: Normal development

Imm: Up to date

SHx: Lives with mother, father, and 3-year-old sister

VS: Temp 38.4°C (101.1°F) rectally, HR 134, BP 78/42, RR 24, SaO_2 100% on RA

PE: *General:* Healthy-appearing infant; fussy. *HEENT:* Anterior and posterior fontanelles soft; conjunctiva clear; decreased tearing; TM within normal limits bilaterally; oropharynx dry, no pharyngeal erythema or lesions; no rhinorrhea. *Neck:* Supple; no nuchal rigidity; no lymphadenopathy. *CV:* S_1, S_2; regular; no murmurs; pulses intact. *Chest:* Clear bilaterally. *Abd:* Soft; nontender; nondistended; bowel sounds present. *GU:* No rashes or lesions. *Extr:* Warm; no rashes. *Neuro:* Alert; interactive.

THOUGHT QUESTIONS

- What is the initial management for this patient?
- What is the differential diagnosis for fever in an infant?
- How are infants with fever treated based on their age?
- Which infants with fever should be hospitalized?

Immediate Actions:
Start IV; give NS bolus of 20 mL/kg; send CBC with differential, blood culture, urinalysis, and urine culture.

Discussion:
Any fever greater than 38.0°C (100.4°F) is worrisome in an infant less than 3 months old because of the concern for serious bacterial infection (SBI), which at this age group includes UTI, pneumonia, meningitis, bacteremia, and sepsis. Infants localize infection poorly, and a simple UTI that is untreated may quickly progress to bacteremia and meningitis or sepsis, both of which have devastating outcomes at this age. Neonates from 0 to 28 days old with a fever greater than 38.0°C are admitted to the hospital for IV antibiotics until blood, urine, and CSF cultures are negative. There are varying practices for infants between 1 and 3 months of age. More commonly these children are evaluated in the ED with a CBC with differential, urinalysis, and blood and urine cultures. If the infant appears ill, or if the WBC is greater than 15 (15,000/mm^3), a lumbar puncture is done and the child is admitted for IV antibiotics. If the child appears well, and the WBC is less than or equal to 15, the child receives ceftriaxone 50 mg/kg IM and is discharged with follow-up the next day with the child's pediatrician; the child receives a second shot of ceftriaxone 24 hours later. This practice has drastically reduced admissions while maintaining a low number of missed serious bacterial infections (<1%). Children between 3 months and 3 years of age are better able to localize infection and are treated less conservatively. Blood and urine cultures are obtained for

(Continued)

a fever greater than 39.0°C (102.2°F) if the WBC is greater than 15. Otherwise, lumbar puncture and chest x-ray are obtained based on the child's symptoms and exam. Any child who appears ill or dehydrated, or who is not tolerating liquids, regardless of temperature or WBC count, needs admission for rehydration and observation. Guidelines for management of the febrile infant are summarized in Table 42-1.

TABLE 42-1 Management of Infant with Fever >38.0°C (100.4°F) and No Obvious Source of SBI

Age	Pathogens	Tests	Treatment
0–30 days	Group B streptococcus, E. coli, Listeria monocytogenes	Blood, urine, and CSF cultures	All are admitted for IV antibiotics until cultures are negative
1–3 mo	S. pneumoniae, N. meningitidis, H. influenzae	Blood and urine cultures, LP if toxic-appearing or WBC > 15	If nontoxic and WBC < 15: Ceftriaxone 50 mg/kg IM and follow-up in 24 hours with pediatrician for second dose of ceftriaxone and to check on culture results. Toxic-appearing or SBI: Admit for IV antibiotics
3 mo–3 yr	S. pneumoniae, N. meningitidis, H. influenzae	Blood culture if temp >39.0°C (102.2°F) and WBC >15; otherwise urine culture, CXR, and LP indicated based on symptoms	Most can go home with close follow-up. Toxic-appearing: Admit

 CASE CONTINUED

The child perks up after her fluid bolus. The labs show a WBC of 18.6 (18,600/mm³) with 90% polys. The urinalysis shows 80 WBCs/hpf, 10 RBCs/hpf, and many bacteria. She is admitted to the hospital and given gentamicin 7.5 mg/kg/day divided for every 8 hours. The next day, the urine cultures grow *Escherichia coli*. The blood culture remains negative on the second day, and she is discharged home with a 14-day course of trimethoprim-sulfamethoxazole (Bactrim), based on the culture sensitivities.

QUESTIONS

42-1. A 22-day-old infant is brought in by his aunt who says the baby seems feverish and isn't taking the bottle today. The baby was acting normally yesterday as far as she knows. The mother has been at work all morning and has been unreachable by phone. The aunt thinks the baby was full term and to the best of her knowledge, had an unremarkable delivery. There was no thermometer at the house, so she has not checked a temperature. Which of the following is the most reliable representative of the baby's actual body temperature?

    A. Axillary temperature
    B. Oral temperature
    C. Rectal temperature
    D. Temporal artery temperature
    E. Tympanic membrane temperature

42-2. A 2-month-old boy presents to the ED with fever and decreased oral intake for one day. He was born at 35 weeks gestation after an induction for intrauterine growth restriction which led to a cesarean delivery for nonreassuring fetal heart rate tracing. He did not need to stay in the neonatal intensive care unit and has otherwise had an unremarkable 2 months of life. His mother reports that her 3-year-old son who attends daycare is just getting over a vomiting and diarrhea "bug." There are no other sick contacts in the household, but the mother says her friend had read an article about meningitis recently and told her that her baby could die. The mother is very worried that her baby might have meningitis. Which of the following would be a reassuring sign for this mother?

    A. Nuchal rigidity
    B. Inconsolability
    C. Vomiting
    D. Sunken fontanelles
    E. Irritability that decreases when the infant is laid down

42-3. A 6-month-old girl, a 12-month-old boy, and a 20-month-old boy are all admitted to the hospital after presenting to the ED with high fever, decreased oral intake, and toxic appearance. Each child is started on IV antibiotics after appropriate cultures have been sent. Which one organism is most commonly responsible for bacteremia in patients of this age range?

A. Group B *Streptococcus*
B. *Streptococcus pneumoniae*
C. *Haemophilus influenzae*
D. *Neisseria meningitidis*
E. *Escherichia coli*

42-4. A 10-week-old infant boy is seen in the emergency department for fever of 38.0°C (100.4°F). He is still nursing and is still having wet diapers, roughly the same number as usual. After appropriate workup, the infant is discharged home with a prescription for antibiotics. Based on that information alone, which of the following bacterial infections does this child likely have?

A. Meningitis
B. Cellulitis
C. Urinary tract infection
D. Otitis media
E. Bacteremia

ANSWERS

42-1. **C. The rectal temperature is the most reliable representative of actual core body temperature.** Oral temperatures are generally 0.6°C (1°F) lower than rectal temperatures, while axillary temperatures are approximately another 0.6°C lower than oral temperatures. Tympanic membrane temperatures are more variable and less reproducible than the other methods described. Temporal artery thermometers are a relatively new technique for measuring temperature. A temperature of 38°C (100.4°F) rectally is generally considered a fever warranting further evaluation.

42-2. **D. Bulging fontanelles, rather than sunken fontanelles, are associated with meningitis in an infant.** Other characteristics suggestive of meningitis in an infant include nuchal rigidity, inconsolability, vomiting, and irritability that increases when the infant is held. Febrile seizure is also suggestive of meningitis in an infant. Nuchal rigidity and other classic signs such as Kernig and Brudzinski signs may not be apparent in infants and children up to 2 years of age who have meningitis.

42-3. B. *Streptococcus pneumoniae* **is the most common cause of bacteremia in infants from 3 to 24 months of age.** Patients not receiving antibiotics for pneumococcal bacteremia can develop complications such as meningitis, cellulitis, pneumonia, or sepsis. Bacteremia is also often caused by *Neisseria meningitidis* or *Haemophilus influenzae* (the latter decreasing in incidence with widespread use of the *H. influenzae* vaccine). Signs of bacteremia include toxic appearance, petechiae, fever greater than 40°C (104°F), WBC greater than 15 (15,000/mm³), and greater than 5% bands. Group B streptococcus, *Escherichia coli*, and *Listeria monocytogenes* are the most common bacterial pathogens in infants younger than 1 month.

42-4. D. Infants younger than 3 months with serious bacterial infections have a high incidence of developing bacteremia and sepsis if not treated with IV antibiotics. Therefore, these infections must be aggressively sought and treated. Otitis media is the only possible exception. In infants younger than 28 days, however, otitis media may represent hematogenous spread of gram-negative bacilli or *Staphylococcus aureus*, so these children require admission for a septic workup regardless of fever.

 SUGGESTED ADDITIONAL READINGS

Bonsu BK, Harper MB. Identifying febrile young infants with bacteremia: is the peripheral white blood cell count an accurate screen? Ann Emerg Med 2003;42:216–225.

Colletti JE, Homme JL, Woodridge DP. Unsuspected neonatal killers in emergency medicine. Emerg Med Clin North Am 2004;22:929–960.

Galetto-Lacour A, Zamora SA, Gervaix A. Bedside procalcitonin and c-reactive protein tests in children with fever without localizing signs of infection seen in a referral center. Pediatrics 2003;112:1054–1060.

Rosman NP. Evaluation of the child who convulses with fever. Paediatr Drugs 2003;5:457–461.

Barking Cough in a Child

CC: 18-month-old girl with barking cough and stridor

HPI: B.C. is an 18-month-old girl who is brought to the ED by her parents because she is having coughing fits with difficulty breathing. Three days ago she developed a runny nose and a dry cough. Last night in bed she began to make noisy inspiratory sounds. Today her cough became harsh, brassy, and staccato, similar to a barking seal. Her breathing became more labored during coughing fits. She has had low-grade fevers but has been eating and drinking well.

PMHx: None

Meds: None

ALL: None

DevHx: Meeting all developmental milestones

SHx: Lives with mother, father, and 5-year-old sister

VS: Temp 38.0°C (100.4°F), HR 134, BP 78/46, RR 38, SaO_2 93% on RA

PE: *General:* Nontoxic; moderate respiratory effort with audible inspiratory stridor. *HEENT:* Conjunctiva clear; clear nasal discharge; oropharynx clear. *Neck:* No adenopathy. *CV:* S_1, S_2; no murmurs. *Chest:* Good air movement; inspiratory stridor; intercostal retractions. *Abd:* Soft; nontender; bowel sounds present. *Extr:* Well-perfused; no rashes. *Neuro:* Alert, sitting upright, interactive.

THOUGHT QUESTIONS

- What is the initial management for this child?
- What are causes of stridor in a young child?
- Which organism is likely responsible for this child's illness?
- Does this child need to be admitted to the hospital?

Immediate Actions:
Administer blow-by oxygen by face mask; place on cardiac monitor and continuous pulse oximetry; administer nebulized racemic epinephrine 5 mL in 2.5 mL of normal saline; administer dexamethasone 1 mg/kg IM; obtain chest and soft-tissue neck x-rays.

Discussion:
Stridor in a young child is evidence of upper airway obstruction and should be taken very seriously. The diameter of the trachea at the level of the cricothyroid membrane is only several millimeters in young children, so a small amount of airway edema can result in significant airway obstruction. Causes of stridor in children include epiglottitis, viral croup, bacterial tracheitis, peritonsillar abscess, foreign body aspiration, and severe allergic reaction (see Table 43-1).

(*Continued*)

TABLE 43-1 Comparison of Croup, Epiglottitis, and Bacterial Tracheitis

	Peak Age	Classic Organism	Signs	X-ray	Management
Croup	6 mo–3 yr	Parainfluenza	URI symptoms, hoarse voice, barking cough, inspiratory stridor	Steeple sign (see Figure 43-1)	Steroids, racemic epinephrine, humidification
Epiglottitis	3–7 years	H. influenzae	High fever, toxic-appearing, drooling, stridor, muffled "hot potato" voice	Thumb sign (see Figure 43-2)	Intubation in OR, admit, IV antibiotics (cefuroxime, cefotaxime, or ceftriaxone)
Bacterial tracheitis	3–5 years	S. aureus	High fever, toxic-appearing, purulent cough, stridor	Shaggy tracheal mucosa	Admit, IV antibiotics (wide-spectrum, including antistaphylococcal)

This child has viral croup, which can be diagnosed based on the history and clinical findings. Viral croup is most often caused by parainfluenza virus; it occurs in fall and early winter. The illness is characterized by subglottic tracheal swelling that causes stridor and the characteristic seal-like barking cough. The subglottic tracheal narrowing can also be seen on an AP soft-tissue neck x-ray as the "steeple sign," (Figure 43-1) although x-rays are not necessary to make the diagnosis. X-rays are obtained in the stridorous young child to look for the "thumb sign," (Figure 43-2) which represents epiglottitis. In contrast to children with epiglottitis, who are toxic with a high fever, children with croup appear relatively well and typically have a low-grade fever.

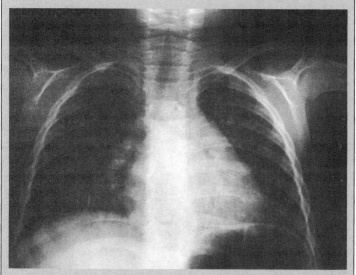

FIGURE 43-1 Soft-tissue neck radiograph depicting the "steeple sign" of croup. (*Image reprinted with permission from Harwood-Nuss A, Wolfson AB, et al. The Clinical Practice of Emergency Medicine, 3rd Ed. Philadelphia: Lippincott Williams & Wilkins, 2001.*)

(Continued)

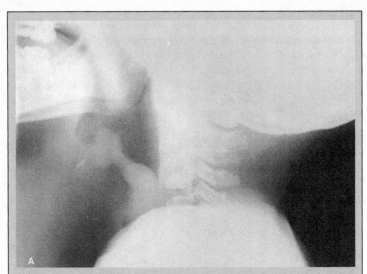

FIGURE 43-2 Inspiratory soft-tissue lateral neck radiograph showing the "thumb sign" of epiglottitis. (*Image reprinted with permission from Harwood-Nuss A, Wolfson AB, et al. The Clinical Practice of Emergency Medicine, 3rd Ed. Philadelphia: Lippincott Williams & Wilkins, 2001.*)

Children with croup can have a significant amount of respiratory distress, especially during coughing spells or when upset and crying. Relief can often be achieved with nebulized saline alone. Administration of dexamethasone 1 mg/kg IM has been shown to significantly reduce the duration of symptoms. Dexamethasone is preferred over oral prednisone because of its long half-life of 48 hours. If the child is in moderate to severe respiratory distress, nebulized racemic epinephrine is useful. Its effect is obtained through vasoconstriction of edematous airway tissue. These treatments are usually effective and children are able to be discharged from the ED with follow-up with their primary pediatricians within 24 hours. Home humidifiers are recommended at night while the child is sleeping.

CASE CONTINUED

The child's breathing becomes less labored with administration of nebulized racemic epinephrine. The soft-tissue AP neck x-ray shows a "steeple sign" (see Figure 43-1). Because the child received epinephrine, she is observed in the ED for 2 hours to ensure that a rebound effect does not occur as the medication wears off. She is discharged with plans to see her primary pediatrician the next day.

QUESTIONS

43-1. It has been shown that antibiotics are overprescribed in children. The emphasis in teaching today is to prescribe antibiotics only when absolutely indicated. A child with which of the following diagnoses should be given supportive care and medication other than antibiotics?

A. Epiglottitis
B. Croup
C. Exudative pharyngitis
D. Tracheitis
E. Peritonsillar cellulitis

43-2. A 3-year-old boy presents with a fever to 41.0°C (105.8°F), a muffled voice, inability to swallow his secretions, and stridor. What is the next step in this child's management?

A. Examine his oropharynx
B. Start an IV and give fluids and antibiotics
C. Take the child to the OR for intubation
D. Obtain soft-tissue neck x-rays
E. Administer nebulized racemic epinephrine

43-3. A 3-year-old boy is brought to the ED for one day of cough, especially at night. There have been a number of children presenting to the ED with the same symptoms in the past month. Which of the following is characteristic of viral croup?

A. Expiratory wheezes
B. Supraglottic tracheal edema
C. High fever
D. Typically RSV infection
E. Seal-like barking cough

43-4. Your pediatric ED rotation is in January and February and you are told to brush up on your knowledge of bronchiolitis because of its prevalence during those months. Which of the following is a characteristic of bronchiolitis?

A. May respond to antibiotics
B. Age 2 to 5 years
C. Parainfluenza infection
D. Upper respiratory tract involvement
E. May respond to β-agonist nebulizers

ANSWERS

43-1. B. Epiglottitis is classically caused by *Haemophilus influenzae,* and therefore a third-generation cephalosporin, such as ceftriaxone, is indicated. The incidence of childhood epiglottitis has decreased significantly over the past decade due to the *H. influenzae* vaccine. Children with pharyngitis should be treated with antibiotics based on the result of a positive rapid antigen detection test or culture. Penicillin is the recommended agent to cover *Streptococcus.* Oral penicillin V potassium for 7 days or benzathine penicillin IM once are both acceptable. Bacterial tracheitis is a clinical diagnosis in a toxic-appearing child with a high fever, cough, and copious amounts of purulent sputum. Antibiotic coverage for *Staphylococcus aureus* and *Streptococcus* is required. Peritonsillar cellulitis, which can progress to peritonsillar abscess, requires antibiotics; penicillin is the antibiotic of choice. **Croup is a viral laryngotracheobronchitis caused most often by parainfluenza virus type I and therefore does not warrant antibiotics. Racemic epinephrine and dexamethasone would be the treatment for croup.**

43-2. C. Epiglottitis in a young child is a true emergency. A child with stridor, muffled voice, and drooling has severe airway obstruction and requires immediate intubation in the OR, where a skilled pediatric surgeon or ENT specialist is ready to perform a tracheostomy if the anesthesiologist is unable to secure an airway. Any attempt to disturb the child (e.g., a tongue blade or attempted venipuncture) can result in total airway obstruction such that orotracheal intubation is impossible. Soft-tissue neck x-rays will show the "thumb sign" of a swollen epiglottis; however, this is not necessary for the diagnosis and should not delay going to the OR. Racemic epinephrine is contraindicated in children with epiglottitis because of its possible rebound effect.

43-3. E. Viral croup is an infection of the subglottic trachea by a virus that causes tracheal edema and narrowing, which results in a seal-like barking cough, inspiratory stridor, and respiratory distress. The offending agent is typically parainfluenza, although adenovirus, influenza, and RSV are implicated as well. Symptomatic treatment is usually achieved with cool vaporized mist and can be done at home. More severe cases may require nebulized racemic epinephrine and dexamethasone. Croup is usually preceded by 2 to 3 days of upper respiratory symptoms such as runny nose, cough, or low-grade fever.

43-4. E. Bronchiolitis is a viral lower respiratory tract infection in infants younger than 15 months occurring between December and March. The causative agent is respiratory syncytial virus (RSV). The syndrome is characterized by low-grade fever, runny nose, cough, and wheezing. Signs of bronchiolar inflammation and edema include tachypnea, nasal flaring and accessory muscle use, diffuse rales, and expiratory wheezes. **Nebulized β-agonists (e.g., albuterol) are sometimes helpful.** Corticosteroids and antibiotics have no role in bronchiolitis.

SUGGESTED ADDITIONAL READINGS

Hammer J. Acquired upper airway obstruction. Paediatr Respir Rev 2004;5:25–33.

Johnson D. Croup. Clin Evid 2005;(14):310–327.

Rotta AT, Wiryawan B. Respiratory emergencies in children. Respir Care 2003;48:248–258.

Ward MA. Emergency department management of acute respiratory infections. Semin Respir Infect 2002;17:65–71.

Dyspnea in a Child

 CC: 2-year-old boy with sudden-onset dyspnea

HPI: D.C. is a 2-year-old boy who is brought to the ED by his parents because he developed difficulty breathing. He had been doing well, playing at a family gathering, when he was found coughing and gasping, then began to cry. He has not had recent fever, cough, or any illness. He is developing appropriately for his age, currently very curious and putting everything in his mouth. There were peanuts and chips on the table and the parents wonder if he may have inhaled a peanut.

PMHx: Prior otitis media and bronchiolitis

Meds: None

ALL: None

SHx: Lives with mother, father, and 5-year-old sister

VS: Temp 36.7°C (98.1°F), HR 106, BP 82/46, RR 28, SaO$_2$ 100% on RA

PE: *General:* Alert, playful, mildly dyspneic. *HEENT:* Oropharynx clear; no stridor. *Neck:* No adenopathy. *CV:* S$_1$, S$_2$; no murmurs. *Chest:* Mild expiratory wheeze on right side. *Abd:* Soft; nontender; bowel sounds present. *Extr:* Well-perfused; no rashes. *Neuro:* Normal gait.

THOUGHT QUESTIONS

- At what level do aspirated foreign bodies usually lodge?
- When is the Heimlich maneuver indicated in children and how should it be done?
- How can you confirm the diagnosis of aspirated foreign body?
- What is the management for inhaled foreign bodies?

Discussion:

Foreign body aspiration is common in infants and young children. Most episodes are unwitnessed and are recognized by fits of coughing, stridor, wheezing, or dyspnea. Sometimes it goes unrecognized and the child develops secondary pneumonia several days later. Aspirated foreign body must be considered in any child who presents with stridor, dyspnea, or wheezing and who has no evidence of other infectious etiologies such as epiglottitis, croup, or bronchiolitis. In children younger than 12 months, a foreign body is more likely to lodge at the level of the larynx or the cricopharyngeus muscle. Children older than 15 months are likely to aspirate foreign bodies into the trachea or bronchi. Hot dogs and bread are common causes of upper airway obstruction in older children.

As a rule, if the child is coughing or vocalizing, the Heimlich maneuver should not be performed because the force created with coughing is much greater than any external maneuver. Also, blind finger probing of the oropharynx should not be done because a foreign body could be pushed into the trachea and cause total airway obstruction. If the child is not breathing, not vocalizing, or unresponsive, then external maneuvers are indicated. For infants younger than 12 months, back blows, chest thrusts, and attempts at ventilation should be done. For children older than 12 months, abdominal thrusts and back blows can be attempted. If these maneuvers fail, then needle cricothyrotomy should be done as a temporizing measure until the child can be taken to the OR for definitive airway management and rigid bronchoscopy or open bronchotomy.

For children who present with mild dyspnea or wheezing, a soft-tissue neck x-ray and chest x-ray should be done. Many foreign bodies, such as peanuts, are not radiopaque and must be inferred from secondary findings. A peanut in a bronchus will often act as a one-way valve and only let inhaled air pass. Therefore, the chest x-ray will often show hyperinflation and diaphragm flattening on the affected side, especially if taken during total exhalation. If the object entirely obstructs the bronchus, then atelectasis, volume loss, and mediastinal shift toward the affected side will occur. Treatment for a tracheal or bronchial foreign body is bronchoscopic removal under general anesthesia.

CASE CONTINUED

A chest x-ray shows hyperinflation of the right lung. The patient's respiratory status remains stable. He is taken to the OR and intubated under general anesthesia. A bronchoscope is passed into the right mainstem bronchus; a peanut is found and extracted with a suction catheter. The child is observed overnight and discharged home in good condition the next day.

QUESTIONS

44-1. A 4-year-old child is brought to the ED by his parents with episodes of choking after eating lunch. He appears to be slightly uncomfortable but has good skin coloration and a normal oxygen saturation. What is an appropriate first step in this child's management?

A. Obtain soft-tissue neck x-rays.

B. Finger sweep into the oropharynx in order to locate the foreign body.

C. Examine oropharynx and attempt removal of foreign body with forceps if visualized.

D. Do not examine the child's oropharynx until an ENT surgeon is present.

E. Give racemic epinephrine nebulizer treatment.

44-2. A 2-year-old girl is brought to the ED by her father with mild respiratory distress. She had been in her usual state of good health until she started coughing and crying at the dinner table. Her father says she was eating lasagna and fruit salad. If food were causing total bronchial obstruction on one side, which of the following chest x-ray findings would be expected?

A. Hyperlucency

B. Diaphragm flattening

C. Atelectasis and mediastinal shift

D. Bronchial dilatation

E. Hyperexpansion

44-3. A 3-year-old girl presents to the ED with stridor and a hoarse cough that began the evening before. Mom is not sure whether the child has had a fever or not. The child was full-term at birth and has had an unremarkable first 3 years of life. Both older brothers currently have coughs and nasal congestion. The girl's symptoms seem to have started after a fit of coughing at the dinner table. Which of the following might the doctor most likely misdiagnose this patient as having?

A. Acute epiglottitis
B. Croup
C. Bronchiolitis
D. Reactive airway disease
E. Pneumonia

44-4. A 15-month-old child is observed placing a 1-cm screw into her mouth. Mom tries to make the child spit it out but she seems to have swallowed it. She has no respiratory distress. An x-ray shows the screw in her stomach. What is the most appropriate management?

A. Ipecac to induce vomiting
B. GI consult to remove endoscopically
C. Whole bowel irrigation
D. Discharge home with follow-up
E. Admit for observation

ANSWERS

44-1. C. A 4-year-old with episodic choking likely has a piece of food lodged at the level of the larynx or just distal to the vocal cords. If the object is proximal to the vocal cords, it may be directly visualized in the oropharynx. If so, it can be removed with forceps. If it cannot be visualized, you should be prepared in case the object suddenly causes total airway obstruction. Preparation should include needle cricothyrotomy and intubation equipment in the room. Any radiographs should be done in the room. An ENT surgeon should then be consulted to take the child to the OR for bronchoscopy. Racemic epinephrine nebulizer treatment is not indicated in foreign body airway obstruction.

44-2. C. Aspirated foreign bodies are often radiolucent and therefore must be diagnosed on chest x-ray by inferential findings. **Total bronchial obstruction causes atelectasis, volume loss, and mediastinal shift.** Partial obstruction often causes a one-way valve effect resulting in unilateral hyperexpansion (sometimes only seen as relative lucency compared with the unaffected side) or diaphragm flattening. These findings are accentuated during the expiratory phase of respiration. Bronchial dilatation is not seen.

44-3. B. Children with an aspirated foreign body are often misdiagnosed because most aspiration events are unwitnessed. Laryngeal or subglottic foreign bodies can be misdiagnosed as epiglottitis; however, the latter is usually associated with a high fever, and the child usually appears toxic. **A tracheal foreign body can mimic croup, causing stridor and a barking, croup-like cough.** Again, croup is usually associated with a fever and preceded by several days of upper respiratory symptoms. Bronchiolitis and reactive airway disease are both associated with generalized wheezing. In contrast, wheezing associated with a foreign body is usually focal, or confined to a certain area in the chest.

44-4. D. Once a swallowed foreign body passes through the esophagus into the stomach, there is a very high chance that it will spontaneously pass through the GI tract. Therefore, no intervention is necessary. The only exception is for sharp objects, such as razor blades or pins, which have a 25% chance of causing perforation; these objects should be endoscopically removed. Esophageal foreign bodies also need to be removed endoscopically because they are likely large enough so they will not pass spontaneously and after time will result in esophageal ischemia and perforation. The child in this question should return in one month for a repeat x-ray if the screw is not found in her stools. If it remains in the stomach at that time, it should be endoscopically removed.

 SUGGESTED ADDITIONAL READINGS

Hayes NM, Chidekel A. Pediatric choking. Del Med J 2004;76: 335–340.

Holmes RL, Fadden CT. Evaluation of the patient with chronic cough. Am Fam Physician 2004;69:2159–2166.

Lima JA, Fischer GB. Foreign body aspiration in children. Paediatr Respir Rev 2002;3:303–307.

Rafanan AL, Mehta AC. Adult airway foreign body removal. What's new? Clin Chest Med 2001;22:319–330.

V

Patients Presenting with Abdominal or Gastrointestinal Complaints

Abdominal Pain Followed by Unconsciousness

CC: 68-year-old woman with severe abdominal pain followed by unconsciousness

HPI: A.P. is a 68-year-old woman with a history of chronic atrial fibrillation on warfarin (Coumadin) who began experiencing severe left flank pain radiating to the back today. She went to sit on the toilet; her husband then heard her groan and found her unconscious on the floor. EMS was called and found her tachycardic with a faint pulse and systolic blood pressure of 60 mm Hg. She was intubated and transferred to the ED. Medical history is obtained from her husband.

PMHx: AF, hypertension

Meds: Coumadin 5 mg PO QD, metoprolol (Lopressor) 50 mg PO BID

ALL: NKDA

SHx: Lives with husband; tobacco 1 ppd × 40 years; occasional alcohol; no drugs

VS: Temp 37.1°C (98.9°F), HR 128, BP 80/42, RR 12 intubated, SaO_2 97% on 100% F_iO_2

PE: *General:* Intubated; cool and pale. *HEENT:* Atraumatic; ETT secured; pupils 3 mm and reactive. *CV:* Tachycardic without murmurs. *Chest:* Clear bilaterally. *Abd:* Soft, mildly distended; no palpable masses. *GU:* Guaiac-negative; normal tone. *Extr:* Mottled and cool; no edema; thready radial pulses. *Neuro:* Withdraws all extremities to pain.

THOUGHT QUESTIONS

- Which immediate actions should be taken for this patient?
- What is the differential diagnosis for abdominal pain and hypotension?
- Which diagnostic tests, if any, should be performed?
- What are the criteria for immediate operative intervention?

Immediate Actions:
Endotracheal tube and mechanical ventilation are already established; place two 14-gauge IVs and send blood for CBC, PT/PTT, chem 7, LFTs, and lipase; hang 2 liters wide-open NS, wide-open uncrossmatched O-positive blood (O-negative for women of childbearing age or younger), and fresh frozen plasma; obtain 12-lead EKG and, if available, bedside abdominal ultrasound.

Discussion:
The differential diagnosis for sudden-onset abdominal pain and hypotension is short. Ruptured abdominal aortic aneurysm (AAA) should be considered first and ruled out with a bedside abdominal ultrasound. Other potential etiologies include peptic ulcer with massive GI bleed or perforation, other sources of perforated viscous, or mesenteric ischemia. Ruptured AAA is classically associated with abdominal or low back pain, pulsatile abdominal mass, and hypotension. Hemodynamically unstable patients with abdominal pain should go emergently to the OR; radiologic studies will only cause unnecessary delay. Stable patients can undergo plain films and an abdominal CT scan to better define the etiology of the pain.

CASE CONTINUED

The patient remains hypotensive despite fluids and blood; therefore, a dopamine drip is started. A bedside ultrasound shows an 8-cm AAA with evidence of a retroperitoneal hematoma. The patient is taken emergently to the OR. In the OR, an exploratory laparotomy is performed. A large amount of gross blood is found in the intraperitoneal cavity, and the patient suddenly loses her pulses and blood pressure. The retroperitoneum is entered and an attempt is made to cross-clamp the aorta proximally. This is unsuccessful and the patient dies on the table. An autopsy shows a ruptured AAA.

QUESTIONS

45-1. A 36-year-old woman with a history of von Willebrand's disease, sickle-cell disease, and Marfan's syndrome presents to the ED with low abdominal cramping and vaginal discharge. On physical exam you note an epigastric pulsatile mass, which you find curious in this patient despite the fact that she is thin. Which of the following is a risk factor for AAA in this patient?
  A. Von Willebrand's disease
  B. Young age
  C. Female gender
  D. Marfan's syndrome
  E. Sickle-cell anemia

45-2. A 64-year-old man presents to the ED with several weeks of abdominal fullness and mid-back discomfort. You palpate an epigastric pulsatile mass and are concerned about an AAA. He has normal femoral pulses. His vital signs are normal. What is the best modality for assessing this patient?
  A. Ultrasound
  B. CT scan
  C. Angiography
  D. MRI
  E. Abdominal radiograph

45-3. A 57-year-old man presents to the ED with right flank pain and hematuria. A CT scan of the kidney and ureter reveals a 3-mm right UVJ kidney stone. In addition, it reveals a 4.0-cm AAA. He is discharged to follow-up with his primary doctor and given a referral to a surgeon. What is the average rate of expansion of an AAA over a one-year period?

    A. 0 to 0.25 cm
    B. 0.25 to 0.50 cm
    C. 0.50 to 0.75 cm
    D. 0.75 to 1.0 cm
    E. 1.0 to 1.25 cm

45-4. A 64-year-old woman presents to the ED with abdominal discomfort. On exam, a pulsatile mass is palpated in the left epigastrium. Her vital signs are normal. A CT scan of the abdomen shows a 6-cm AAA. At what size is an aneurysm considered a significant risk for rupture and elective operative repair indicated?

    A. 3 cm
    B. 4 cm
    C. 5 cm
    D. 6 cm

 ANSWERS

45-1. D. **Increased risk of AAA has been associated with male gender, age over 60 years, family history of AAA, Marfan's disease, history of other aneurysms or peripheral arterial disease, and atherosclerotic risk factors.** Von Willebrand's disease is a hereditary bleeding disorder due to a deficiency or abnormality of von Willebrand factor, which is a glycoprotein that allows platelets to adhere to damaged endothelium and that carries factor VIII in the plasma. Von Willebrand's disease is not known to be a risk factor for AAA. Sickle-cell anemia is a hereditary hemolytic anemia due to a single point mutation on the β-chain of hemoglobin, leading to hemoglobin S, which tends to polymerize when deoxygenated, causing a sickle shape of the red blood cells. These sickled cells cause obstruction in the microcirculation. Sickle-cell anemia is not known to be associated with AAA.

45-2. B. An ultrasound is essentially 100% sensitive for making the diagnosis of AAA when performed by an experienced operator. However, it is not as useful for identifying whether the AAA has ruptured. **Therefore, in a hemodynamically stable patient a CT**

scan is the optimal study in the ED. **In addition to making the diagnosis of AAA, the CT scan is very sensitive for detecting periaortic free blood.** MRI is often used to follow the growth of a known AAA over a period of months or years. Angiography is not indicated in making a diagnosis of AAA acutely because the lumen is usually narrowed by mural thrombus and may appear falsely normal. An enlarged, calcific aorta can sometimes be detected by plain abdominal radiograph, especially on a cross-table lateral view; however, the sensitivity is low.

45-3. B. On average, an aortic aneurysm expands 0.25 to 0.50 cm per year. The 5-year rupture rate for AAAs smaller than 4.0 cm in diameter is 2%, while for AAAs 5.0 to 5.9 cm in diameter, the rate is 25%. The 5-year rupture rate for AAAs larger than 7.0 cm in diameter is 75%.

45-4. C. The normal size of the abdominal aorta distal to the renal arteries is approximately 2 cm. A diameter of 3 cm is used to define AAA. **There is a significant increase in the risk of rupture when an abdominal aneurysm is greater than 5 cm in diameter.** As an aneurysm becomes larger, the expanding force on the aortic wall applied by the blood flow becomes greater, as described by Laplace's law. Therefore, a larger aneurysm will expand more rapidly and is at greater risk for rupture.

 SUGGESTED ADDITIONAL READINGS

Anderson LA. Abdominal aortic aneurysm. J Cardiovasc Nurs 2001;15:1–14.

Kozuch PL, Brandt LJ. Review article: diagnosis and management of mesenteric ischaemia with an emphasis on pharmacotherapy. Aliment Pharmacol Ther 2005;21:201–215.

Sakalihasan N, Limet R, Defawe OD. Abdominal aortic aneurysm. Lancet 2005;365:1577–1589.

Lower Abdominal Pain

CC: 28-year-old woman with lower abdominal pain

HPI: L.P. is a healthy 28-year-old woman who had vegetable pizza and ham for dinner, went to sleep, and awoke several hours later with a vague, low, periumbilical abdominal pain. The pain has been constant since its onset a couple of hours earlier. She denies nausea, vomiting, diarrhea, recent urinary symptoms, or vaginal discharge. Her last menstrual period was 3 to 4 weeks ago; she has no history of sexually transmitted infections (STIs) and is monogamous with her husband of several years. Her husband ate the same food for dinner and does not have any symptoms.

PMHx: None; $G_0 P_0$

Meds: None

ALL: NKDA

FHx: None

SHx: Married for 3 years; denies tobacco, alcohol, or drug use

VS: Temp 37.2°C (99.0°F), HR 108, BP 127/72, RR 16, SaO$_2$ 100% on RA

PE: *General:* Healthy-appearing young woman in no apparent distress. *HEENT:* Moist mucous membranes. *CV:* S$_1$, S$_2$; slightly tachycardic; no murmurs; good pulses throughout. *Chest:* Clear to auscultation. *Abd:* Soft; nondistended; mild tenderness in suprapubic, RLQ, and LLQ regions with some voluntary guarding; hypoactive bowel sounds; equivocal rebound tenderness. *Pelvic:* External exam normal; speculum exam unremarkable with closed os; no cervical motion tenderness or adnexal tenderness; no discharge. *GU:* Guaiac-negative; nontender; normal tone. *Extr:* Warm; no rashes or lesions. *Neuro:* Alert and oriented.

THOUGHT QUESTIONS

- What is the initial management for this patient?
- What is the differential diagnosis for this patient?
- Which diagnostic tests, if any, should be performed?
- How should this patient be managed if a diagnosis is not clear after initial workup?

Immediate Actions:
Establish IV; send CBC with differential, chem 7, urinalysis, urine βhCG; keep NPO; hang 1 liter NS.

Discussion:
The differential diagnosis for low abdominal pain in a young woman includes both abdominal and pelvic pathology, with ectopic pregnancy and acute appendicitis being the most concerning possibilities. Ovarian torsion is also an important consideration, but usually presents with sudden onset of excruciating adnexal pain and tenderness. Other possibilities include gynecologic disorders (e.g., PID, tubo-ovarian abscess, ruptured ovarian cyst), GI disorders (e.g., gastroenteritis, inflammatory bowel disease, intestinal obstruction, mesenteric adenitis), urologic disorders (e.g., UTI, renal colic), and incarcerated inguinal hernia.

If the patient has a positive urine βhCG, a quantitative serum βhCG and pelvic ultrasound are indicated. An IUP should be visualized with pelvic ultrasound if the serum βhCG is greater than 1,500 mIU/mL. If no IUP is identified in a βhCG-positive woman with low abdominal pain, then ectopic pregnancy must be suspected. If these patients do not appear ill, they may be discharged with close gynecologic follow-up in 48 hours to confirm an appropriate doubling in serum βhCG. If they appear ill, they require gynecologic admission and possibly exploratory laparoscopy or laparotomy. If the urine βhCG is negative, an abdominal CT scan is helpful if appendicitis or any other abdominal process is suspected. A pelvic ultrasound is indicated in a woman with significant adnexal tenderness, which may be evidence

(Continued)

of a ruptured ovarian cyst, torsion, or abscess. Many women with low abdominal pain of unclear etiology can simply be observed for several hours with repeat abdominal exams and then sent home with instructions to return immediately if symptoms worsen.

CASE CONTINUED

While waiting for lab results, the patient begins complaining of mild nausea and worsening pain. Upon reexamination, her pain has mostly localized to the right lower quadrant, approximately one-third the distance from the anterior superior iliac spine to the umbilicus (McBurney's point). Repeat abdominal exam is also significant for rebound tenderness, involuntary guarding in the RLQ, and referred RLQ pain with palpation of the LLQ. Her labs return with a WBC count of 14 (14,000/mm³) with 90% polys, negative urine βhCG, and normal urinalysis. A CT scan is obtained, which shows a thickened appendix that does not fill with contrast, consistent with appendicitis (Figure 46-1). Surgery is consulted; she is kept NPO and given IV

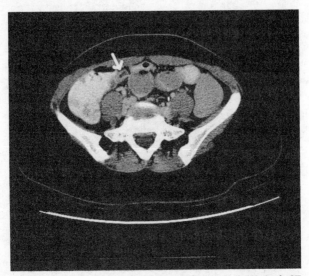

FIGURE 46-1 Oral and IV contrast-enhanced abdominal CT scan shows a nonfilling, thickened appendix (white arrow) located adjacent to the contrast-filled cecum, consistent with acute appendicitis. (*Image courtesy of Massachusetts General Hospital, Boston.*)

fluids and cefoxitin 2 g IV. She is taken to the OR, where an inflamed but nonperforated appendix is found and removed without incident.

QUESTIONS

46-1. A 21-year-old man presents to the ED with severe right lower quadrant abdominal pain. On examination, he has a lot of pain when you internally rotate his right hip while he is supine with the hip flexed. What is the name of the sign that is positive?

A. McBurney
B. Rovsing
C. Murphy
D. Obturator
E. Psoas

46-2. A 31-year-old man complains of abdominal pain that started about 12 hours prior to presentation. He has no past medical history and was well until last night, when he started feeling nauseated with an "upset stomach;" his symptoms were constant throughout the night, with no periods of relief. This morning, he woke up with right-sided flank pain and anorexia. He denies dysuria, hematuria, or frequency. He is uncomfortable during palpation of his abdomen, but with no particular worsening at McBurney's point. CT scan shows a nonfilling appendix. What is likely going on?

A. Right-sided kidney stone
B. Right-sided infectious colitis
C. Retrocecal appendicitis
D. Pelvic appendicitis
E. Malingering

46-3. A 40-year-old woman with history of high cholesterol and cholecystectomy presents with right lower abdominal pain for the past hour. She reports feeling sweaty and feverish, but denies vomiting or diarrhea. She has had no appetite all day long. She denies vaginal discharge, dyspareunia, dysuria, frequency, or urgency. On exam, she appears pale and uncomfortable, with significant rebound tenderness at McBurney's point. Pelvic exam is unremarkable, with no cervical motion tenderness or adnexal tenderness. Which symptom is the most sensitive and specific for her condition?

A. Diaphoresis
B. Fever
C. Diarrhea
D. Anorexia
E. Pallor

46-4. A 29-year-old woman with past medical history significant only for asthma presents to the ED with several days of abdominal pain and anorexia. Initially her pain was vague and in the epigastric region; later, her pain was worst on the right lower side. Last night she thought her pain improved somewhat, but this morning she presents for worsening again. Which of the following is most suggestive of perforated appendicitis?

    A. WBC greater than 10,000/mm³
    B. Temperature higher than 39°C (102.2°F)
    C. Slightly elevated heart rate
    D. Slightly elevated urine WBC
    E. Soft abdomen without guarding or rebound but with significant tenderness at McBurney's point

ANSWERS

46-1. D. The described test is the obturator sign, in which the patient is supine with right hip flexed; passive internal rotation of the hip eliciting pain is a positive test for appendicitis and is due to an inflamed appendix irritated by stretch of the obturator internus muscle. McBurney's point is the classic location of maximum tenderness to palpation in the RLQ—one-third the distance from the anterior superior iliac crest to the umbilicus—in patients with an anterior appendix. Rovsing's sign refers to pain in the RLQ elicited by palpation/pressure in the LLQ. Murphy's sign refers to pain causing cessation of respiration during palpation of the RUQ and is seen in acute cholecystitis. The psoas sign for appendicitis is tested by having the patient lie on his or her left side; pain caused by passive right thigh extension (inflamed appendix irritated by stretch of the iliopsoas muscle) is a positive test result.

46-2. C. This patient has appendicitis but his appendix is likely retrocecal; approximately 15% of appendices are retrocecal. The importance of knowing that there are different anatomic locations of the appendix lies in realizing there are different possible presentations of acute appendicitis. With a retrocecal appendix, pain may be more pronounced in the right flank. With a pelvic appendix, pain may be more pronounced in the suprapubic region or right pelvis. For this reason, adnexal tenderness should not dissuade you from considering the diagnosis of appendicitis.

46-3. D. Appendicitis is characterized by abdominal pain, usually beginning as a vague, constant pain in the epigastric or periumbilical region and localizing to the RLQ. The pain is typically associated with anorexia, nausea or vomiting, or low-grade fever. Anorexia is the most common of these symptoms and is usually the first of these to appear. The initial pain of appendicitis is thought to be due to distention of the appendiceal lumen, triggering visceral afferent pain fibers; these fibers enter the spinal cord at the tenth thoracic vertebra, resulting in a patient's perception of vague epigastric or periumbilical pain. As the appendicitis worsens, inflammation of the appendix and surrounding structures triggers somatic pain fibers, resulting in a patient's perception of RLQ pain. Diarrhea is not typically associated with acute appendicitis, though it is present in some patients.

46-4. B. Normal temperature or low-grade fever is common in uncomplicated (nonperforated) acute appendicitis, whereas temperature greater than 39°C (102.2°F) is more typical of a ruptured appendix. WBC greater than 10,000/mm^3, normal or slightly elevated heart rate, and normal or slighted elevated urine WBCs are also typical of uncomplicated appendicitis. Urine may contain WBCs due to appendiceal inflammation extending to the ureter. Acute appendicitis is often misdiagnosed as UTI; therefore, caution must be used when making a diagnosis of UTI by urine WBCs in the absence of bacteria or nitrite. A patient with a perforated appendix would likely display peritoneal signs, including abdominal guarding and rebound.

 SUGGESTED ADDITIONAL READINGS

Cardall T, Glasser J, Guss DA. Clinical value of the total white blood cell count and temperature in the evaluation of patients with suspected appendicitis. Acad Emerg Med 2004;11:1021–1027.

Simpson J, Speake W. Appendicitis. Clin Evid 2004;(11):544–551.

Yu J, Fulcher AS, Turner MA, et al. Helical CT evaluation of acute right lower quadrant pain: part I, common mimics of appendicitis. AJR Am J Roentgenol 2005;184:1136–1142.

Yu J, Fulcher AS, Turner MA, et al. Helical CT evaluation of acute right lower quadrant pain: part II, uncommon mimics of appendicitis. AJR Am J Roentgenol 2005;184:1143–1149.

Right Upper Quadrant Abdominal Pain

CC: 52-year-old man with right upper quadrant abdominal pain

HPI: R.Q. is a 52-year-old man who developed severe upper abdominal pain following lunch 2 days ago. The pain came in waves and was associated with bloating and nausea. The pain has been getting progressively worse and is now localized to the right upper quadrant. The pain is associated with nausea but not vomiting or diarrhea. He denies fever, chills, sweats, chest pain, or shortness of breath. He has felt similar pain a few times in the past couple years, but those episodes were brief and resolved on their own.

PMHx: Hypercholesterolemia; s/p tonsillectomy

Meds: None

ALL: Penicillin–rash

FHx: Noncontributory

SHx: Tobacco 1 ppd; 2 beers per day

VS: Temp 37.2°C (99.0°F), HR 99, BP 117/77, RR 16, SaO$_2$ 99%

PE: *General:* Well-appearing, in no distress. *HEENT:* Nonicteric; oropharynx moist. *Neck:* Supple; no JVD. *CV:* Normal rate, regular rhythm, no murmurs. *Chest:* Clear bilaterally. *Abd:* Soft, nondistended; tender in RUQ with guarding, made worse with deep inspiration causing patient to catch his breath (positive Murphy's sign); no hepatosplenomegaly. *GU:* Guaiac-negative brown stool; nontender prostate. *Extr:* No edema; 2+ radial and DP pulses bilaterally; no rashes.

THOUGHT QUESTIONS

- What is the initial management for this patient?
- What is the differential diagnosis for upper abdominal and RUQ pain?
- Which diagnostic tests should be performed?

Immediate Actions:

Place on oxygen; obtain 12-lead EKG; establish IV access; send blood for CBC with diff, PT/PTT, chemistries including LFTs and lipase, clot to blood bank; obtain urinalysis.

Discussion:

The differential diagnosis for upper abdominal and RUQ pain is extensive, including processes involving any organ or structure in the vicinity (e.g., gallbladder, pancreas, stomach, liver, kidney, heart, lungs, aorta, intestines). The most common etiology of RUQ pain is biliary (e.g., cholelithiasis, cholecystitis, or rarely cholangitis). Biliary disease can also present with epigastric pain and is difficult to distinguish clinically from GI pathology (gastritis, peptic ulcer disease, gastroesophageal reflux) or pancreatitis. More serious conditions can also present with pain to this region and must be considered and excluded as well (e.g., cardiac ischemia, aortic dissection, aortic aneurysm). In women of childbearing age, ectopic pregnancy and other gynecologic etiologies must be considered. Pulmonary disease (e.g., pneumonia or pulmonary effusion) can sometimes present with RUQ abdominal pain.

A specific diagnosis is made based on the history, physical, blood work, and imaging studies. Often, no imaging is required and a presumptive diagnosis of PUD can be made (e.g., epigastric pain in a young person with NSAID use, no Murphy's sign, and normal LFTs and lipase). If the history and physical are consistent with biliary colic, ultrasound is the test of choice. If there is a history of fever or cough, a chest x-ray is warranted. In elderly patients, more serious conditions should be considered, such as cardiac ischemia, neoplasm, and aortic pathology. In these patients, a 12-lead EKG and abdominal CT scan are advisable.

CASE CONTINUED

An EKG shows no evidence of ischemia. Labs show WBC 11.3 with 90% polys, Hct 39.0%, and normal LFTs, amylase, and lipase. An ultrasound reveals multiple gallstones with mild gallbladder wall thickening and a small amount of pericholecystic fluid (Figure 47-1). The common bile duct measures 4 mm (normal < 5 mm). A sonographic Murphy's sign (pain with compression over the gallbladder with the ultrasound probe) is present, and the diagnosis of cholecystitis is confirmed. He receives 2 liters NS, cefoxitin 2 g IV, and hydromorphone (Dilaudid) 2 to 4 mg for pain. He is admitted for IV antibiotics and undergoes a laparoscopic cholecystectomy the next day. He recovers uneventfully.

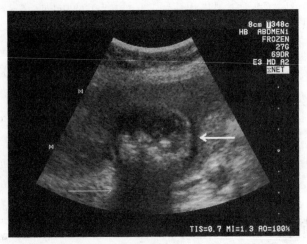

FIGURE 47-1 Abdominal ultrasound of the gallbladder in cross-section shows the gallbladder lumen filled with stones (the thin arrow points to the ultrasonographic shadow cast by these stones), and a mildly thickened gallbladder wall with a small amount of surrounding fluid (large arrow). These findings in conjunction with a sonographic Murphy's sign suggest acute cholecystitis. (*Image courtesy of Massachusetts General Hospital, Boston.*)

QUESTIONS

47-1. A 67-year-old thin man with hypertension and diabetes presents to the ED with right upper quadrant pain for 8 hours. He developed the pain after lunch and has vomited twice. He denies fever, diarrhea, hematuria, or dysuria. Which of the following is considered a risk factor for cholecystitis and cholelithiasis?

A. Male gender
B. Older age (>65 years)
C. Diabetes
D. Hypertension
E. Underweight

47-2. A 64-year-old man presents to the ED with 2 days of high fever, upper abdominal pain, vomiting, and anorexia. His temperature is 39.3°C (102.8°F), HR is 124, BP is 104/74, and oxygen saturation is 98% on room air. The patient appears ill. His abdomen is tender in the epigastrium with guarding. Which one of the following is part of Charcot's triad?

A. Fever
B. Nausea
C. LUQ pain
D. Vomiting
E. JVD

47-3. A 46-year-old woman presents to the ED with severe, constant, midepigastric pain radiating to the back. Her serum lipase is elevated. What is the most likely diagnosis?

A. Cholecystitis
B. Hepatitis
C. Peptic ulcer disease
D. Pancreatitis
E. Ascending cholangitis

47-4. A 30-year-old alcoholic presents to the ED with RUQ pain, tachycardia, fever, nausea, and moderately elevated AST and ALT (AST greater than ALT). Bilirubin and alkaline phosphatase are normal. What is the most likely diagnosis?

A. Cholecystitis
B. Hepatitis
C. Peptic ulcer disease
D. Pancreatitis
E. Ascending cholangitis

ANSWERS

47-1. C. The classic risk factors for biliary disease include the four Fs: **fat, female, forty, and fertile (multiparous).** Other risk factors include **diabetes**, OCP use, family history, prolonged fasting, significant weight loss, cystic fibrosis, and intestinal malabsorption syndromes.

47-2. A. Charcot's triad is indicative of ascending cholangitis and includes fever, jaundice, and RUQ pain. However, it is present in only 25% of patients with ascending cholangitis. Ascending cholangitis is an infection of the biliary tract usually caused by organisms from the GI tract (typically *Escherichia coli* and anaerobic organisms). These patients become rapidly septic and therefore require broad-spectrum IV antibiotics and aggressive evaluation for an inciting source of infection. A CT scan should be obtained to identify an abscess, mass, or biliary obstruction.

47-3. D. Acute pancreatitis is the most likely diagnosis. Characteristic pain of pancreatitis is severe, constant, boring pain in the mid-epigastrium radiating to the back or flanks. Serum amylase and lipase levels are usually elevated. The most common causes of acute pancreatitis include gallstones and alcohol. Ranson's criteria on admission (age > 55 years, blood glucose level > 200 mg/dL, WBC > 16 k/mm^3, SGOT > 250 IU/L, LDH > 350 IU/L) and at 48 hours (Hct decrease > 10%, BUN increase > 5 mg/dL, calcium < 8 mg/dL, PaO$_2$ < 60 mm Hg, fluid sequestration > 6 liters, base deficit > 4 mEq/L) are used for predicting mortality risk from acute pancreatitis. Chronic pancreatitis is most often caused by chronic alcohol abuse and can present with normal amylase and lipase levels. The treatment for pancreatitis includes IV fluids, parenteral pain medication, and bowel rest.

47-4. B. Alcoholic hepatitis is the most likely diagnosis. Alcohol, metabolized in the liver, can cause liver injury when chronically consumed in excess. Patients may complain of nausea, vomiting, and RUQ pain. They typically are tachycardic with a low-grade fever. AST and ALT are usually moderately elevated, with AST greater than ALT. Treatment is supportive and includes correction of fluid and electrolyte imbalances, as well as administration of glucose, thiamine, magnesium and/or antiemetics if necessary. Admission is warranted if the patient cannot tolerate liquids by mouth, or if there is evidence of fulminant hepatic failure (e.g., elevated PT/INR, altered mental status, elevated ammonia levels, or hypotension). Otherwise, patients should be referred to an alcohol treatment program.

SUGGESTED ADDITIONAL READINGS

Browning JD, Horton JD. Gallstone disease and its complications. Semin Gastrointest Dis 2003;14:165–177.

Margenthaler J, Schuerer D, Whinney R. Acute cholecystitis. Clin Evid 2004;571–580.

Peter NG, Clark LR, Jaeger JR. Fitz-Hugh-Curtis syndrome: a diagnosis to consider in women with right upper quadrant pain. Cleve Clin J Med 2004;71:233–239.

Schirmer BD, Winters KL, Edlich RF. Cholelithiasis and cholecystitis. J Long Term Eff Med Implants 2005;15:329–338.

Left Lower Quadrant Abdominal Pain

CC: 61-year-old woman with LLQ abdominal pain

HPI: L.Q. is a 61-year-old woman who developed gradual onset of left lower quadrant abdominal pain 3 days prior to presentation. She describes the pain as steady and deep and has had anorexia for the past 2 days. She also complains of being constipated for 2 days; she usually is regular with two bowel movements per day. She denies nausea, vomiting, diarrhea, fever, chills, vaginal bleeding or discharge, black or bloody stools, or weight loss. She saw her primary care physician yesterday, who gave her an antibiotic and let her go home. Her pain has gotten worse today despite the medication.

PMHx: Hypertension

Meds: Metoprolol (Lopressor) 50 mg PO BID, unknown antibiotic × 1 d

ALL: NKDA

FHx: Father with CAD

SHx: Lives alone; no tobacco, alcohol, or drug use

VS: Temp 37.5°C (99.5°F), HR 70, BP 130/75, RR 14, SaO$_2$ 99% on RA

PE: *General:* Elderly woman, mildly obese, nontoxic-appearing, in minimal distress. *HEENT:* Slightly dry mucous membranes; non-icteric sclerae. *CV:* S$_1$, S$_2$; regular; no murmurs; 2+ pulses throughout. *Chest:* Clear bilaterally. *Abd:* Soft; mildly obese; mild tenderness LLQ, left flank, left back; bowel sounds hypoactive. *Rectal:* Trace guaiac-positive brown stool; nontender; mildly decreased tone. *Pelvic:* External exam normal; speculum exam unremarkable with closed os; no discharge; no cervical motion tenderness or adnexal tenderness. *Extr:* Warm; intact; no lesions; no edema. *Neuro:* Alert, nonfocal.

THOUGHT QUESTIONS

- What is the initial management for this patient?
- What is the differential diagnosis for this patient?
- Which diagnostic tests, if any, should be performed?
- What is the treatment for this disorder?
- What are potential complications of her condition?

Immediate Actions:
Obtain IV access and start 1 liter NS; order CBC with differential, chem 7, urinalysis; obtain CT scan with oral and IV contrast.

Discussion:
In an elderly woman with several days of LLQ pain, the most likely diagnosis is diverticulitis, although low-grade fever may be expected. Other considerations include sigmoid volvulus, low-grade obstruction caused by a pelvic or abdominal mass, ischemic colitis, UTI, renal colic, or simply constipation. The most helpful lab test is the urinalysis, which will mostly exclude UTI or renal colic (up to 5% to 10% of patients with renal colic, however, can have absence of RBCs on urinalysis). A plain KUB will be diagnostic for sigmoid volvulus or other bowel obstruction (Figure 48-1), although low-yield in this patient who has no clinical evidence for obstruction. An abdominal CT scan with oral and IV contrast will differentiate between renal and bowel pathology, in addition to showing diverticulitis, ischemic bowel, obstruction, or abdominal and pelvic masses.

(Continued)

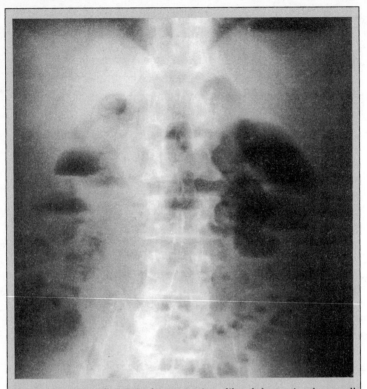

FIGURE 48-1 Upright KUB demonstrating dilated loops in the small bowel, with numerous air–fluid levels, consistent with small bowel obstruction. (*Image reprinted with permission from Harwood-Nuss A, Wolfson AB, et al. The Clinical Practice of Emergency Medicine, 3rd Ed. Philadelphia: Lippincott Williams & Wilkins, 2001.*)

Treatment for acute diverticulitis includes IV rehydration, bowel rest (i.e., NPO followed by liquid diet, then low-residue diet), and broad-spectrum antibiotics. Patients who appear well and can tolerate fluids can be discharged home with oral antibiotics and close follow-up with their primary care physician. Patients who have failed outpatient therapy, or who have signs or symptoms of systemic infection or localized peritonitis, need inpatient therapy with IV fluids, IV antibiotics, and surgical consultation. Complications of diverticulitis include perforation, abscess formation (Figure 48-2), and obstruction. As the infected

(Continued)

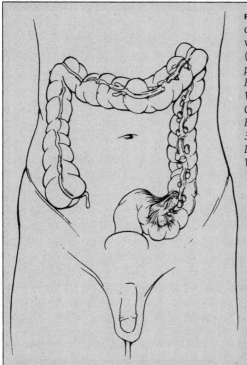

FIGURE 48-2 Drawing depicting diverticullitis with abscess formation. *(Image reprinted with permission from Harwood-Nuss A, Wolfson AB, et al. The Clinical Practice of Emergency Medicine, 3rd Ed. Philadelphia: Lippincott Williams & Wilkins, 2001.)*

diverticulum becomes inflamed, its lumen is occluded and it commonly perforates. This is referred to as a microperforation because it does not communicate directly with the intraluminal bowel. Macroperforation with subsequent peritonitis, however, is also possible; this requires emergent surgery. Microperforations usually become walled off by an inflammatory response. Occasionally, this may develop into an abscess, which requires drainage either percutaneously or surgically. The inflammatory scar tissue can also envelop the bowel and result in obstruction. Surgery is then indicated for a partial colectomy to remove the obstructing piece of bowel.

CASE CONTINUED

Significant labs include WBC 10.9, Hct 38%, and normal basic chemistry panel. CT scan of the abdomen and pelvis with oral and IV contrast reveals sigmoid diverticulitis with stranding and bowel wall thickening, without evidence of (macro-)perforation. Because the patient has already failed a trial of outpatient oral antibiotics, she is admitted to the hospital for IV fluids and IV antibiotics. She is started on ampicillin 2 g IV, gentamicin 400 mg (5 mg/kg) IV, and metronidazole (Flagyl) 1 g IV.

QUESTIONS

48-1. A 64-year-old woman with abdominal cramping and diarrhea for several days does not improve with IV ampicillin. Which of the following colonic pathogens is likely responsible for her symptoms?

A. *Escherichia coli*
B. *Klebsiella*
C. *Peptostreptococcus*
D. *Enterobacter*
E. *Listeria monocytogenes*

48-2. An 85-year-old woman presents to the ED with 2 days of constant left lower abdominal pain. She is status post hysterectomy and bilateral oophorectomy, but otherwise is very healthy with no other significant past medical history. She lives alone, walks one mile daily, does not smoke, drinks one glass of red wine daily, and visits her primary care doctor yearly. After appropriate examination and workup, you tell her she has diverticulitis. She becomes extremely upset, stating that she has always been in perfect health and was never told she even had diverticulosis in the past, let alone diverticulitis. She asks you what percentage of 85-year-olds have diverticulosis?

A. 5%
B. 33%
C. 66%
D. 75%
E. 95%

48-3. A 71-year-old man with past medical history significant for hypertension, constipation, MI status post CABG, Alzheimer's dementia, adult-onset diabetes, benign prostatic hypertrophy, and high cholesterol, presents with 3 days of abdominal pains, nausea, vomiting, and worsening constipation. His vital signs are normal. He clutches his left lower quadrant when you palpate his abdomen, which is otherwise soft without guarding. Rectal exam is unremarkable. His wife denies any major weight loss or night sweats on his review of systems. What is the diagnostic test of choice?

   A. Ultrasound
   B. Colonoscopy
   C. CT scan
   D. Plain radiograph
   E. Barium enema

48-4. A 55-year-old man complains of 2 days of constipation, low-grade fever, nausea, and left-sided low abdominal pain. He has a history of CAD, CHF, hypertension, kidney stones, urinary tract infections, and chronic renal insufficiency. On examination, he has moderate tenderness to palpation of the left lower quadrant, with some voluntary guarding and equivocal rebound. He is guaiac-negative. Abdominal CT scan shows multiple small colonic outpouchings with bowel wall thickening and a small abscess adjacent to the area. Which of the following may be protective against developing his condition?

   A. High-cholesterol foods
   B. Constipation
   C. High intraluminal pressure
   D. High-residue diet
   E. Colonic wall weakness

ANSWERS

48-1. C. Ampicillin is effective against aerobic organisms, including the predominant colonic aerobes *Escherichia coli*, *Klebsiella*, and *Enterobacter*. Ampicillin is also effective against the bacterial pathogen *Listeria monocytogenes*, a gram-positive bacillus that has aerobic and facultative anaerobic characteristics, and which is typically a food-borne organism. **Ampicillin is not effective against anaerobic organisms, such as *Peptostreptococcus*, a predominant colonic anaerobe.** The other predominant colonic anaerobes include *Bacteroides fragilis* and *Clostridium* species; metronidazole or clindamycin is used to treat these.

48-2. C. It is estimated that roughly one-third, or 33%, of the population develops diverticulosis by age 50, while roughly two-thirds, or 66%, of the population develops diverticulosis by age 85. Of those patients with diverticulosis, approximately 10% to 25% will have an episode of diverticulitis. Diverticulitis is much less common in younger patients, although those who develop it at a young age tend to have more severe episodes than the older population.

48-3. C. CT scan is the diagnostic study of choice for diverticulitis. Abdominal CT is very useful because it can detect diverticulosis, peridiverticular abscess, inflammation of pericolic fat, and bowel wall thickening. Although ultrasound can be helpful, it is not specific for diverticulitis and is very operator-dependent. Plain x-rays may show a partial small-bowel obstruction or free air due to perforation, but no findings are specific to diverticulitis. A barium contrast study is useful for showing diverticulosis, but will not provide information regarding diverticulitis. Barium under pressure may further cause colonic perforation in diverticulitis. Colonoscopy (or sigmoidoscopy) is the diagnostic study of choice for diagnosing *colon cancer*.

48-4. D. A high-residue diet (e.g., fiber, vegetables) may be protective against developing diverticulosis. Low-residue diets (e.g., fatty foods), high intraluminal pressures, and colonic wall weakness are thought to be associated with diverticular disease. The exact pathophysiology of diverticulosis is unknown, but it is hypothesized that high intraluminal pressures (e.g., caused by straining with bowel movements) cause outpouchings in the colonic wall where natural weaknesses are already present. Diverticulitis (i.e., infection/inflammation of a diverticulum) is characterized by abdominal pain (most frequently in the LLQ but also possible in other areas such as the RLQ) and change in bowel habits (diarrhea or constipation); tenesmus is also common. Urinary symptoms (frequency, dysuria, pyuria) may also be present if the area of inflammation is near to and irritates the bladder or ureters.

 SUGGESTED ADDITIONAL READINGS

Dang C, Aguilera P, Dang A, et al. Acute abdominal pain. Four classifications can guide assessment and management. Geriatrics 2002;57:30–32, 35–36, 41–42.

Hendrickson M, Naparst TR. Abdominal surgical emergencies in the elderly. Emerg Med Clin North Am 2003;21:937–969.

Simpson J, Spiller R. Colonic diverticular disease. Clin Evid 2004;(12):599–609.

Diffuse Abdominal Pain with Nausea and Vomiting

CC: 71-year-old man with abdominal pain, nausea, and vomiting

HPI: N.V. is a 71-year-old man who presents to the ED with diffuse, crampy abdominal pain that began one hour after lunch today. The pain has been going on intermittently for 8 hours with increasing severity. He also complains of nausea and chills, and vomited once on his way to the ED. He has had neither a bowel movement nor flatus since the pain began. He denies fever, chest pain, shortness of breath, weight loss, diarrhea, bloody stools, dysuria, or urinary frequency.

PMHx: Prostate cancer s/p TURP; basal cell cancer s/p resection; appendectomy 30 years ago; left total hip replacement 10 years ago; left iliac artery aneurysm s/p repair 5 years ago; incisional hernia repair 4 years ago; irritable bowel syndrome; lactose intolerance

Meds: Simethicone (Gas-X) PRN

ALL: NKDA

SHx: Lives with wife; occasional alcohol; no tobacco or drug use

VS: Temp 35.6°C (96.1°F), HR 52, BP 153/92, RR 16, SaO$_2$ 99% on RA

PE: *General:* Healthy-appearing, pleasant, older gentleman in mild distress. *HEENT:* No scleral icterus; moist mucous membranes. *CV:* S$_1$, S$_2$; slightly bradycardic; no murmurs; intact pulses. *Chest:* Clear bilaterally. *Abd:* Moderate distention; intermittent high-pitched bowel sounds; diffuse tenderness with guarding and maximal tenderness in periumbilical region; no rebound tenderness. *Rectal:* Normal prostate; brown, heme-negative stool. *Back:* No CVA tenderness. *Extr:* Warm; well-perfused; no rashes or lesions. *Neuro:* Alert and oriented; grossly intact.

321

THOUGHT QUESTIONS

- What is the initial management for this patient?
- What is the differential diagnosis for this patient?
- Which radiographic tests, if any, should be performed?
- Which patients with bowel obstruction need to go emergently to the OR?

Immediate Actions:
Obtain IV access and start NS at 250 mL/hr; place NG tube; order CBC, chem 7, type and screen, urinalysis; obtain upright chest x-ray, KUB supine and upright.

Discussion:
This patient has evidence for bowel obstruction, including a history of diffuse abdominal pain with vomiting and lack of flatus, and a physical exam that includes distention and high-pitched bowel sounds. Obstruction can be either functional or mechanical. Functional obstruction, or adynamic ileus, occurs secondary to an inflammatory process (e.g., diverticulitis, inflammatory bowel disease, appendicitis, ischemic bowel, postsurgical bowel), resulting in decreased motility. The symptoms of functional obstruction are less pronounced and include constipation, abdominal distention, decreased bowel sounds, pain related to the underlying process, and eventually vomiting. Mechanical obstruction [e.g., small-bowel obstruction (SBO), intussusception, incarcerated hernia, volvulus] tends to be more rapid in onset, resulting in abdominal distention, high-pitched tinkling bowel sounds, bilious or feculent vomiting, and absence of flatus.

In a patient with suspected bowel obstruction, an upright chest x-ray and supine and upright abdominal x-rays should be obtained to look for subdiaphragmatic free air, dilated bowel loops, and air-fluid levels. Further imaging and treatment depends on the type of obstruction. For example, in a patient with a history of multiple

(Continued)

abdominal surgeries and an SBO, adhesions would be the most likely etiology for obstruction, and treatment would first be conservative with NG suction, NPO, and IV hydration. In a patient with large-bowel obstruction (LBO) without evidence of volvulus, a CT scan may be indicated to look for a diverticular mass or a cancerous mass causing obstruction. Sigmoid volvulus can often be reduced by rigid sigmoidoscopy or simply by insertion of a rectal tube. If this is unsuccessful, then operative reduction is indicated. Patients with signs of gangrenous or perforated bowel (e.g., localized or rebound tenderness, toxic appearance, hypotension) or with evidence of a closed-loop obstruction, incarcerated hernia, or cecal volvulus require immediate surgical intervention and preoperative broad-spectrum antibiotics.

CASE CONTINUED

Labs are significant for a WBC of 12,000/mm³. Chest x-ray is unremarkable; abdominal plain films reveal dilated small-bowel loops (Figure 49-1) consistent with SBO. An abdominal CT with oral and IV contrast reveals dilated small bowel, decompressed terminal ileum, and evidence of an incarcerated left inguinal hernia. Cefotaxime 2 g IV and metronidazole (Flagyl) 1 g IV are given; he is then taken urgently to the OR for exploratory laparotomy, which reveals small bowel incarcerated in a left inguinal hernia. Approximately 5 feet of small bowel is resected, with reanastomosis of the proximal jejunum and ileum. The left inguinal hernia is repaired by closing the internal ring. The patient's recovery is uneventful.

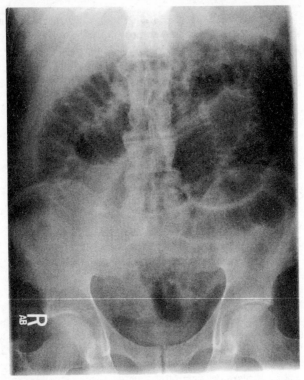

FIGURE 49-1 Supine abdominal x-ray shows markedly dilated loops of small bowel in the midabdomen, consistent with small-bowel obstruction. (*Image courtesy of Massachusetts General Hospital, Boston.*)

 QUESTIONS

49-1. A 54-year-old woman with a history of abdominal surgeries presents to the ED with a 6-hour history of abdominal distention, diffuse colicky pain, and vomiting feculent material. An upright KUB shows several loops of dilated small intestine and multiple air–fluid levels. What percentage of acute surgical admissions does her likely diagnosis account for in the United States?

A. 5%
B. 10%
C. 20%
D. 33%
E. 50%

49-2. A 60-year-old man presents to the ED with vomiting. On exam, he has a distended abdomen and intermittent high-pitched bowel sounds. What is the most common cause of his likely diagnosis in adults?

A. Diverticulitis
B. Bezoar
C. Adhesion
D. Neoplasm
E. Incarcerated hernia

49-3. A 76-year-old man presents to the ED with diffuse abdominal pain and vomiting. On exam, his abdomen is distended and tympanitic to percussion. His bowel sounds are absent. A KUB shows a massively-dilated large bowel loop. What is the most common cause of his diagnosis in adults?

A. Diverticulitis
B. Bezoar
C. Adhesion
D. Neoplasm
E. Incarcerated hernia

49-4. An elderly man who is bedridden and on multiple medications presents to the ED for failure to thrive. On exam, he has a distended abdomen with few bowel sounds. A KUB is obtained to rule out bowel obstruction, which shows multiple dilated loops of large bowel. Which one of the following is characteristic of Ogilvie's syndrome?

A. Can be caused by anticholinergics
B. Increased motility
C. Air–fluid levels on upright abdominal x-ray
D. Large amounts of gas in small bowel
E. Surgery often indicated

ANSWERS

49-1. C. In the United States, small-bowel obstruction accounts for 20% of acute surgical admissions. In the elderly, the mortality rate for SBO ranges from 14% to 45%. Causes of increased mortality include misinterpretation of radiographic studies and delays in going to the OR.

49-2. C. The most common cause of small-bowel obstruction in adults is adhesions due to previous surgery, followed by incarceration of an inguinal hernia. Intussusception, lymphoma, and stricture are less common causes of SBO. Bezoars, neoplasm, and gallstone ileus are possible causes of SBO, though uncommon. Diverticulitis is not known to cause SBO. The most common cause of SBO in children (ages 3 months to 6 years) is intussusception, with ileocolic intussusception being the most prevalent cause.

49-3. D. The most common cause of large-bowel obstruction is neoplasm, followed by secondary obstruction (stricture, abscess) due to diverticulitis, then sigmoid volvulus. Fecal impaction, ulcerative colitis, intussusception, and pseudo-obstruction are also common causes of LBO. Adhesions and hernias, the most common causes of SBO, are uncommon causes of large-bowel obstruction.

49-4. A. Ogilvie's syndrome, also known as intestinal pseudo-obstruction, is caused by decreased motility in a segment of bowel; any segment can be affected, but low colonic obstruction is the most common type. Decreased motility can be caused by medications such as anticholinergics, narcotic analgesics, antidepressants, or antihypertensives. This condition is common in people who are chronically debilitated, bedridden, or institutionalized. Large amounts of gas in the colon or large bowel are common, but air-fluid levels on upright abdominal x-ray are not (due to very little fluid being present in the colon). The x-ray is often remarkable and can be easily mistaken for large-bowel obstruction. Approach to treatment involves digital rectal exam followed by colonoscopy; barium studies and surgery are not indicated.

 SUGGESTED ADDITIONAL READINGS

Dang C, Aguilera P, Dang A, et al. Acute abdominal pain. Four classifications can guide assessment and management. Geriatrics 2002;57:30–32, 35–36, 41–42.

Marincek B. Nontraumatic abdominal emergencies: acute abdominal pain: diagnostic strategies. Eur Radiol 2002;12:2136–2150.

Suleiman S, Johnston DE. The abdominal wall: an overlooked source of pain. Am Fam Physician 2001;64:431–438.

Weakness and Vomiting

CC: 30-year-old man with weakness and vomiting for 5 days

HPI: R.S. is a 30-year-old man with history of Type 1 diabetes mellitus who recalls having eaten some bad seafood 5 days earlier. He has been vomiting since, unable to keep down solids or liquids, and has felt progressively weaker. He has been nauseated and very thirsty, but has managed to continue his insulin injections. He recently cut down on his evening NPH dose due to a few episodes of hypoglycemia. His weakness and malaise were so profound today that he called his sister for help, and she brought him to the ED.

PMHx: Type 1 DM × 12 years, mild hypercholesterolemia

Meds: NPH 16 QAM, 16 QPM; insulin lispro (Humalog) with meals; atorvastatin (Lipitor) 5 mg PO QD

ALL: NKDA

FHx: CAD

SHx: No tobacco or drug use; rare alcohol intake (1 to 2 drinks per year)

VS: Temp 37.7°C (99.8°F), HR 120, BP 127/60, RR 30, SaO$_2$ 100% on RA

PE: *General:* Well-developed young man who appears acutely ill. *HEENT:* Nonicteric sclerae; fruity breath odor; dry mucous membranes. *CV:* S$_1$, S$_2$; tachycardic; regular rhythm; no murmurs. *Chest:* Clear bilaterally. *Abd:* Soft; nontender; nondistended; bowel sounds present. *Extr:* Pulses 1 to 2+ throughout; no edema. *Neuro:* Lethargic but conversant and appropriate; motor and sensory grossly intact.

THOUGHT QUESTIONS

- What is the initial management for this patient?
- Which two regulatory hormones play the largest roles in the pathophysiology of diabetic ketoacidosis (DKA)?
- What is the diagnostic triad for DKA?
- What are the three key components of treatment for DKA?

Immediate Actions:
Place on oxygen by nasal cannula and cardiac monitor; place two large-bore IVs and administer 2 liters normal saline over 30 minutes; check fingerstick blood sugar, urine dip, and EKG; send chem 7, Ca, Mg, PO$_4$, CBC, and venous blood gas; place Foley; obtain portable chest x-ray.

Discussion:
The first consideration in a Type 1 diabetic patient with intractable vomiting is DKA. DKA is characterized by an absolute deficiency of circulating insulin and an overabundance of glucagon, which alters normal metabolism from an anabolic to a catabolic state. This results in release of hepatic glucose (via glycogenolysis and gluconeogenesis) and inhibition of glucose uptake into peripheral tissues that have insulin-dependent transporters (muscle and adipose). With the excess of the regulatory hormone glucagon, adipose cells convert triglyceride into free fatty acids (FFAs), which are released into circulation. Again in the presence of glucagon, FFAs are converted to ketoacids in the liver, which results in a metabolic ketoacidosis. Hyperglycemia results in a hyperosmolar diuresis and profound dehydration, which further exacerbates metabolic acidosis. The diagnostic triad for DKA is hyperglycemia, metabolic acidosis, and ketosis (Figure 50-1).

(Continued)

Diagnostic Triad of Diabetic Ketoacidosis

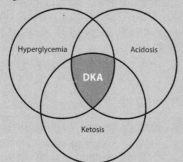

FIGURE 50-1 Hyperglycemia, acidosis, and ketosis are three essential components for the diagnosis of DKA. (*Illustration courtesy of Massachusetts General Hospital, Boston.*)

The three keys to the treatment of DKA are fluid replacement, insulin administration, and potassium replacement. Insulin is crucial in reversing the catabolic metabolism of FFAs into ketoacids and thus reversing DKA. It is important to know that insulin drives potassium into cells. Therefore, in DKA (an insulin-deficient state), potassium accumulates extracellularly, which initially causes hyperkalemia. However, with significant diuresis in DKA, this potassium is lost and leads to an overall *hypokalemic* state. Insulin administration will rapidly drive potassium into the cells, further exacerbating hypokalemia, which can be fatal. Therefore, potassium replacement is required for any level less than 5.0 mEq/dL.

CASE CONTINUED

EKG shows sinus tachycardia without evidence of ischemia. IVs are placed and NS infusion begun. Fingerstick glucose is 521 mg/dL, and urine dip is positive for glucose and ketones. Labs are significant for Na 132 mEq/L, K 5.6 mEq/L, Cl 92 mEq/L, CO_2 16 mEq/L, BUN 24 mg/dL, Cr 1.4 mg/dL, Ca 9.7 mg/dL, Mg 1.8 mEq/L, PO_4 3.4 mg/dL, anion gap 24 mEq/L, and a venous pH 7.05. Insulin is started after the first liter of NS as a 0.1 U/kg bolus (7 U) followed by a 0.1 U/kg/hr drip (7 U/hr). Electrolytes are repeated every 2 hours and KCl 20–40 mEq is added to each liter of fluid once repeat potassium level is less than 5.0 mEq/L. After 2 liters of NS over the first hour, the fluid is changed to ½ NS, the rate is decreased to 250 mL/hr to prevent cerebral and pulmonary edema, and urine output is maintained greater than 1.0 mL/kg/hr. The patient is admitted to the ICU, where his fluids are changed to D5 ½ NS once the glucose is between 250 and 300 mg/dL. At that time, he is administered 10 U regular insulin SC and 20 U NPH insulin SC, and the insulin drip is stopped.

 QUESTIONS

50-1. A 17-year-old girl with a history of Type 1 diabetes mellitus, asthma, and eczema, presents to the ED with complaint of several days of abdominal pain, nausea, vomiting, dysuria, and urinary frequency. She typically uses insulin glargine (Lantus) 24 units SC QHS and counts carbohydrates during the day to decide how much insulin lispro (Humalog) to use SC QID PRN. She has not been able to keep down any foods or liquids, so has not taken any Humalog in the past couple of days. Her labs are significant for a blood sugar of 440 mg/dL and anion gap of 22 mEq/L. Which of the following represents a proper sequence of events in the pathophysiology of her illness?

   A. Increased insulin/glucagon ratio; decreased GFR; anion gap metabolic acidosis; osmotic diuresis; ketone formation

   B. Increased glucagon/insulin ratio; lipolysis; osmotic diuresis; vomiting; hyperglycemia

   C. Decreased glucagon/insulin ratio; lipolysis; ketone formation; anion gap metabolic acidosis

   D. Increased glucagon/insulin ratio; hyperglycemia; osmotic diuresis; decreased GFR; dehydration

   E. Decreased insulin/glucagon ratio; protein breakdown; ketonuria; volume depletion; glycosuria

50-2. A 35-year-old woman with type 1 diabetes presents to the ED with nausea, weakness, polydipsia, and polyuria. She has no other past medical history and denies chest pain or abdominal pain. She also denies fever, cough, dysuria, diarrhea, sore throat, or rhinorrhea. Her last menstrual period was 1 week ago. On exam, she is afebrile and has 5/5 motor strength bilaterally in the arms and legs. EKG is normal. Her urinalysis is positive for glucose and ketones, with 0 to 2 WBCs per high-power field. Which of the following is the likely precipitant of her acute condition?

   A. Stroke

   B. Pregnancy

   C. Infection

   D. Myocardial infarction

   E. Inadequate administration of insulin

50-3. A 65-year-old man with DKA in the setting of myocardial infarction is admitted to the hospital for treatment. Which of the following is the most likely complication of his treatment?
  A. Central pontine myelinolysis
  B. Hypokalemia
  C. ARDS
  D. Hyperglycemia
  E. Hyperphosphatemia

50-4. A 22-year-old woman with Type 1 diabetes and hyperemesis gravidarum presents to the ED with weakness and malaise. She is found to have a blood sugar of 565 mg/dL with hypomagnesemia, hypokalemia, hypophosphatemia, and severe acidosis. An arterial blood gas returns with a pH of 7.02. Which of the following is most likely to help reverse her acidosis?
  A. Magnesium
  B. Potassium
  C. Insulin
  D. Phosphate
  E. Bicarbonate

ANSWERS

50-1. D. This patient has DKA. **The pathophysiology of DKA begins with a relative insulin deficiency or catabolic hormone excess. This can result in increased gluconeogenesis and cellular underutilization of glucose, leading to hyperglycemia. Once the level of hyperglycemia exceeds the capacity of the glomeruli, glycosuria results, leading to an osmotic diuresis and then decreased GFR; this in turn leads to more severe hyperglycemia and dehydration. Relative insulin deficiency also causes lipolysis, with fatty acids transported to hepatocytes and oxidated to ketoacids.** Ketoacids are apparent as an anion gap metabolic acidosis and lead to vomiting (causing worse dehydration) and ketonuria. Finally, relative insulin deficiency also leads to protein breakdown and muscle wasting. (Choice C would also be a correct sequence of events if the initial step were listed as *increased* instead of decreased glucagon/insulin ratio.)

50-2. E. DKA is triggered by a relative insulin deficit. This can occur when a patient does not take the recommended insulin dose or when the insulin requirement is increased, such as occurs with underlying illness. Stroke, pregnancy, infection, and myocardial infarction are all common precipitating causes of DKA. However, in

25% of patients with DKA, no precipitant is found. **Noncompliance (or inadequate administration of insulin) and infection are the two most common identifiable precipitants of DKA.** Other possible precipitants include surgery, PE, pancreatitis, hyperthyroidism, and any other stressful event. **This patient has no evidence of infection, stroke, or MI. Her LMP one week earlier would suggest that she is not pregnant. The most likely precipitant of her DKA is thus inadequate administration of insulin.**

50-3. **B. Hypokalemia, cerebral edema, ARDS, hypoglycemia, and hypophosphatemia are potential complications of DKA treatment. Of these, hypokalemia and hypoglycemia are the most common.** Hypokalemia can be insidious, because the initial serum potassium values are typically normal or high, despite total body potassium depletion. This is a result of acidosis, which drives potassium out of cells. This potassium is subsequently cleared by the kidneys, such that when normal pH is later restored, hypokalemia ensues. Therefore, potassium repletion is recommended for initial potassium levels of 4.0 mEq/L or less after the first 2 liters of normal saline have been given and once an insulin drip has been initiated.

50-4. **C. Insulin is absolutely critical for correction of DKA (recall, though, that replacement of fluid is first and foremost in importance for treatment of DKA).** In DKA, osmotic diuresis causes total body loss of potassium, phosphate, and magnesium, in spite of initial blood levels, which may reflect intracellular to extracellular shifts. Replacement of potassium early is vital to avoid consequences of hypokalemia. Phosphate and magnesium can usually be replaced orally once the patient is able to tolerate POs. Although DKA represents a state of acidosis, bicarbonate use in DKA treatment has not been shown beneficial and its use is not recommended. **Acidosis in DKA is reversed by stopping ketogenesis, which can only be achieved by administering insulin.**

 SUGGESTED ADDITIONAL READINGS

Charfen MA, Fernandez-Frackelton M. Diabetic ketoacidosis. Emerg Med Clin North Am 2005;23:609–628, vii.

Wallace TM, Matthews DR. Recent advances in the monitoring and management of diabetic ketoacidosis. QJM 2004;97:773–780.

Yared Z, Chiasson JL. Ketoacidosis and the hyperosmolar hyperglycemic state in adult diabetic patients. Diagnosis and treatment. Minerva Med 2003;94:409–418.

Episodic Irritability and Vomiting in an Infant

CC: 9-month-old boy with episodic crying and vomiting

HPI: I.V. is a 9-month-old boy who is brought to the ED by his parents because of episodes of crying associated with vomiting. He has recently recovered from gastroenteritis, during which he had 3 days of watery diarrhea. Today he was doing well until he suddenly curled up and began to cry. He pulled away from his mother when she reached out to pick him up. The episode lasted for about 2 minutes, and then he seemed fine again. This happened two more times during the day, and in the last episode he vomited twice. He has had no fever and he has been feeding well. He had a stool earlier today with a small amount of blood mixed in.

PMHx: None

Meds: None

ALL: NKDA

DevHx: Meeting all developmental milestones

SHx: Lives with mother and father

VS: Temp 37.0°C (98.6°F), HR 148, BP 72/48, RR 24, Sao$_2$ 100% on RA

PE: *General:* Well-developed infant who appears ill; lethargic; irritable. *HEENT:* Conjunctivae clear; oropharynx clear. *Neck:* No adenopathy. *CV:* S$_1$, S$_2$; no murmurs. *Chest:* Clear to auscultation bilaterally. *Abd:* Firm; cries with palpation; decreased bowel sounds. *Rectal:* Stool with dark red blood. *Extr:* Well-perfused; no rashes.

THOUGHT QUESTIONS

- What is the initial management for this child?
- What are common causes of rectal bleeding in an infant?
- Which test is both diagnostic and therapeutic for this child?
- When is surgery indicated for this condition?

Immediate Actions:
Establish IV access; send blood for CBC, chem 7, LFTs, lipase; give NS bolus of 20 mg/kg; obtain abdominal x-ray; order barium enema study; consult surgery.

Discussion:
Abdominal pain in infants is often difficult to discern because infants are unable to verbalize their pain. Often the only evidence of abdominal pain is irritability, decreased oral intake, or vomiting. Common causes of lower GI bleeding in infants include anal fissures, protein-induced enterocolitis (e.g., from cow's milk or soy-based formulas), and infectious colitis (e.g., *Shigella*, *Salmonella*). In conjunction with irritability and vomiting, abdominal pathology must be considered, such as intussusception, midgut volvulus, incarcerated hernia, Meckel's diverticulum, or appendicitis (see Table 51-1 for a summary of abdominal emergencies in children). In this case, intussusception is suspected based on the episodic nature of the infant's pain. This illness is characterized by a piece of bowel, usually the terminal ileum, telescoping into the bowel ahead of it. This often reduces spontaneously, accounting for the episodic nature of the pain. However, if reduction does not occur, the bowel wall begins to swell. This leads to local bowel ischemia, causing epithelial sloughing and bleeding. The resultant rectal bleeding is referred to as "currant jelly stool." A mechanical bowel obstruction also occurs. The area of intussusception can sometimes be palpated as an abdominal mass. Plain abdominal

(Continued)

radiographs may show a dense mass and proximal dilated loops of small bowel. A barium or air-insufflation enema under fluoroscopy is both diagnostic and therapeutic. It will show the area of intussusception and in most cases will result in reduction. If reduction does not occur, if the child's symptoms have lasted longer than 12 hours, or if the child has evidence of peritonitis, then surgical repair should be undertaken immediately.

(Continued)

TABLE 51-1 Abdominal Emergencies in Children

	Typical Age	Signs	Diagnosis	Treatment
Necrotizing enterocolitis	Premature newborn	Anorexia, abdominal distention, vomiting, heme-positive stool, toxic-appearing	X-ray shows dilated small-bowel loops and air-fluid levels	IV hydration, NPO, NG suction, antibiotics, parenteral nutrition
Pyloric stenosis	2–6 wks	Projectile vomiting, hypochloremic hypokalemic alkalosis, olive-shaped mass in epigastrium	Ultrasound	Pyloromyotomy
Midgut volvulus	1–2 mos	Bilious vomiting, abdominal distention, heme-positive stool, toxic-appearing	Upper GI series	Immediate laparotomy
Intussusception	5–12 mos	Intermittent colic, vomiting, inconsolable, tender abdomen, currant jelly stool	Air-contrast enema or barium enema	Air-contrast enema or barium enema
Appendicitis	Adolescents	RLQ pain, anorexia, vomiting	CT scan	Appendectomy

CASE CONTINUED

The child undergoes a barium enema under fluoroscopy that shows an ileocolic intussusception as a filling defect within the hepatic flexure surrounded by spiral mucosal folds (Figure 51-1). As more barium is added, the area undergoes reduction. The child is admitted to the surgical service and observed overnight with IV hydration, broad-spectrum antibiotics, and bowel rest. Over the next 2 days, he is advanced to clear liquids, and then formula, and is able to go home.

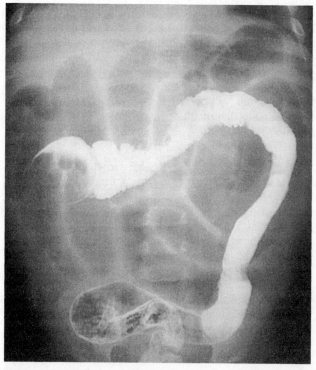

FIGURE 51-1 Barium enema shows the intussusception as the filling defect within the hepatic flexure surrounded by spiral mucosal folds. Significant distended small bowel represents distal small bowel obstruction. (*Image reprinted with permission from Fleisher GR, Ludwig S, Baskin MN. Atlas of Pediatric Emergency Medicine. Philadelphia: Lippincott Williams & Wilkins, 2004.*)

QUESTIONS

51-1. A 12-month-old infant presents to the ED with abdominal pain, anorexia, and heme-positive stools. Which of the following can easily be ruled out?
   A. Pyloric stenosis
   B. Sepsis
   C. Intussusception
   D. Midgut volvulus
   E. Appendicitis

51-2. A 14-month-old boy is brought to the ED by his parents for intermittent colic and inconsolability that lasts for several minutes and then abruptly resolves. The parents state that he had a viral illness last week with low-grade fever, rhinorrhea, and diarrhea. Given this history, you consider the possibility of intussusception. Which of the following is the most likely lead point for intussusception in this child?
   A. Enlarged Peyer's patches
   B. Intestinal lymphoma
   C. Meckel's diverticulum
   D. Intestinal polyp
   E. Cystic fibrosis

51-3. A 6-week-old boy is brought to the ED with multiple episodes of vomiting. At triage his vitals are HR 158, BP 68/42, RR 48, and oxygen saturation 96%. You are asked to come to triage to take a look at the child. He looks very pale and listless. Amongst other concerning possibilities, including meningitis, you consider midgut volvulus as a possible diagnosis. Which of the following would be expected in midgut volvulus?
   A. Presentation between 6 and 12 months of age
   B. Profuse watery diarrhea
   C. Point of obstruction classically at pyloric outlet
   D. Embryologic malrotation
   E. Spontaneous reduction

51-4. A newborn presents to the ED with her parents for anorexia, abdominal distention, and vomiting. The baby appears listless. A rectal exam reveals heme-positive stool. An x-ray shows distended loops of bowel with air–fluid levels. Which of the following statements regarding necrotizing enterocolitis is accurate?

    A. Ninety percent of cases occur in infants 6 to 12 months old.
    B. Anorexia, abdominal distention, and vomiting are uncommon.
    C. Antibiotics are not indicated.
    D. Surgery is usually required.
    E. KUB usually shows dilated loops of bowel with air–fluid levels.

ANSWERS

51-1. A. Abdominal pain, anorexia, vomiting, and heme-positive stool should raise the suspicion for a surgical emergency such as intestinal obstruction, appendicitis, intussusception, Meckel's diverticulum, or an incarcerated hernia. Any of these conditions can also subsequently lead to sepsis if left untreated. A Meckel's diverticulum is the remnant of the omphalomesenteric duct and is an outpouching from the ileum. It occurs in 2% of the population and typically remains clinically silent. Heterotopic tissue within this pouch can include acid-producing gastric mucosa, which can lead to ulceration, bleeding, scarring, and obstruction. This tissue can also act as a lead point for intussusception. **Pyloric stenosis causes gastric outlet obstruction in newborns from 2 to 6 weeks old. It is characterized by projectile vomiting and hypochloremic hypokalemic alkalosis. Sometimes an olive-shaped mass can be palpated in the epigastrium. Treatment consists of a surgical pyloromyotomy.**

51-2. A. In those children who require surgery for intussusception, only 10% have an identifiable lead point. **Viral illnesses, particularly adenovirus, have been implicated in activating intestinal lymph nodes to create a lead point (i.e., enlarged Peyer's patches).** Other sources include Meckel's diverticulum, intestinal polyps, lymphoma, and cystic fibrosis.

51-3. D. Midgut volvulus is a surgical emergency that occurs within the first month of life in 75% of cases. **It is caused by an embryonic malrotation of the small intestine, which results in a long segment of small bowel attached to narrow-based mesentery. This allows the bowel to easily twist upon itself and create**

obstruction and mesenteric ischemia. This must be considered in infants with bilious vomiting who appear ill. Bowel ischemia, sepsis, and death will ensue rapidly if the condition is left undiagnosed. If suspected, a nasogastric tube should be placed to decompress the stomach and duodenum. Water-soluble contrast (e.g., Gastrograffin) should be infused through the NG tube, and an upper GI series obtained. Classic findings include a point of obstruction in the distal third of the duodenum to the right of the spine. The intestine distal to the obstruction wraps around the superior mesenteric vessels, creating a corkscrew appearance. Treatment consists of IV hydration, broad-spectrum antibiotics, and prompt surgical repair.

51-4. E. Necrotizing enterocolitis (NEC) is a disease of newborns, most of whom were born prematurely or have significant cardiovascular or pulmonary disease. **NEC is characterized by erosive intestinal mucosa and functional ileus that results from bowel wall invasion by intestinal microbes.** The neonate presents with anorexia, abdominal distention, and vomiting. On exam the neonate appears ill and may be listless and poorly perfused. The abdomen is distended and variably tender, while rectal exam is typically heme-positive. **A plain abdominal x-ray will show dilated loops of bowel and air–fluid levels consistent with a functional ileus.** Treatment includes NG suction, NPO, parenteral nutrition, and antibiotics. Surgery is indicated only in cases of perforation, frank peritonitis, and gangrenous bowel.

 SUGGESTED ADDITIONAL READINGS

D'Agostino J. Common abdominal emergencies in children. Emerg Med Clin North Am 2002;20:139–153.

Hammond P, Curry J. Paediatric acute abdomen. Hosp Med 2004;65:686–689.

McCollough M, Sharieff GQ. Abdominal surgical emergencies in infants and young children. Emerg Med Clin North Am 2003;21:909–935.

Sorantin E, Lindbichler F. Management of intussusception. Eur Radiol 2004;14 Suppl 4:L146–154.

Vomiting Blood

CC: 51-year-old man presents vomiting blood

HPI: V.B. is a 51-year-old man who presents to the ED after one episode of vomiting blood this morning. Yesterday he had intermittent epigastric pain throughout the day. Today he was driving to work when he felt nauseated and lightheaded, after which he vomited approximately a cup of bright red blood. He has been taking ibuprofen daily for a number of months for chronic low back pain. For the past 2 months, he has noted dark, blackish stools intermittently, but has had no other change in bowel habits and has otherwise felt well. He denies ingestion of iron, bismuth, or beets (all of which can turn the stool black). He has no history of hematemesis, hemoptysis, abdominal pain, or weight loss.

PMHx: HTN; back surgery 2 years prior and again 6 months prior to presentation

Meds: Hydrochlorothiazide 12.5 mg PO QD; ibuprofen (Motrin) 800 mg PO TID

ALL: Mint (causes throat tightening)

SHx: Lives with family; denies tobacco use; occasional alcohol intake (1 to 2 drinks per week)

VS: Temp 36.9°C (98.4°F), HR 98, BP 130/85, RR 16, Sao$_2$ 99% on RA

PE: *General:* Awake, alert, healthy appearing; in no apparent distress. *HEENT:* Nonicteric; pink conjunctivae; moist mucous membranes; oropharynx clear. *CV:* S$_1$, S$_2$; regular rate and rhythm; no murmurs; pulses normal and equal bilaterally. *Chest:* Lungs clear to auscultation bilaterally; no respiratory distress. *Abd:* Soft; nondistended; mildly tender to palpation in epigastric region; bowel sounds present; no masses or organomegaly. *Back:* No CVA tenderness. *Rectal:* Heme-positive black stool; nontender prostate; normal tone. *Extr:* Good pulses throughout. *Skin:* Intact; warm; no spider angiomata or jaundice; no petechiae or purpura.

THOUGHT QUESTIONS

- Which immediate actions should be taken for this patient?
- What is the differential diagnosis for upper GI bleeding?
- What is the differential diagnosis for lower GI bleeding?
- Which patients should be admitted to the hospital?

Immediate Actions:
Administer oxygen while placing a cardiac monitor and two 16-gauge IVs. Bolus with 1 liter NS, and hang second liter. Send blood for CBC, chemistries including LFTs and lipase, coags, and type and hold. NG lavage should be performed to assess the presence and extent of upper GI bleeding.

Discussion:
The differential diagnosis for a patient presenting with symptoms of an upper GI bleed, such as hematemesis or melena, includes peptic ulcer disease, erosive gastritis, esophagitis, esophageal and gastric varices, Mallory-Weiss syndrome, and ENT sources of bleeding (e.g., epistaxis). Less common causes of upper GI bleed include arteriovenous malformations, malignancy, and aortoenteric fistulas. The differential diagnosis for lower GI bleeding includes hemorrhoids, diverticulosis, angiodysplasia, and malignancy. Less common causes of lower GI bleed include inflammatory bowel disease, polyps, and infectious gastroenteritis.

Patients with GI bleeding as evidenced by history, examination, positive NG lavage, low Hct, or abnormal vital signs need to be admitted to the hospital for endoscopy to identify the source of bleeding. All patients with GI bleeding should have at least two large-bore IVs for fluid (and potential PRBC) resuscitation. If upper GI bleeding is significant, airway protection needs to be addressed. Patients on warfarin (Coumadin) can be given fresh frozen plasma to reverse their anticoagulation; patients on aspirin or NSAID therapy can be given a platelet transfusion. In certain conditions, such as bleeding esophageal varices, specific pharmacologic therapy (e.g., octreotide) may be useful.

CASE CONTINUED

Pertinent lab results are Hct 40.0%, plt 298 k/mm³, PT 12.1, and PTT 28.6. LFTs and lipase are normal. An NG tube is placed with return of dark, maroon-colored coffee grounds that do not clear after irrigation with 500 mL NS. The patient is begun on ranitidine (Zantac) 50 mg IV and octreotide (a somatostatin analogue that is thought to act by constricting splanchnic capillary beds and limiting the extent of upper GI bleeding) 50 mg/hr IV with a 50 mg bolus. He is then sent for an upper GI endoscopy, which shows esophagitis in the lower esophagus as well as a gastric ulcer in the body of the stomach. At the base of the ulcer is a slowly oozing vessel, which is endoscopically electrocoagulated without complication. The patient is admitted for observation, does not have any further hematemesis, and maintains a stable hematocrit. He is discharged home a day later on omeprazole (Prilosec) 20 mg PO QD, with follow-up in the gastroenterology clinic in 1 week.

QUESTIONS

52-1. An 86-year-old woman on warfarin (Coumadin) with a history of CHF, CAD, and AF presents to the ED with weakness and dyspnea of several days. Her physical exam is only remarkable for bibasilar pulmonary crackles and heme-positive brown stool. Her abdominal exam is unremarkable. Her hematocrit is 30.6% and her INR is 1.9. Her CXR shows mild pulmonary congestion. She is admitted to hold her Coumadin, get blood transfusion, and undergo endoscopy. What is the most likely cause of this patient's GI bleeding?

A. Erosive gastritis
B. Diverticulitis
C. Hemorrhoids
D. Carcinoma
E. Esophageal varices

52-2. A 55-year-old alcoholic with a history of bleeding esophageal varices 3 years earlier, presents to the ED after vomiting a "very, very large" amount of bright red blood. On initial evaluation of this new-onset large GI bleed, which of the following would you expect?
- A. Normal hematocrit
- B. Metabolic alkalosis
- C. Increased pulse pressure
- D. Bradycardia
- E. Respiratory acidosis

52-3. A 16-year-old girl with history of bulimia is brought to the ED after an episode of bright red hematemesis. What is the most likely cause of this patient's upper GI bleed?
- A. Factitious disorder
- B. Mallory-Weiss syndrome
- C. Stress ulcer
- D. Boerhaave's syndrome
- E. Erosive gastritis

52-4. A 76-year-old woman presents to the ED after three episodes of bright red hematemesis, which she describes as "enough to fill a wash-basin." Which of the following is useful both diagnostically and therapeutically to evaluate her bleeding?
- A. Endoscopy
- B. Scintigraphy
- C. Barium contrast study
- D. Angiography
- E. Plain radiography

ANSWERS

52-1. D. The greatest concern of painless, heme-positive stool in the elderly is carcinoma. Diverticulosis causing bleeding is also painless and more common in the elderly, and may cause massive bleeding; diverticulitis (which denotes infection and inflammation of the diverticular sac), however, usually causes left lower quadrant abdominal pain and fever without bleeding. Erosive gastritis is generally associated with upper GI bleeding signs and symptoms, such as dark stools and epigastric tenderness. Although hemorrhoids are a common cause of lower GI bleeding, they are more likely to present with blood on the toilet paper as opposed to brown heme-positive stool. Esophageal varices cause vomiting of blood and black, tarry stools.

52-2. A. With significant GI bleeding, rapid volume loss leads to an increase in catecholamines, which results initially in a reflex tachycardia and increased diastolic blood pressure, and thus a narrowed or decreased pulse pressure (i.e., the difference between systolic and diastolic blood pressure). **An initial hematocrit is often normal after a brisk bleed because re-equilibration of third-space fluid into the vascular space has not yet occurred.** With further volume loss, tissue hypoperfusion occurs, with a resulting lactic acidosis. This leads to a physiologic tachypnea in an attempt to counter the acidosis with a compensatory respiratory alkalosis. Frank hypotension is the last sign of hypovolemic shock and indicates a life-threatening blood loss.

52-3. B. Mallory-Weiss syndrome refers to a longitudinal mucosal tear in the esophagus causing bright red hematemesis, usually following repeated retching. Mallory-Weiss syndrome is the most likely cause of this patient's symptoms because her history of bulimia suggests that she is having episodes of self-induced vomiting. In contrast, Boerhaave's syndrome is a full-thickness distal esophageal tear usually induced by alcohol-related retching that causes a chemical mediastinitis and rapid sepsis. The latter condition requires broad-spectrum antibiotics and immediate surgical repair.

52-4. A. Endoscopy (upper GI or colonoscopy) can be very useful both diagnostically and therapeutically (e.g., band ligation, injection sclerotherapy, or electrocoagulation). It is usually the treatment of choice for significant upper GI bleeding. Scintigraphy with technetium-labeled red cells can help localize bleeding when the source is not identified by endoscopy and the bleeding rate is relatively low (0.1 mL/min). Angiography can be useful to detect a bleeding site when the bleeding rate is greater than 0.5 to 2.0 mL/min; angiography can also permit transcatheter arterial embolization or sclerotherapy. Barium studies are useful in diagnosing peptic ulcer but have limited use for emergent evaluation of GI bleeding. Plain radiography is unlikely to be useful in evaluation of GI bleeding.

 SUGGESTED ADDITIONAL READINGS

Farrell JJ, Friedman LS. Review article: the management of lower gastrointestinal bleeding. Aliment Pharmacol Ther 2005;21:1281–1298.

Palmer K. Management of haematemesis and melena. Postgrad Med J 2004;80:399–404.

Rivkin K, Lyakhovetskiy A. Treatment of nonvariceal upper gastrointestinal bleeding. Am J Health Syst Pharm 2005;62:1159–1170.

CASE **53**

Buttock Pain

CC: 23-year-old woman with buttock pain

HPI: B.P. is a 23-year-old woman who has had a boil on her buttock cheek for one week that has gotten progressively bigger and more painful. She saw her PCP 3 days ago for this and was given an antibiotic that she can't recall the name of, but takes twice a day. There has been no drainage from the boil, and no improvement with antibiotics. She had something similar 6 months ago that resolved with antibiotics alone. She denies fever, chills, nausea, vomiting, diarrhea, dysuria, frequency, vaginal discharge, or blood in her stools.

PMHx: Bipolar disorder, endometriosis s/p laparoscopy 3 weeks ago

Meds: Nortriptylline, citalopram (Celexa), lorazepam (Ativan), birth control pills, antibiotics PO BID

ALL: NKDA

SHx: Smokes 1 ppd, drinks alcohol socially, lives with boyfriend, denies recreational drugs.

VS: Temp 36.1°C (96.9°F), HR 133, BP 114/80, RR 24, Sao$_2$ 97% on room air

PE: *General:* Well-developed, well-nourished, moderate discomfort with any movement involving her buttocks. *CV:* S$_1$, S$_2$; regular; no murmurs; 2+ radial and DP pulses bilaterally. *Chest:* Clear bilaterally. *Abd:* Soft; nondistended, mild tenderness periumbilically at the recent laparascopy site. *Skin:* Upper buttocks left side with 2.5 cm × 2 cm area of erythema, tenderness, and fluctulance surrounded by induration. *Rectal:* No masses or tenderness.

THOUGHT QUESTIONS

- What are the immediate actions for this patient?
- Which process is common with ingrown hairs at the sacrococcygeal region?
- Which other types of abscesses occur in the buttocks?
- What is the approach to management for these conditions?

Immediate Actions:
Give adequate analgesia, often requiring IV narcotics in preparation for incision and drainage (I&D); prepare for I&D, including 5 to 10 mL lidocaine 1% solution, syringe and needle, sterile preparation with iodine, scalpel, forceps, and iodiform gauze for packing.

Discussion:
A pilonidal cyst, or pilonidal abscess, occurs at the upper buttocks in the gluteal fold, often due to ingrown hairs. The predisposition to pilonidal cyst formation is thought to be due to the blockage of a congenital pilonidal sinus. Other abscesses that occur in the buttock region, collectively termed perirectal abscesses, come in four types: perianal, ischiorectal, supralevator (pelvirectal), and intersphincteric abscesses (Figure 53-1). These are thought to arise from fistulous tracts originating in anal crypts, where mucous-secreting anal glands are located. These abscesses most often contain mixed aerobic and anaerobic species. Patients with perirectal abscesses tend to be adults, more frequently male. There are sometimes associated predisposing conditions such as diabetes mellitus or inflammatory bowel disease. Perianal abscesses are the most common of the perirectal abscesses and are usually easy to diagnose. On the contrary, deep abscesses that have no involvement near the skin may only present with deep buttock or rectal pain, or tenderness on rectal exam. The diagnosis may only be possible with CT scan or ultrasound. Pilonidal cysts, perianal abscesses, and possibly very small ischiorectal abscesses

(Continued)

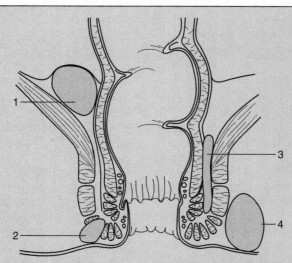

FIGURE 53-1 Depiction of different types of perirectal abscesses: 1, supralevator abscess. 2, perianal abscess. 3, intersphincteric abscess. 4, ischiorectal abscess. (*Image reprinted with permission from Blackbourne LH. Advanced Surgical Recall, 2nd Ed. Baltimore: Lippincott Williams & Wilkins, 2004.*)

that are near the skin can be treated in the ED. ED management for these abscesses consists of I&D after local anesthesia with or without intravenous analgesia. Conscious sedation may be required for larger abscesses. A "wick" (packing) should be placed to promote abscess drainage, with instructions for frequent sitz baths beginning 24 hours after the incision procedure; packing should be changed by a health care professional every 2 days until the abscess cavity heals. Antibiotics for simple perianal or pilonidal abscesses are indicated for those with surrounding cellulitis or signs of systemic involvement such as fever, malaise, or leukocytosis. Supralevator abscesses, intersphincteric abscesses, large and/or deep ischiorectal abscesses, and abscesses with deep sinus tracts, frequent recurrences, or other complexities require surgical intervention in the operating room for definitive treatment. Complications of undiagnosed or inadequately treated deep perirectal abscesses include local extension of cellulitis, deep-tissue infections such as fasciitis, or systemic spread with sepsis and even death.

CASE CONTINUED

The patient has a pilonidal cyst. She is given 100 µg of fentanyl IV for pain. The area surrounding the abscess is prepped with Betadine and draped. The abscess itself is anesthetized with approximately 5 mL of 1% lidocaine with epinephrine. The wound is incised with a #11 scalpel with return of about 5 mL of pus. The cavity is irrigated with normal saline and then packed with iodiform gauze. She is instructed to do sitz baths 3 times daily and return for a wound check and repacking in 2 days. She is discharged with a work note and a prescription for Percocet. She is also advised not to smoke cigarettes while using birth control pills due to increased likelihood for developing deep venous thromboses.

QUESTIONS

53-1. A 30-year-old man complains of a dull, aching pain in the rectal area for the past week. On exam, he has no obvious lesions near his anorectal area, including no fluctulance or tenderness to palpation externally. On digital rectal exam, you feel a soft, tender, sausage-shaped mass above the anorectal ring. Which of the following is most likely?
   A. Pilonidal abscess
   B. Perianal abscess
   C. Pelvirectal abscess
   D. Intersphincteric abscess
   E. Ischiorectal abscess

53-2. A 24-year-old man complains of fever, chills, and malaise for the past several days, and pain in the rectal area. Examination is notable for erythema and induration of the perianal tissue on the left side. Digital rectal exam is remarkable for large, tense, tender swellings above the anorectal ring on both sides of the anal canal. Of the following options, which is the best management plan?
   A. Local anesthesia and then incision and drainage in the ED
   B. Oral analgesia plus local anesthesia, and then incision and drainage in the ED
   C. IV procedural sedation for incision and drainage in the ED
   D. IV antibiotics in the ED followed by a 14-day course of oral antibiotics
   E. CT scan, surgical consult, and drainage in the OR

53-3. A 43-year-old woman complains of throbbing buttock pain for the past several days, worse with sitting, movement, coughing, or trying to have a bowel movement. On examination, she appears nontoxic and has a small area adjacent to the anus that is swollen, very tender, indurated, and red. Digital rectal exam seems uncomfortable overall but is otherwise unremarkable. What is the best treatment approach for her?

- A. Oral antibiotics for mixed bowel flora as an outpatient for 14 days
- B. Incision and drainage using a single linear incision over the most fluctuant area
- C. Incision and drainage using an elliptical incision enveloping the most indurated area
- D. Extensive debridement in the OR
- E. IV antibiotics for mixed bowel flora in the hospital for 24 hours followed by operative incision and drainage

53-4. A 20-year-old hirsute woman complains of severe pain in the sacrococcygeal area for the past couple days. She has had this twice in the past couple years, each time resolved by antibiotics alone. She asks how she can best avoid having to go through this again once this episode has been treated. Which of the following is a reasonable answer?

- A. Prophylactic antibiotics QOD
- B. Sitz baths QID
- C. Shaving of the hair in that area at least every 3 weeks
- D. Elective surgical excision
- E. Incision and drainage

ANSWERS

53-1. D. This patient's digital rectal examination is consistent with an intersphincteric abscess. These are much less common than perianal abscesses and are located between the internal and external anal sphincters. Patients classically complain of a dull, aching pain in the rectal area, with digital rectal exam revealing a soft, tender, sausage-shaped mass above the anorectal ring. These should be managed surgically in the OR.

53-2. E. This patient's history and examination—including fever, chills, malaise, rectal pain, perianal erythema and induration, and tense, tender swellings above the anorectal ring—are consistent with an ischiorectal abscess involving the bilateral ischiorectal spaces. Ischiorectal abscesses should be managed in

the operating room; therefore, only answer E provides an appropriate management choice. Choices A, B, and C involve incision and drainage in the ED, which is only appropriate for pilonidal cysts, perianal abscesses, and possibly very small ischiorectal abscesses that are near the skin. The ischiorectal abscesses described in this patient, however, are large, bilateral, and not limited to the superficial areas given they are palpable above the anorectal ring. Choice D consists of antibiotics alone, without abscess drainage, which is not an adequate treatment regimen for ischiorectal abscesses.

53-3. B. This patient's history and examination are consistent with a simple perianal abscess, which can be treated in the ED with a single linear incision over the most fluctuant area after appropriate analgesia. The wound is then packed with iodiform gauze and the patient discharged home without antibiotics. Instructions should include sitz baths after 24 hours 3 or 4 times daily for 15 to 20 minutes each time to help promote drainage and keep the incision from closing prematurely. The patient should return every 2 days for wound checks and packing replacement until the abscess cavity resolves. Antibiotics, whether oral or IV, are insufficient for treatment of abscesses. Elliptical incisions are classically taught for excision of thrombosed external hemorrhoids.

53-4. D. This patient has a pilonidal abscess, which is more common in hirsute individuals and usually affects young adults, men more than women. There is a recurrence rate of 40% for pilonidal abscesses. Recurrences can be avoided by elective surgical excision of the remnant sinus tract in the area after the acute abscess has subsided. Prophylactic antibiotics have no role in preventing recurrences. Incision and drainage is the treatment for the acute abscess, but not for prevention of recurrences. Shaving the hair in the region may also help to decrease recurrences.

 SUGGESTED ADDITIONAL READINGS

Chandwani D, Shih R, Cochrane D. Bedside emergency ultrasonography in the evaluation of perirectal abscess. Am J Emerg Med 2004;22:315.

Gerdom LE, Dixon D, Diplama JA. Hemorrhoids, genital warts, and other perianal complaints. JAAPA 2001;14:37–39, 43–44, 47.

McClane SJ, Rombeau JL. Anorectal Crohn's disease. Surg Clin North Am 2001;81:169–183, ix.

Nisar PJ, Scholefield JH. Managing haemorrhoids. BMJ 2003; 327:847–851.

VI

Patients Presenting with Genitourinary or Gynecologic Complaints

Scrotal Pain

CC: 38-year-old man with left scrotal pain

HPI: S.P. is a 38-year-old man who has left scrotal pain that started somewhat suddenly this morning after showering. He later masturbated and noted a small amount of blood in his semen. The pain has been present and worsening since onset 6 hours ago. He has had one episode of dysuria today, but denies urinary frequency, urethral discharge, fevers, chills, nausea, vomiting, diarrhea, abdominal or flank pain, or any other symptoms. He has a history of gonorrhea 7 years ago, and was tested HIV-negative one year ago. He adds that he had a sexual encounter a couple weeks ago involving anal intercourse in which the condom broke.

PMHx: Gonorrhea 7 years ago; arthroscopic left knee surgery 10 years ago

Meds: None

ALL: NKDA

SHx: Lives alone; 1 ppd tobacco; occasional alcohol; occasional marijuana

VS: Temp 37.5°C (99.5°F), HR 93, BP 144/98, RR 20, Sao$_2$ 99% on RA

PE: *General:* Healthy-appearing man in minimal to no apparent distress. *HEENT:* No oral lesions. *CV:* S$_1$, S$_2$; regular; no murmurs; pulses intact. *Chest:* Clear bilaterally. *Abd:* Soft; nontender; nondistended; bowel sounds present. *GU:* No urethral discharge; moderate left testicular tenderness; left scrotal erythema, edema; left epididymal tenderness, edema; left testicle riding slightly higher than right testicle upon standing though not clearly horizontal; right testicle, epididymis, and scrotum unremarkable; cremasteric reflex present bilaterally; no inguinal hernias; guaiac-negative; prostate nontender. *Extr:* Warm; intact; no rashes or lesions; no edema. *Neuro:* Alert, oriented.

THOUGHT QUESTIONS

- What is the initial management for this patient?
- What is the differential diagnosis of acute scrotal pain?
- Which diagnostic tests, if any, should be performed?
- When is an operation indicated?

Immediate Actions:
Send urinalysis; send urethral swab for *Chlamydia* and gonorrhea cultures; obtain color Doppler ultrasound.

Discussion:
The most concerning diagnosis in the differential for acute scrotal pain is testicular torsion. Other possible diagnoses include epididymitis, epididymo-orchitis, torsion of the testicular appendages, orchitis, hernia, hydrocele, and testicular tumor. Testicular torsion is a urologic emergency that can lead to ischemia and infarction of the involved testis. If the diagnosis is clearly testicular torsion, an attempt can be made at the bedside to detorse the testicle by rotating it externally like opening the cover of a book. If this is unsuccessful, the patient should be taken by urology to the OR for surgical exploration, detorsion, and bilateral orchiopexy. If the diagnosis is not clear, color Doppler ultrasound can quickly establish whether or not blood flow to the painful side is present, absent, decreased, or increased; ultrasound in addition has the advantage of being able to evaluate for other etiologies of the pain. Radionuclide scintigraphy is also theoretically useful for diagnosing testicular torsion, but is not readily available as a tool in the ED. Torsion of the appendix testis is usually managed with conservative care, with symptoms resolving in 7 to 10 days. Patients suspected of having a testicular tumor should be referred to a urologist.

CASE CONTINUED

Urinalysis shows 5 to 10 WBCs per high power field, 5 to 10 RBCs per high power field, and few bacteria. Color Doppler ultrasound shows increased flow to the left testicle consistent with epididymitis, and normal flow to the right testicle. The patient is diagnosed with bacterial epididymitis, presumed to be sexually acquired. A urethral swab is performed and sent for gonococcal and *Chlamydia* cultures. He is given ceftriaxone 125 mg IM to cover for gonorrhea. The patient is discharged with ofloxacin 300 mg PO BID for 14 days for chlamydial and enteric coverage. He is given instructions to use scrotal support, take acetaminophen or ibuprofen for discomfort, and have his sexual partner seek medical care. He is further instructed not to resume intercourse until both he and his partner have completed their treatment regimens.

QUESTIONS

54-1. A 19-year-old man presents to the ED with complaint of sudden-onset left-sided scrotal pain since 2 hours earlier. He also complains of nausea, mild abdominal discomfort, and low-grade fever. He has no medical problems, but has had occasional scrotal pain in the past that was less severe and that always resolved on its own. He denies any new sexual partners or penile discharge. On physical examination, he is afebrile and has a soft, nontender, and nondistended abdomen. He has no penile discharge or rashes, and his left testicle, which appears elevated compared with the right side, is painful to palpation. There is mild scrotal erythema. The epididymis is nontender bilaterally. Which of the following is associated with increased likelihood of his condition?
    A. Undescended testis
    B. Older age
    C. Fixed testis
    D. Short spermatic cord
    E. Past history of epididymitis

54-2. An 11-month old male infant is brought to the ED for persistent crying and irritability. He was the product of a full-term gestation and normal spontaneous vaginal delivery without complications. In his first 11 months of life, he has not had any major medical problems; his shots are up to date. Mom denies any sick contacts at home, and the infant does not attend daycare. On examination, he is afebrile but irritable and inconsolable. He has normal tympanic membranes and no pharyngeal erythema. He has clear nares and bilateral clear lung sounds, with a soft abdomen that is nontender to palpation. On urologic examination, he has a high-riding testicle on the right side, with absent cremasteric reflex on the right side. There is also some scrotal swelling and erythema. Which one of the following is commonly associated with his condition?

A. Lack of history of similar symptoms
B. Diarrhea
C. Occurrence during sleep
D. Urinary frequency
E. Gradual onset of symptoms

54-3. A 69-year-old man with history of hypertension, CAD status post CABG, BPH, and prior stroke, presents with complaint of pain with urination, feeling like he is not fully emptying his bladder, nausea, subjective fever, and right-sided scrotal pain and swelling. He denies any penile discharge, and is monogamous with his wife of 42 years. On examination, he has a benign abdominal exam, with urologic examination notable for right-sided scrotal erythema, edema, and tenderness. He reports that his pain is lessened upon elevating the right scrotum. Which of the following is true of his condition?

A. Most commonly occurs during puberty
B. Most common reason for days lost from military service
C. Uncommon intrascrotal inflammatory disease
D. Usually due to hematogenous spread of bacterial pathogens
E. Average age of occurrence is 50 years

54-4. A 32-year-old man with no past medical history presents with left-sided testicular pain for the past couple days. On ultrasound, an intra-testicular mass is seen on the left side, with heterogenous echoes surrounding the mass. Which of the following statements about testicular cancer is true?

    A. Embryonal cell cancers are the most common testicular cancer.

    B. Testicular cancers are painless.

    C. CT scan is the initial diagnostic imaging study.

    D. Cisplatin has been effective in improving survival rates from testicular cancer.

    E. Testicular tumors comprise approximately 10% of cancers in men.

ANSWERS

54-1. A. Testicular torsion is more common in the first year of life and at puberty (not with older age), although it can occur at any age. Testicular torsion is more common with an undescended testicle or with underlying bilateral maldevelopment of the testicular fixation mechanism. The latter leads to a mobile testis, redundant spermatic cord, and a "bell-clapper deformity" (named because of the resemblance of the testis dangling low in the scrotum to a bell clapper).

54-2. C. Urinary symptoms (e.g., frequency, dysuria) are not commonly reported in testicular torsion. Many patients have had a previous similar episode of pain (or symptoms, in the case of a preverbal infant) that resolved spontaneously. The pain of testicular torsion is usually described as sudden in onset and can be associated with nausea and vomiting. **Testicular torsion often occurs during sleep, or following strenuous physical activity or trauma.**

54-3. B. Epididymitis is the most common intrascrotal inflammatory disease as well as the number one reason for days lost from military service, with an average age of occurrence at 25 years. It is not particularly common during puberty (whereas testicular torsion is) and is rare before puberty. Epididymitis is usually due to retrograde ascent of pathogens from the urethra or bladder and is rarely due to hematogenous spread. In men under age 35, *Chlamydia* and *Neisseria gonorrhoeae* are the usual cause of bacterial epididymitis, whereas in men age 35 and older, *Escherichia coli* is usually the culprit. Treatment for sexually acquired epididymitis can be accomplished with one-time ceftriaxone and 10 days of doxycycline, tetracycline, or ofloxacin; treatment for nonsexually acquired epididymitis can be accomplished with 14 days of trimethoprim-sulfamethoxazole (Bactrim). Ciprofloxacin or ofloxacin can also be used for epididymitis (single dose for sexually acquired, 14-day course for nonsexually acquired).

54-4. D. Testicular tumors are the most common cancer of young men (average age 32 years), comprising approximately 1% of cancers in all men, with seminomas being the most common testicular cancer. Following seminomas, embryonal cell cancers and teratomas are most frequent among testicular tumors. Although testicular tumors are usually painless, 10% present with pain, usually due to acute hemorrhage into the tumor. The initial diagnostic imaging study is usually color Doppler ultrasound to identify an intratesticular mass. CT scan can be useful for staging or looking for metastases. Management of seminomas includes radical orchiectomy, radiation, and/or chemotherapy with cisplatin. **Cisplatin has helped to improve survival rates in patients with seminomas.**

 SUGGESTED ADDITIONAL READINGS

Blaivas M, Brannam L. Testicular ultrasound. Emerg Med Clin North Am 2004;22:723–748.

Cole FL, Vogler R. The acute, nontraumatic scrotum: assessment, diagnosis, and management. J Am Acad Nurse Pract 2004;16: 50–56.

Marcozzi D, Suner S. The nontraumatic, acute scrotum. Emerg Med Clin North Am 2001;19:547–568.

Vaginal Spotting and Pelvic Pain in Pregnancy

CC: 26-year-old woman at 7 weeks' gestation with vaginal spotting and pelvic pain

HPI: V.S. is a 26-year-old woman now 7 weeks into her current pregnancy dated by her last menstrual period. She had a positive self-administered urine pregnancy test about 2 weeks ago. She had been doing well until this evening, when she started having some lower abdominal cramping. About an hour later, she had vaginal spotting and her pelvic pain increased slightly. She has mild nausea and vomiting at baseline. She denies fever, chills, changes in bowel or bladder activity, or anorexia.

PMHx: None

Meds: Prenatal vitamins

ALL: NKDA

**OB/
GynHx:** First trimester therapeutic abortion (TAB) 3 years ago; regular menses every 29 to 30 days; no STIs; no pelvic surgery; no infertility

SHx: Lives with boyfriend; no domestic violence; no tobacco or recreational drugs; occasional alcohol (but not while pregnant)

VS: Temp 37.1°C (98.8°F), HR 84, BP 118/72, RR 16, Sao$_2$ 100% on RA

PE: *General:* Comfortable; no apparent distress. *HEENT:* Non-icteric; oropharynx clear and moist. *Neck:* Supple. *CV:* S$_1$, S$_2$; no murmurs. *Chest:* Clear bilaterally. *Abd:* Soft, nondistended, nontender. *GU:* Cervix closed, small amount of blood coming from os.

BME: Uterus about 4- to 5-week size and slightly tender; no CMT; no palpable adnexal masses.

Labs: Urine hCG (+), Hct 37.4%, βhCG 384 mIU/mL, blood type A–

THOUGHT QUESTIONS

- What is the differential diagnosis of first trimester vaginal bleeding and pain?
- How does the quantitative βhCG value aid in this patient's management?
- How should this patient be managed if an intrauterine pregnancy is not seen by ultrasound?

Immediate Actions:
Establish IV; send CBC, βhCG, and blood type and screen; get urinalysis; obtain pelvic ultrasound.

Discussion:
The differential diagnosis for this patient includes ectopic pregnancy, spontaneous abortion (SAB), and threatened abortion. She has no risk factors for ectopic pregnancy, but this remains the most dangerous possible diagnosis. It is estimated that approximately 15% to 20% of known pregnancies result in SAB (referred to by the layperson as a miscarriage). An SAB is any pregnancy that terminates itself prior to 20 weeks' gestation. In a woman who has vaginal bleeding in the first trimester, the following definitions are used: 1) threatened abortion—bleeding, no tissue passage, os closed; 2) missed abortion—nonviable gestation based on absent fetal heart motion or absent fetal pole when one should be present based on gestational age or βhCG, os closed; 3) inevitable abortion—bleeding, no tissue passage, os open; 4) incomplete abortion—bleeding, partial tissue passed or tissue in cervix; 5) complete abortion—entire pregnancy has passed through the cervix.

(Continued)

The percentage of all pregnancies that result in SAB is probably even higher than those recognized and diagnosed, as many pregnancy failures likely occur at 4 to 5 weeks' gestation. The primary etiology for a first trimester SAB is abnormal karyotype, one of the most common of these being 45XO, Turner's syndrome. Other known etiologies for first trimester SAB include uterine abnormalities (e.g., bicornuate uterus, submucosal fibroids), luteal phase defect (believed to be due to corpus luteum progesterone production that is inadequate to maintain pregnancy), thrombophilias (e.g., antiphospholipid antibody syndrome, SLE), infections (e.g., CMV, VZV, HSV), and balanced translocation of a chromosome in one of the parents. Despite these numerous possible etiologies as well as extensive testing, most SABs are idiopathic, meaning that their etiology is never discovered.

The quantitative βhCG can be helpful in a variety of ways to the clinician. First, in the acute setting, the βhCG level indicates whether an intrauterine pregnancy (IUP) should be visualized by ultrasound. With transvaginal ultrasound, an IUP can be seen with a βhCG of 1,500 to 2,000 mIU/mL (Table 55-1). Thus, in V.S., who has a βhCG of 384 mIU/mL, visualizing a normal IUP would not be expected. Pelvic ultrasound is needed nevertheless to look for adnexal masses (i.e., an ectopic pregnancy) or an abnormal IUP. A patient in whom an IUP is not visualized can be discharged with ectopic precautions (i.e., instructions to return if pain or bleeding worsens) provided that the ultrasound is otherwise normal and that she is reliable, hemodynamically stable, and able to take oral liquids. The second important use of the quantitative βhCG is to follow patients in whom ectopic pregnancy needs to be ruled out. Because most normal-pregnancy βhCG levels will increase by at least 65% every 48 hours, serial βhCG values can be used to determine whether a pregnancy is normal. Once the βhCG has risen above 1,500 mIU/mL, a transvaginal ultrasound can be repeated to see if there is an IUP. If the βhCG does not rise normally, the patient is offered a dilation and curettage (D&C) to see if the pregnancy was indeed intrauterine and to test for genetic anomalies.

TABLE 55-1 Ultrasound Findings in Pregnancy Based on βhCG Levels

βhCG Level	Transvaginal US	Transabdominal US
<1,500 mIU/mL	IUP not seen	IUP not seen
1,500–2,000 mIU/mL	IUP usually seen	IUP not seen
5,000–6,000 mIU/mL	Cardiac activity seen	IUP seen

CASE CONTINUED

The pelvic ultrasound shows a left ovarian 1.5-cm cyst consistent with a corpus luteum, no intrauterine pregnancy or gestational sac, no other adnexal masses, and no free fluid. Given these findings, the diagnosis is threatened abortion and possible ectopic pregnancy. Because she is having vaginal bleeding and is Rh-negative, she is given RhoGAM 1 vial (300 μg) IM. RhoGAM will bind to fetal hemoglobin antigen that might be introduced to the mother's blood; this prevents the development of anti-Rh antibodies. She is discharged with gynecologic follow-up in 48 hours for a repeat serum βhCG. She returns for follow-up testing at 96 hours instead, and her repeat hCG is 1,854 mIU/mL.

QUESTIONS

55-1. What is the next step in the management of this patient?
A. Follow-up in 48 hours for βhCG
B. D&C
C. Ultrasound
D. Methotrexate
E. Routine prenatal care

55-2. If the βhCG is now 668 mIU/mL at 48 hours and she has had no heavy bleeding, but continues with LLQ pain, what should be the next step in management?
A. Follow-up in 48 hours for βhCG
B. D&C
C. Ultrasound
D. Methotrexate
E. Routine prenatal care

55-3. If the patient had not returned to the ED for a week and had presented with the ultrasound described above but with free intra-abdominal fluid (Figure 55-1), an acute abdomen, BP 70/40, and tachycardia, what would be the likely diagnosis?
A. Complete abortion
B. Incomplete abortion
C. Ectopic pregnancy
D. Threatened abortion
E. Missed abortion

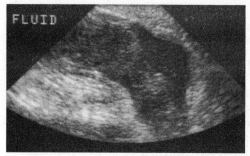

FIGURE 55-1 In this transvaginal image, there is no intrauterine pregnancy seen, but there is a moderate amount of free fluid in the posterior cul-de-sac. (*Image provided by the Departments of Radiology and Obstetrics & Gynecology, University of California, San Francisco.*)

55-4. A patient presents with a βhCG of 4,160 mIU/mL, hematocrit of 36%, vaginal spotting, and moderate LLQ pain, but no peritoneal signs. Her ultrasound shows no IUP or adnexal masses. Assuming she has an ectopic pregnancy, what would be the next step in her management?

    A. Exploratory laparotomy
    B. Exploratory laparoscopy
    C. Methotrexate
    D. Misoprostol
    E. Expectant management

ANSWERS

55-1. C. As discussed in the case, the key to following patients with a diagnosis of rule-out ectopic pregnancy is to measure their quantitative βhCG and see if it rises appropriately. In general, it should approximately double every 48 hours, or rise by at least 65% during that time. In this patient, whose βhCG rose from 384 mIU/mL to 1,854 mIU/mL in 96 hours, the rise is entirely normal. **Furthermore, with a βhCG above 1,500 mIU/mL, there is a high likelihood that the pregnancy can now be visualized by ultrasound.**

55-2. B. Now, her βhCG has risen inappropriately. There is no doubt that this pregnancy is abnormal. However, it is unclear whether the pregnancy is intrauterine or extrauterine. **Obtaining a sample of the intrauterine contents in this case is both diagnostic and possibly therapeutic. If this is indeed a blighted ovum or missed abortion, then there should still be trophoblastic tissue**

on D&C. **If the pregnancy is ectopic, the D&C findings will be negative.** At that point, with a negative pathology report, the patient can be treated with methotrexate for presumed ectopic pregnancy.

55-3. C. Although a patient undergoing SAB may rarely present with shock, it would be unlikely for such a patient to have free intra-abdominal fluid. **Therefore, this patient is more likely to have a ruptured ectopic pregnancy and requires an immediate laparotomy to control the bleeding and remove the ectopic tissue.**

55-4. C. This patient likely has an ectopic pregnancy based on the high level of βhCG and the absence of an IUP. However, no ectopic pregnancy is clearly identified by ultrasound. Thus, the ectopic pregnancy is likely small and therefore amenable to methotrexate therapy. In this setting, because the pregnancy is clearly abnormal, often a D&C is performed to verify that the pregnancy is indeed extrauterine. Once there is no microscopic evidence that the pregnancy is intrauterine, the patient can be treated with methotrexate for ectopic pregnancy. Contraindications for methotrexate include moderate to large amounts of free fluid, baseline liver disease, adnexal mass greater than 3 cm, positive ectopic fetal heart rate, or βhCG greater than 5,000 mIU/mL (occasionally, up to 10,000 mIU/mL is used). The last three findings are suggestive of a gestation that is likely beyond the age at which methotrexate would be successful.

SUGGESTED ADDITIONAL READINGS

Coppola PT, Coppola M. Vaginal bleeding in the first 20 weeks of pregnancy. Emerg Med Clin North Am 2003;21:667–677.

Della-Giustina D, Denny M. Ectopic pregnancy. Emerg Med Clin North Am 2003;21:565–584.

Munoz M, Usatine RP. Abdominal pain in a pregnant woman. J Fam Pract 2005;54:665–668.

Sharp HT. The acute abdomen during pregnancy. Clin Obstet Gynecol 2002;45:405–413.

Sexual Assault

CC: 19-year-old woman presents to the ED complaining of sexual assault

HPI: S.A. is a 19-year-old woman who was at a campus party two nights (36 hours) ago. At the party she drank more alcohol than she is accustomed to and passed out. She awoke the next morning in someone's bed naked but alone. She dressed, went home, and showered. A day later she discussed what happened with a friend who recommended that she go to the ED. She is concerned that she may have been raped while she was unconscious and now wants the "morning after pill," as well as help in determining whether she was really raped. She has no bruises, no musculoskeletal pain, no vaginal or anal soreness, no bleeding or discharge. She states that she had vaginal intercourse with her boyfriend on the night before the incident, and that they had used a condom.

PMHx: Mild asthma

Meds: PRN inhaler

ALL: Penicillin—anaphylaxis

OB/ GynHx: Uncomplicated TAB 2 years ago; regular menses; sexually active since age 16; has had two different male sexual partners over the past 4 months; uses condoms for birth control

SHx: College sophomore; lives with one other woman on campus; smokes tobacco 1 ppd; social alcohol with no previous episodes of blacking out and no use of illicit drugs

VS: Temp 36.2°C (97.2°F), HR 88, BP 118/66, RR 24, Sao$_2$ 100% on RA

PE: *General:* No acute distress, but patient appropriately concerned. *HEENT:* No ecchymoses or lesions. *Neck:* Supple, nontender. *CV:* S$_1$, S$_2$; regular; no murmurs. *Chest:* No bruises; clear lungs.

Abd: Soft; nondistended; nontender. *Back:* No bruises; nontender spine. *GU:* Normal external genitalia; no obvious bruising or evidence of trauma; pubic hair is combed out to collect samples. Swabs of vagina and cervix are taken for cultures and for the rape kit; no particular discharge noted. *BME:* No evidence of CMT; no adnexal masses or tenderness; uterus is normal size.

THOUGHT QUESTIONS

- Will you be able to help this patient determine whether she was raped?
- Which particular aspects need to be focused on during the physical examination?
- Which tests should be sent in addition to the cultures collected?

Immediate Actions:
This patient is medically stable; however, many EDs have specially trained nurses, physicians, or social workers who will counsel and/or examine patients who have been sexually assaulted. If so, they should be contacted immediately upon the patient's arrival to the ED. If not, one-on-one nursing should be arranged in the short term, and a quick assessment made of the acute risks to the patient from either her assailant or herself.

Discussion:
It may be difficult to determine whether this patient has been raped for several reasons. One is the amount of time that has passed since the event and another is that she has showered several times. If there had been forced intercourse, there might be visual evidence of trauma in and around the vagina or anus; however, some of this evidence resolves over time. In addition, there can be hair and other DNA evidence that can collect in her pubic hair, vagina, or anus that may have been washed away. If there was ejaculation, the evidence can be present commonly up to 24 hours, but dissipates with time. Finally, it is important to know whether she has had any other episodes of sexual intercourse recently.

(Continued)

The physical examination of a victim of sexual assault must be performed in a systematic manner. Most EDs have a "rape kit," a collection of instructions on how to proceed with evidence collection, which includes shaking out the victim's clothing, collecting tissue from under her fingernails, and combing her pubic hair to collect foreign hair. In addition to evidence collection, cultures of any possible exposure should be collected. If the patient has been physically assaulted, photographic evidence should be collected as well. In this patient, though it is unclear, the same approach should be utilized to collect any possible information that may remain. If she hasn't washed the clothing she wore the night in question, she should bring them in to be examined. In addition, to help answer the question of whether nonconsensual intercourse occurred, anal and vaginal swabs as well as a careful examination should be performed.

In this patient who may have been exposed to an unknown assailant, there is no test that can be performed immediately to determine whether she has been exposed to or infected with an STI. However, vaginal and cervical cultures or DNA tests for gonorrhea and *Chlamydia* can be performed, which will usually return in 48 to 72 hours. Baseline serum testing for other STIs should also be offered to establish that she is negative, with a plan for follow-up testing in 2 to 4 weeks to determine whether she has been infected. Thus, baseline serum testing for hepatitis B, hepatitis C, HIV, and RPR are commonly performed. A serum pregnancy test is also sent to establish a baseline.

CASE CONTINUED

You offer the patient the testing mentioned above and she agrees. She also asks again about the morning after pill and whether it is now too late. You discuss this issue with her (see below) and offer prophylactic medications against possible STIs.

QUESTIONS

56-1. A 15-year-old girl presents to the ED asking for the "morning after pill." She says that she had been having intercourse with her boyfriend 3 days prior, when the condom broke. She had been too embarrassed to come in sooner, but now says she'll be in bigger trouble if she gets pregnant. For how many hours after intercourse is postcoital contraception still effective and indicated?

A. 12 hours
B. 24 hours
C. 48 hours
D. 72 hours
E. 96 hours

56-2. A 20-year-old woman with past medical history significant only for appendectomy presents to the ED asking for the "morning-after pill," after having had unprotected sexual intercourse the night before. She has no allergies to medications and takes no medications. Which of the following is commonly used as postcoital contraception?

A. Ethinyl estradiol/levonorgestrel (Ovral) two tablets given twice 12 hours apart
B. Any two contraceptive pills given twice 12 hours apart
C. IUD
D. Depo-Provera (medroxyprogesterone acetate) injection
E. Vaginal misoprostol

56-3. A 41-year-old woman presents to the ED after alleged sexual assault by an ex-boyfriend. She has a past medical history significant for diabetes mellitus, endometriosis, and motor vehicle accident. Her allergies include penicillin and seafood, both of which cause anaphylaxis. She does not drink or use illicit drugs, but smokes one pack per day of cigarettes. She appears to be in no apparent distress and has an unremarkable examination. After a sexual assault evidence collection kit is performed, you provide her with STI prophylaxis. Which of the following medications would be appropriate?

A. Ceftriaxone 125 mg IM × 1 for *Neisseria gonorrhoeae*
B. Azithromycin 1 g PO × 1 for *Chlamydia trachomatis*
C. Azithromycin 2 g PO × 1 for HIV
D. Ofloxacin 400 mg PO × 1 for HIV
E. Ciprofloxacin 500 mg PO × 1 for hepatitis B

56-4. A 22-year-old woman is seen in the ED after a possible sexual assault by an unknown assailant that occurred the night before at a college fraternity party. She is a second-year medical student and says she has recently been learning about sexually transmitted infections; she is extremely anxious about possible infections. Which of the following is she still at risk for contracting if she takes appropriate prophylactic medications?

A. *Chlamydia trachomatis*
B. *Neisseria gonorrhoeae*
C. HIV
D. Hepatitis B
E. Hepatitis C

ANSWERS

56-1. D. 56-2. A. The postcoital form of contraception, named the Yuzpe method after its founder, consists most commonly of two Ovral pills given in two doses 12 hours apart. It has been shown to be effective up to 72 hours after intercourse, with decreased efficacy thereafter. Ovral is a combination of ethinyl estradiol 50 μg and norgestrel 0.5 mg. Most contraceptive pills today vary between 20 μg and 35 μg of ethinyl estradiol and may have a different progestin; therefore, equivalent postcoital dosing would require three to five pills given 12 hours apart. An IUD placed postcoitally will work as contraception (though not commonly used in the United States). In the setting of possible exposure to STIs, however, this is not a good option because of the risk of PID. Vaginal misoprostol can be used as an abortifacient early in pregnancy, but it is not effective in the periconceptual period.

56-3. B. Given the potential cross-reactivity between cephalosporins and penicillin, it is not wise to give a cephalosporin to this patient, who has a history of anaphylaxis to penicillin. Ceftriaxone 125 mg IM is typically used to cover *Neisseria gonorrhoeae*, but alternatives include one-time doses of ofloxacin 400 mg PO or ciprofloxacin 500 mg PO. Azithromycin 1 g PO single dose or doxycycline 100 mg BID for 7 days effectively covers *Chlamydia trachomatis*. HIV prophylaxis is also offered if the assailant is unknown or if it was an otherwise high-risk exposure. A typical regimen includes zidovudine (AZT) 300 mg PO BID for 28 days and lamivudine (Epivir) 150 mg PO BID for 28 days. An antiemetic is typically prescribed with zidovudine and lamivudine because these medications commonly cause nausea and vomiting.

56-4. E. Hepatitis C is transmitted sexually, vertically, and through exposure to blood products. Unfortunately, there is no specific medication to prevent its transmission other than barrier methods (e.g., condoms). HIV, chlamydia, and gonorrhea can all be prevented with prophylactic antivirals and antibiotics, as discussed previously. The recommendation for hepatitis B virus prophylaxis for a nonimmunized person is to initiate the first immunization and follow-up for 2-month and 6-month immunizations. Hepatitis B immune globulin is only recommended if the assailant is known to have acute or chronic hepatitis B infection.

SUGGESTED ADDITIONAL READINGS

Cantu M, Coppola M, Lindner AJ. Evaluation and management of the sexually assaulted woman. Emerg Med Clim North Am 2003;21:737–750.

Mein JK, Palmer CM, Shand MC, et al. Management of acute adult sexual assault. Med J Aust 2003;178:226–230.

Patel M, Minshall L. Management of sexual assault. Emerg Med Clin North Am 2001;19:817–831.

Wiese M, Armitage C, Delaforce J, et al. Emergency care for complainants of sexual assault. J R Soc Med 2005;98:49–53.

Acute Lower Abdominal Pain in a Young Woman

CC: 19-year-old woman with 3 hours of severe RLQ pain

HPI: A.P. is a 19-year-old woman who reports pain in her right lower abdomen that started earlier in the day and has become increasingly more severe. She developed nausea shortly after the pain began and vomited twice before arriving to the ED. She has never had similar pain in the past. She has not eaten since lunch and is not hungry. She denies fever, chills, dysuria, back pain, diarrhea, constipation, or unusual vaginal discharge.

PMHx: None

Meds: None

ALL: NKDA

**OB/
GynHx:** G_0; LMP 3 weeks ago; regular menses every 28 days; no STIs; sexually active, uses condoms for contraception

VS: Temp 37.2°C (99.0°F), HR 98, BP 124/78, RR 16, Sao_2 99% on RA

PE: *General:* Appears uncomfortable; lying flat on her back; very still on the gurney. *Abd:* Nondistended; diffusely tender, worse in RLQ; localized rebound in RLQ. *GU:* No vaginal discharge seen. *BME:* Uterus normal size; tenderness in RLQ with manipulation of cervix and uterus; difficult to assess adnexa because of pain. *Rectal:* Tender with palpation; guaiac-negative.

Labs: WBC 10.1 k/mm³, 75% polys, Hct 38.3%, urinalysis and urine hCG negative

THOUGHT QUESTIONS

- What is the initial management for this patient?
- What are the chief diagnoses to be considered in this woman?
- Which lab test provides a branch point for different gynecologic pathologies?
- Which imaging study would be most helpful in this patient?

Immediate Actions:
Establish IV access; send blood for CBC with diff, basic chemistries, LFTs, lipase, and blood-bank sample; get urinalysis and urine hCG; start NS 1 liter over 1 hour.

Discussion:
It is useful to think of the differential diagnosis by system and consider more serious etiologies first (Table 57-1). Abdominal pathology includes both inflammatory processes (e.g., acute appendicitis, inflammatory bowel disease, diverticulitis, mesenteric adenitis) and structural processes (e.g., incarcerated hernia, small-bowel obstruction). Of these conditions, appendicitis is the most likely, given the location of pain, short duration of symptoms, and lack of clinical evidence for obstruction. Urologic etiologies include UTI and ureteral stone. Lack of urinary symptoms, lack of hematuria, and presence of a normal urinalysis will for the most part exclude these possibilities. Pelvic pathology includes ruptured ectopic pregnancy, ovarian torsion, PID or tubo-ovarian abscess (TOA), ruptured corpus luteum cyst, and endometriosis. A negative urine βhCG will exclude ectopic pregnancy. The next most concerning possibility is ovarian torsion, which is typically acute in onset, sometimes waxing and waning if intermittent, and often associated with nausea and vomiting. PID and TOA are typically associated with signs of infection, including fever, chills, and malodorous vaginal discharge, although the onset of symptoms may be acute in the setting of TOA rupture.

(Continued)

TABLE 57-1 Serious Causes for Acute Lower Abdominal Pain in Young Women

	Symptoms and History	Exam
Appendicitis	Generalized, then localized RLQ; onset <48 hr; low-grade fever; nausea; anorexia	RLQ tender, ± peritoneal; adnexal or cervical tenderness not typical
Ectopic pregnancy	Severe, sharp, lateral pelvic pain; vaginal spotting; missed period; risk factors (previous ectopic pregnancy, infertility, IUD, PID)	Variable, ± adnexal mass and CMT, sometimes peritoneal; high suspicion if hCG-positive
Ovarian torsion	Acute, severe, lateral pelvic pain; onset <48 hr; nausea and vomiting	Exquisite adnexal and cervical tenderness, focal peritonitis
PID/TOA	PID pain bilateral, dyspareunia, subacute onset, fever, vaginal discharge	Cervical tenderness, pus from os, adnexa full and tender if TOA, often bilateral low abdominal tenderness
Ruptured corpus luteum cyst	Acute, lateral pelvic pain; abrupt onset; dizziness	Hypotension, mild abdominal distention, adnexal tenderness, often peritonitis, hemoperitoneum by bedside ultrasound

A ruptured corpus luteum cyst may occur late in the menstrual cycle or early in pregnancy and causes abrupt lateral abdominal pain that may be associated with significant hemoperitoneum with hypotension and peritonitis.

It is often difficult to decide whether to do a CT scan or a pelvic ultrasound in a woman with low abdominal pain. A CT scan is ideal for identifying abdominal pathology, particularly appendicitis, but it is suboptimal for evaluating the uterus, adnexae, and ovaries. A pelvic ultrasound is very useful for evaluating ovarian cysts or masses (e.g., simple cysts, hemorrhagic cysts, endometriomas, ovarian tumors), ovarian blood flow, TOAs, pelvic free fluid (i.e., ruptured ovarian cyst), and uterine abnormalities (e.g., fibroids). Often, the decision of whether to obtain a CT scan or ultrasound is

(Continued)

based on the pelvic exam. Significant adnexal tenderness or cervical motion tenderness (CMT) argues for a pelvic ultrasound because of the higher likelihood of pelvic pathology. It is important to remember, however, that an elongated appendix often lies in the pelvis and when inflamed can cause significant pelvic pain and adnexal tenderness as well.

CASE CONTINUED

Because of her significant adnexal tenderness, an ultrasound is obtained, which shows a 6-cm right ovarian mass (Figure 57-1). Color-flow Doppler shows decreased blood flow to the ovary consistent with ovarian torsion. She receives morphine 6 mg IV for pain relief, and gynecology is consulted.

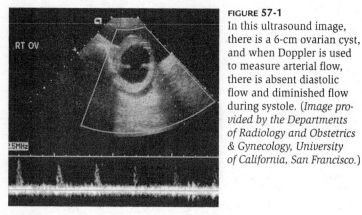

FIGURE 57-1
In this ultrasound image, there is a 6-cm ovarian cyst, and when Doppler is used to measure arterial flow, there is absent diastolic flow and diminished flow during systole. (*Image provided by the Departments of Radiology and Obstetrics & Gynecology, University of California, San Francisco.*)

QUESTIONS

57-1. What is the most appropriate management for this woman with ovarian torsion?
A. Immediate laparoscopic surgery
B. Immediate exploratory laparotomy
C. Admit to gynecology for observation
D. IV antibiotics and operate later once inflammation has abated
E. Discharge and arrange follow-up ultrasound in 2 weeks

57-2. Another young woman presents in a similar fashion to the case presented above, but has a fever of 38.4°C (101.1°F) and an elevated WBC count to 17,000/mm³. A CT scan is obtained, which shows a normal appendix but a right adnexal mass. What is the most likely diagnosis?
A. Fitz-Hugh-Curtis syndrome
B. Tubo-ovarian abscess
C. Appendicitis
D. Ruptured ovarian cyst
E. Diverticulitis

57-3. A 32-year-old woman presents to the ED with severe right lower quadrant pain that suddenly started about an hour ago. She is visibly uncomfortable and vomits twice. She has right pelvic tenderness well below McBurney's point, and pelvic exam reveals exquisite right adnexal tenderness. You suspect ovarian torsion. Which of the following is the most common ovarian neoplasm to undergo torsion?
A. Endometrioid tumor
B. Benign cystic teratoma
C. Cystadenocarcinoma
D. Granulosa cell tumor
E. Corpus luteum

57-4. A 27-year-old woman presents with sudden acute pelvic pain and signs of hypovolemia. What is the most likely cause?
A. Ruptured endometrioma
B. Ruptured cystic teratoma
C. Ruptured corpus luteum cyst
D. Ruptured ovarian follicle
E. Ovarian torsion

ANSWERS

57-1. A. Similar to testicular torsion, ovarian torsion is a diagnosis that needs to be made quickly and operated upon quickly to save the function of the affected organ. Typically a laparoscopic approach is taken. Once the affected ovary is identified, it can be mechanically detorsed. If it still appears to be viable, it is left in place. If the torsion is associated with an ovarian cyst, the cyst is resected to prevent recurrence. Exploratory laparotomy is not unreasonable; however, it is more invasive and associated with greater morbidity than the laparoscopic approach. The other three options, all of which involve waiting, are unacceptable.

57-2. B. In a woman with an elevated temperature and white blood cell count with an adnexal mass, the diagnosis is tubo-ovarian abscess, a complication of PID. Currently, TOAs are treated with aggressive antibiotic therapy; however, if they do not respond to therapy, surgical resection may be required. Fitz-Hugh-Curtis, another sequelae of PID, is a perihepatitis that develops when the pelvic infection spreads throughout the abdomen. A ruptured ovarian cyst is less likely to give both an elevated WBC count and a fever. Missed appendicitis is less likely, given that the sensitivity of CT scan is approximately 95% for acute appendicitis.

57-3. B. Although the corpus luteum is the most likely cyst to undergo torsion, it is not considered a neoplasm. **The most common neoplasm to undergo torsion is the benign cystic teratoma or dermoid cyst. One reason why these benign germ cell tumors may be seen in a higher number of cases of torsion is that they grow slowly and can be in the ovary for years.**

57-4. C. The ruptured corpus luteum cyst can lead to a large-volume hemoperitoneum, hypovolemia, and shock. Thus, a patient who presents in this fashion should receive aggressive fluid resuscitation. If the patient is hemodynamically stable, an ultrasound can be obtained in an attempt to clarify the diagnosis. However, preparations should be in place for the patient to go directly to the OR in case her condition changes. An open rather than laparoscopic approach is often favored because it allows faster evacuation of clot and hemostasis. If the patient is hemodynamically stable, though, even with significant hemoperitoneum, laparoscopy is not unreasonable.

SUGGESTED ADDITIONAL READINGS

Cass DL. Ovarian torsion. Semin Pediatr Surg 2005;14:86–92.

Lambert MJ, Villa M. Gynecologic ultrasound in emergency medicine. Emerg Med Clin North Am 2004;22:683–696.

Lawrence LL. Unusual presentations in obstetrics and gynecology. Emerg Med Clin North Am 2003;21:649–665.

Webb EM, Green GE, Scoutt LM. Adnexal mass with pelvic pain. Radiol Clin North Am 2004;42:329–348.

Abdominal Pain and Vaginal Odor

CC: 20-year-old woman with abdominal pain and vaginal odor

HPI: P.P. is a 20-year-old woman who began having pain in her lower abdomen 4 days ago, which has gradually worsened. She describes the pain as dull, constant, worse on the right but also present on the left. She has had no changes in her bowel habits and has a good appetite. She denies fever, chills, nausea, vomiting, or dysuria. She also denies unusual vaginal discharge or bleeding, but has noted an abnormal vaginal or urine odor. Her last menstrual period was 10 days ago and had normal flow and duration.

PMHx: None

Meds: OCPs

ALL: NKDA

OB/ GynHx: TAB at 9 weeks' gestation 2 years ago, without complications; regular cycles; no STIs; sexually active with new partner; uses OCPs

SHx: No alcohol, drugs, or tobacco

VS: Temp 38.2°C (100.8°F), HR 106, BP 107/68, RR 16, Sao$_2$ 99% on RA

PE: *General:* Uncomfortable, ill-appearing; mild pallor. *HEENT:* Nonicteric; oropharynx moist. *Neck:* Supple. *CV:* S$_1$, S$_2$; regular; mildly tachycardic; no murmurs. *Chest:* Clear bilaterally. *Abd:* Nondistended; diffusely tender, worse in RLQ; mild diffuse rebound tenderness; decreased bowel sounds. *GU:* No external, vaginal, or cervical lesions; os closed; mild creamy, malodorous discharge. *BME:* Marked CMT; uterus normal size, mildly tender to palpation; tenderness in both adnexae (R > L); no appreciable adnexal masses.

Labs: WBC 15.9 k/mm^3, 90% neutrophils, Hct 42.6%, urine hCG negative, urinalysis 0–2 WBCs/hpf, 0–2 RBCs/hpf

THOUGHT QUESTIONS

- What are emergent and nonemergent causes for pelvic pain?
- What is the most likely etiology in this woman?
- How would the presence of an adnexal mass change your management?

Immediate Actions:
Establish IV access; send blood for CBC with differential, basic chemistries, PT/PTT, blood-bank sample; send for urinalysis and urine hCG; send cervical swab for GC and *Chlamydia;* start NS 1 liter over 1 hour; administer cefotetan 2 g IV, doxycycline 100 mg IV.

Discussion:
It is useful to differentiate between acute and chronic pelvic pain. Etiologies for acute pelvic pain tend to be more worrisome and include those listed in Case 57, including appendicitis, ectopic pregnancy, ovarian torsion, TOA, and ruptured corpus luteum cyst. A subacute or gradual onset of pelvic pain in a woman who is hemodynamically stable is less worrisome; however, certain pelvic pathology can lead to long-term sequelae such as infertility and chronic pelvic pain. Therefore, even though definitive diagnosis is not always possible in the ED, it is important that certain etiologies are excluded and that patients have good follow-up with a gynecologist. Other etiologies for pelvic pain include ovarian cysts, mittelschmerz, endometriosis, dysmenorrhea, uterine fibroids, PID, endometritis, and cervicitis.

(*Continued*)

Ovarian cysts are the most common cause of noninfectious pelvic pain, with follicular cysts being the most common type. These cysts may cause chronic pelvic aching as they enlarge or acute exacerbation of pain if they rupture their contents into the peritoneum. Unruptured follicular cysts will typically regress over several months. Their diagnosis in the ED is by ultrasound; treatment should be symptomatic (e.g., NSAIDs for pain), with gynecologic follow-up arranged. A ruptured follicular cyst can cause peritoneal irritation and more significant pain. A short period of observation, monitoring of hemodynamic status, and parenteral narcotics may be warranted.

Many women suffer from dysmenorrhea, which is pain associated with menses. Dysmenorrhea can be primary (associated with menarche) or secondary (associated with infection, fibroids, pelvic adhesions, endometriosis). An infectious etiology is suspected in this patient given her low-grade fever, malodorous vaginal discharge, and toxic appearance. The primary concern is for PID with or without associated TOA. Major criteria for the diagnosis of PID include abdominal, adnexal, and cervical motion tenderness, all of which this patient has. Minor criteria include fever, elevated WBC count or ESR, and malodorous vaginal discharge; these help to support the diagnosis. Imaging is warranted if there is suspicion for an alternative diagnosis (e.g., appendicitis, ovarian torsion) or if TOA is a possibility (e.g., adnexal fullness or tenderness). PID is treated with a second- or third-generation cephalosporin and doxycycline. A stable, nontoxic patient who is able to tolerate oral medications can be treated as an outpatient. Otherwise, admission for IV antibiotics is necessary.

 CASE CONTINUED

The patient feels a little better with IV hydration. Given that she has adnexal tenderness (more on the right), an ultrasound is obtained to rule out TOA; it shows no ovarian or adnexal masses and no pelvic free fluid. A presumptive diagnosis of PID is made based on the presence of low abdominal pain, bilateral adnexal tenderness, and cervical motion tenderness in the presence of low-grade fever, leukocytosis, and vaginal discharge. Given her mildly toxic appearance, she is admitted to the observation unit for IV antibiotics, hydration, and gynecologic consultation.

QUESTIONS

58-1. A patient with an ultrasound-confirmed TOA fails to improve after 2 days of IV cefotetan and doxycycline. What is the appropriate next management step for this patient?
A. Expand antibiotic coverage with ampicillin, gentamicin, and clindamycin
B. Laparoscopy for confirmation of the diagnosis
C. Laparotomy with unilateral salpingo-oophorectomy
D. Laparotomy with hysterectomy and bilateral salpingo-oophorectomy
E. Continue with a longer course of cefotetan and doxycycline

58-2. A 30-year-old prostitute is seen in the emergency department for low abdominal pain, fever, and vaginal discharge. On examination, she has bilateral low abdominal tenderness to palpation, cervical motion tenderness, and bilateral adnexal tenderness. She also has a creamy, thick vaginal discharge. Of the following, which is the most common sequela of her condition?
A. Fitz-Hugh-Curtis syndrome
B. Infertility
C. Toxic shock syndrome
D. Bacterial vaginosis
E. Urinary tract infection

58-3. A 17-year-old woman complains of an abnormal vaginal discharge. A mucopurulent discharge is seen on speculum examination, and a first-stream urine test is positive for *Chlamydia*. What is appropriate treatment for this woman?
A. Dicloxacillin 250 mg QID for 10 days
B. Cephalexin (Keflex) 500 mg QID for 7 days
C. Metronidazole (Flagyl) 750 mg PO single dose
D. Azithromycin 1 g PO single dose plus ceftriaxone 125 mg IM single dose
E. Trimethoprim/sulfamethoxazole (Bactrim) one tablet BID for 14 days

58-4. A 42-year-old female prostitute presents to the ED with complaint of malodorous vaginal discharge. She has a history of several STIs in the past, for which she has taken antibiotics each time. On examination, she is febrile, and has moderate cervical motion tenderness along with a thick, mucopurulent discharge. Which of the following has been shown to be protective against her condition?

A. IUD use
B. Oral contraceptive use
C. Weekly douching with dilute vinegar solution
D. Cigarette smoking
E. Multiple sexual partners

ANSWERS

58-1. A. If the first line of antibiotics fails, the appropriate treatment is to expand coverage to triple antibiotic therapy. Persistent PID can lead to tubo-ovarian abscesses (TOAs) or tubo-ovarian complexes (TOCs). Unlike TOAs, TOCs are pelvic adnexal infections that are not walled off and thus may be more responsive to antibiotic therapy. Finding an adnexal mass on exam should raise concern for a TOA or TOC. A pelvic ultrasound will confirm the diagnosis. Laparotomy and adnexal surgery is reserved for TOAs that are unresponsive to triple antibiotic therapy or that are grossly ruptured. Usually a unilateral salpingectomy is performed for unilateral TOAs. For bilateral TOAs, bilateral salpingectomy or even a concomitant total abdominal hysterectomy may be necessary. Continuing on the same antibiotics when there has been no improvement is inappropriate.

58-2. B. The two most common sequelae of PID are infertility (estimated to occur in 20% of all PID patients) and ectopic pregnancy (10-fold increased risk with history of PID). Fitz-Hugh-Curtis syndrome, an ascending perihepatitis, is an uncommon complication of PID. Toxic shock syndrome (TSS) occurs rarely. It has been associated with menstruation and tampon use and with postpartum and postabortion endometritis. However, neither TSS nor bacterial vaginosis are sequelae of PID.

58-3. D. Both gonorrhea and *Chlamydia* can cause a mucopurulent discharge. Currently, a first-stream urine test is only available for *Chlamydia*. **The treatment for chlamydial cervicitis is doxycycline 100 mg PO BID for 7 days or azithromycin 1 g PO single dose. This patient should also be treated presumptively for gonorrhea with ceftriaxone 125 mg IM single dose.**

58-4. B. This woman has PID. Risk factors for PID include young age, multiple sexual partners, being unmarried, recent history of douching, and cigarette smoking. IUDs have been considered a risk factor for PID as well. With current IUDs, however, it seems this risk only exists around the time of placement. **OCPs have been found to be protective against PID. The mechanism is thought to involve alterations in cervical mucus.** The best protection against PID is provided by barrier contraceptives.

 SUGGESTED ADDITIONAL READINGS

McKinzie J. Sexually transmitted diseases. Emerg Med Clin North Am 2001;19:723–743.

Ross J. Pelvic inflammatory disease. Clin Evid 2005;(13):2031–2037.

Zeger W, Holt K. Gynecologic infections. Emerg Med Clin North Am 2003;21:613–648.

Heavy Vaginal Bleeding

CC: 45-year-old woman with heavy vaginal bleeding

HPI: V.B. states that she is currently completing a menstrual period complicated by heavy bleeding requiring up to 30 pads a day for a 5-day period and now down to 5 pads a day. In total, she has been bleeding for 12 days. Overall, she has had somewhat regular 28- to 34-day cycles, bleeding for 5 to 6 days, using 5 to 6 pads a day. During the past year her periods have become increasingly heavier. She did miss a period 3 months ago, with an ensuing period that was quite heavy. She denies spotting between her menses. She has a history of significant cramping and breast tenderness with her menses, but states that these complaints have gotten better over the past year. She additionally complains of dizziness when she stands but has no nausea or vomiting. She denies having any hot flashes, vaginal dryness, night sweats, or changes in weight over the past 6 months. She further denies fevers, chills, nausea, vomiting, abdominal pain, dysuria, or diarrhea.

PMHx: Hypothyroidism

Meds: Synthroid 0.05 mg PO QD

ALL: NKDA

**OB/
GynHx:** Normal PAP smears, last 6 months ago; SAB × 2; sexually active with husband; wishes to maintain fertility

SHx: No tobacco, alcohol, or drugs; denies domestic violence

VS: Temp 37.0°C (98.6°F), HR 96, BP 107/68, RR 16, Sao$_2$ 99% on RA

PE: *General:* No acute distress; pale. *HEENT:* Nonicteric; pale conjunctivae; oropharynx moist. *CV:* S$_1$, S$_2$; regular; no murmurs. *Chest:* Clear bilaterally. *Abd:* Soft, nontender, nondistended. *Extr:* Warm; well-perfused; delayed capillary refill. *GU:* No vulvar lesions; pink, moist mucous membranes; normal vaginal mucosa, blood clots in vault; cervical os closed with small amount of dark blood oozing. *BME:* Enlarged uterus, 12-week size, no adnexal masses or tenderness.

Labs: WBC 6,000/mm^3, Hct 26.0%, plt 300,000/mm^3, urine hCG negative

THOUGHT QUESTIONS

- What is the initial management for this patient?
- What is the difference between menorrhagia, metror-rhagia, and menometrorrhagia?
- What are the two main phases of the menstrual cycle, and which hormones predominate?
- What is the most common cause of dysfunctional uterine bleeding?

Immediate Actions:
Establish large-bore IV; send blood for CBC, basic chemistries, PT/PTT; type and crossmatch 2 units of PRBCs; administer 2 liters NS over 2 hours; get urinalysis and urine hCG.

Discussion:
Menorrhagia is bleeding at the time of menses that is heavy or prolonged. Metrorrhagia is bleeding between menses. Menometrorrhagia is a combination of the two (i.e., menses that are heavy or prolonged with occasional intermenstrual bleeding). The menstrual cycle consists of the follicular (proliferative) phase and luteal (secretory) phase (Figure 59-1). The follicular phase starts on the first day of menses and continues until ovulation. During this phase, endometrial glands proliferate under the influence of estrogen, primarily estradiol. This phase is characterized by secretion of estrogen by the ovaries, variable length, low basal body temperature, development of ovarian follicles, and vascular growth of the endometrium. The luteal phase begins with ovulation and continues through the onset of menses. Although estrogen is still present during the luteal phase, progesterone is responsible

(Continued)

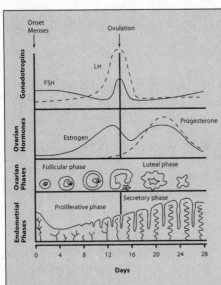

FIGURE 59-1
Hormonal, ovarian, and endometrial changes throughout the normal menstrual cycle. (*Illustration by Shawn Girsberger Graphic Design.*)

for endometrial secretion, which prepares the endometrium for implantation. This phase is characterized by constant duration (usually 14 days), elevated body temperature, formation of the corpus luteum (secretes both progesterone and estrogen), and endometrial gland secretion, stromal edema, and a decidual reaction. In the absence of fertilization and maintenance of the corpus luteum by hCG, both estrogen and progesterone levels fall, causing coiling and constriction of the endometrial arteries. As a result, the endometrial tissue undergoes ischemia and sloughing (i.e., menses).

Dysfunctional uterine bleeding (DUB) is any abnormality in the regular bleeding pattern of the menstrual cycle, as described by the terms menorrhagia, metrorrhagia, and menometrorrhagia. Anovulation is the cause of 90% of DUB. Anovulation, or the failure of the ovary to excrete an ovum, prevents luteinization from occurring, thus preventing progesterone synthesis. In the absence of progesterone, the endometrium continues to proliferate unchecked (endometrial hyperplasia) until it outgrows its blood supply and begins to slough (i.e., abnormal spotting or bleeding). Other causes for DUB include reproductive tract pathology (e.g., endometritis, endometrial polyps, uterine fibroids, endometrial carcinoma), exogenous estrogens (e.g., estrogen supplements, vaginal creams, OCPs), endocrine axis dysfunction (e.g., pituitary adenoma), bleeding disorders (e.g., von Willebrand's disease, cirrhosis), and trauma (e.g., foreign body, IUD).

CASE CONTINUED

The patient's hematocrit is low; however, she currently has little active bleeding and has no immediate need for a blood transfusion. A pelvic ultrasound is obtained, which shows the presence of a large submucosal uterine fibroid (Figure 59-2) but is otherwise normal. Given that she has recently skipped several periods, she is likely experiencing anovulatory bleeding, exacerbated by her uterine fibroids. The only other potential concern for a woman this age is endometrial cancer and thus whether she warrants a biopsy. This is discussed with her primary gynecologist, who recommends starting progesterone-only therapy (Provera) 10 mg PO QD for 10 days. The patient is discharged with plans for gynecology follow-up.

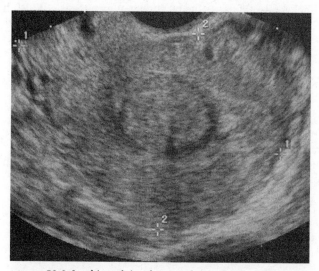

FIGURE 59-2 In this pelvic ultrasound image, the calipers are placed around the enlarged uterus; of note, there is a 2-cm submucosal uterine fibroid in the center of the image. (*Image provided by the Departments of Radiology and Obstetrics & Gynecology, University of California, San Francisco.*)

QUESTIONS

59-1. A 36-year old woman presents with heavy vaginal bleeding for 2 days associated with low abdominal cramps. Her last normal period was about 7 weeks ago. She has a history of irregular periods. What hormone level related to the menstrual cycle would suggest an anovulatory cycle?

   A. Progesterone (day 21) high
   B. Progesterone (day 21) low
   C. Estrogen (day 7) high
   D. Estrogen (day 7) low
   E. FSH low

59-2. A 52-year-old woman presents with irregular menstrual bleeding, hot flashes, and bloating. A urine pregnancy test is negative. She wonders if this is the beginning of menopause. Which hormone abnormality is characteristic of the perimenopausal period?

   A. Elevated estrogen
   B. Elevated progesterone
   C. Decreased LH
   D. Elevated FSH
   E. Decreased GnRH

59-3. A 38-year-old woman is having difficulty conceiving and has been having very heavy menstrual periods. CBC and PT/PTT are normal. An ultrasound shows several large submucosal uterine fibroids. What is the best treatment modality for the reduction or removal of submucosal uterine fibroids?

   A. Oral contraceptive pills
   B. Hysteroscopic resection
   C. D&C
   D. Abdominal myomectomy
   E. Estrogen replacement

59-4. A 45-year-old woman presents with heavy vaginal bleeding and cramping. She has had a week of bleeding during which she has gone through 15 to 20 pads a day. Her last menstrual period was 8 weeks ago. Her pelvic exam is unremarkable except for dark blood in the vault and a small amount coming through the os. Her vital signs are normal and her hematocrit is 32%. Which of the following may help if she is perimenopausal, but would be ineffective for anovulatory bleeding?
- A. Low-dose combination oral contraceptive pills
- B. Cyclic oral progesterone
- C. Endometrial ablation
- D. Continuous hormone replacement therapy
- E. The progestin-only contraceptive pill

ANSWERS

59-1. B. A review of the menstrual cycle demonstrates that after ovulation, progesterone rises dramatically as the corpus luteum develops during the second half of the menstrual cycle. Progesterone makes the endometrium more glandular and secretory in anticipation of possible ovum implantation. **If ovulation does not occur, progesterone levels remain low.** Estrogen levels are less reliable in predicting the presence of an anovulatory cycle because levels are less associated with ovulation.

59-2. D. Perimenopausal women have dramatically elevated levels of FSH. Menopause is characterized by the decreased responsiveness of the remaining ovarian follicles to FSH, decreased maturation of follicles, and decreased excretion of estrogens. A feedback mechanism causes increased levels of GnRH in the hypothalamus, which in turn stimulates the production of FSH in the pituitary gland. Because follicle maturation does not occur, follicular LH receptors do not properly develop, and thus luteinization cannot occur. Abnormal LH levels are not a reliable indicator of menopause.

59-3. B. Submucosal fibroids that cause infertility or menorrhagia are commonly resected. This can be performed via hysteroscopy or abdominal myomectomy. Hysteroscopy is less invasive and utilizes an electrocautery loop to resect the fibroid in a piecemeal fashion. The only hormonal treatment effective for fibroids is leuprolide (Lupron), a GnRH agonist. The continuous action of GnRH interrupts its usual physiologic pulsatile secretion, leading to down-regulation of the GnRH receptors. This essentially results in a state similar to menopause, which may reduce the size of the fibroid but not eradicate it. D&C is not usually adequate to resect submucosal fibroids.

59-4. D. Menorrhagia, which also falls under the category of dysfunctional uterine bleeding, can be treated in many ways, both surgically and medically. Expectant management is reasonable if the occurrence is infrequent. However, a more chronic anovulatory state (i.e., an estrogen-dominant state) can put a patient at risk for developing abnormal hyperplasia or carcinoma; thus, progesterone therapy is recommended. Progesterone therapy can include a combination OCP (usually low dose in a woman aged 45), progestin-only pill, or oral progesterone. **Continuous hormonal therapy may help perimenopausal patients with symptoms; however, it is not particularly effective in the setting of anovulatory bleeding.**

 SUGGESTED ADDITIONAL READINGS

Bryan S. Abnormal vaginal bleeding. Emerg Med (Fremantle) 2003;15:215–218.

Daniels RV, McCuskey C. Abnormal vaginal bleeding in the nonpregnant patient. Emerg Med Clin North Am 2003;21:751–772.

Dubinsky TJ. Value of sonography in the diagnosis of abnormal vaginal bleeding. J Clin Ultrasound 2004;32:348–353.

Farrell E. Dysfunctional uterine bleeding. Aust Fam Physician 2004;33:906–908.

Left Flank Pain

CC: 45-year-old man presents with left flank pain

HPI: F.P. is a 45-year-old man who presents to the ED complaining of occasional "twinges" in the left flank for the past few weeks, approximately once every 2 to 4 days. Today he developed left flank pain that gradually worsened over 3 hours. The pain is sharp, constant, and comes in waves of severe intensity during which he feels the need to move around. The pain radiates into his left groin and he can't find a position that is comfortable. The pain is associated with nausea, but he has not vomited. He has no fever, chills, dysuria, hematuria, frequency, hesitancy, or abdominal pain.

PMHx: Right shoulder surgery

Meds: None

ALL: Amoxicillin

VS: Temp 35.6°C (96.1°F), HR 96, BP 182/93, RR 16, Sao$_2$ 98% on RA

PE: *General:* Healthy-appearing man writhing in pain holding his left side. *HEENT:* Oropharynx is moist. *CV:* S$_1$, S$_2$; regular rate without murmurs; pulses normal and equal bilaterally. *Chest:* Lungs clear bilaterally; no respiratory distress. *Abd:* Soft, nontender, nondistended; bowel sounds present; left flank moderately tender; no bruits or pulsatile masses. *Back:* CVA tenderness on left. *GU:* Normal inspection; nontender testicles; no hernias. *Rectal:* Heme-negative stool; nontender prostate; normal tone. *Skin:* Warm, dry; no rashes. *Neuro:* Alert and oriented.

THOUGHT QUESTIONS

- What is the initial management for this patient?
- What is the differential diagnosis for flank pain?

- Which tests can be useful for narrowing the differential diagnosis?
- Which patients with renal colic can be discharged home and which should be admitted?

Immediate Actions:
Establish an 18-gauge IV and send a CBC, chem 7, and urinalysis; start a 1-liter NS bolus; give ketorolac (Toradol) 30 mg IV and then morphine 2 to 4 mg every 30 minutes if the pain persists.

Discussion:
Ruptured abdominal aortic aneurysm and aortic dissection must be considered in any patient with severe back or flank pain, especially in elderly patients with cardiovascular risk factors and in patients who present with shock. Flank pain is more commonly associated with renal pathology, typically renal calculi or pyelonephritis. Certain abdominal pathology, such as pancreatitis, perforated duodenal ulcer, or retrocecal appendicitis, can occasionally cause back or flank discomfort. Pelvic pathology may, in addition to pelvic pain, also cause low back pain, especially pelvic inflammatory disease, ruptured ovarian cyst, or ectopic pregnancy. Obtaining a urine hCG is important in all women with flank pain. Renal calculus is the most common etiology in a young patient with sudden onset of sharp flank pain radiating to the groin without symptoms of UTI. A urinalysis is most helpful in making this diagnosis, which will show microscopic hematuria in over 90% of patients with a ureteral calculus. A helical CT scan of the ureter without contrast is typically used to assess stone size and location, ureteral obstruction, and hydronephrosis. An added advantage of CT scan over other imaging modalities is that it can assess other organ systems (e.g., aorta, pancreas, bowel) when the diagnosis of renal calculus is not certain. Intravenous pyelogram, used more commonly before the advent of helical CT scan, can assess hydronephrosis and the degree of functional obstruction, but gives no information regarding surrounding organs. A quick bedside ultrasound is also a good way to diagnose hydronephrosis, but cannot detect a stone. In patients with known renal calculi, an abdominal x-ray can be useful in confirming a ureteral stone, 90% of which are radiopaque.

(Continued)

Patients with ureteral stones less than 5 mm in diameter with adequate pain control can be discharged home with oral analgesics and instructed to drink plenty of fluids, run all urine through a strainer to catch passed stones, and follow up with an urologist within 7 days. Urology should be consulted in the ED if the stone is greater than 5 mm because more than half of these will not pass spontaneously. Patients who have underlying structural abnormalities, concomitant stone with UTI, other significant comorbidities, pain uncontrolled by oral analgesics, or intractable emesis require urologic consultation and hospitalization.

 CASE CONTINUED

The patient is given 2 liters IV NS, Toradol 30 mg IV, morphine 4 mg IV, and metoclopramide (Reglan) 10 mg IV for nausea; this provides adequate pain relief. His CBC and serum electrolytes are normal. Urine sediment shows 0 WBCs/hpf, 25 to 30 RBCs/hpf, and 1+ bacteria. Ureter CT reveals a 10-mm stone in the proximal left ureter with hydronephrosis and perinephric stranding (hyperdense strands in the fat tissue surrounding the kidney on CT scan, which is indicative of inflammation and is a common finding with ureteral obstruction). The patient is taken to the OR for cystourethroscopy, urethral dilatation, and basket extraction of the stone. Afterwards, the patient is admitted to urology for rehydration and observation.

 QUESTIONS

60-1. A 31-year-old man presents to the ED with a single episode of painful hematuria this morning. He has no abdominal, flank, or testicular pain. He denies fever, chills, nausea, vomiting, diarrhea, or recent illness. Which of the following is the most likely cause of this patient's symptoms?

    A. Urinary tract infection
    B. Neoplasm
    C. Nephrolithiasis
    D. Urethritis
    E. Prostatitis

60-2. Which of the following patients can appropriately be discharged to home?

    A. A 31-year-old man with history of congenital solitary left kidney who has a 1-mm ureteral kidney stone and whose pain is well controlled with ibuprofen and oxycodone.

    B. A 78-year-old woman with history of diabetes and breast cancer, status post chemotherapy 2 weeks prior, who has a 3-mm right sided ureteropelvic junction (UPJ) stone without hydronephrosis or hydroureter.

    C. A 55-year-old woman with history of hysterectomy and bilateral oophorectomy with a 4-mm left sided ureterovesicle junction (UVJ) stone with mild hydronephrosis on the left; she needs oxycodone every 4 to 6 hours as well as ibuprofen every 6 hours in order to control her pain.

    D. A 24-year-old man with no past medical history who has a 2-mm left UPJ stone; he has had several bouts of vomiting and has not been able to hold down any fluids since pain onset.

    E. A 33-year-old woman with no past medical history whose urinalysis shows 5 to 10 RBCs/hpf, 15 to 20 WBCs/hpf, 3+ bacteria, and 2+ leukocyte esterase, and whose CT scan shows a 4-mm right UVJ stone without hydroureter or hydronephrosis

60-3. A 36-year-old man with a history of kidney stones presents to the ED with an acute onset of right flank discomfort with hematuria. He is given intravenous ketorolac (Toradol) with little relief. Given his history of kidney stones, an upright KUB is obtained in order to locate the size and position of a stone; however, no stone is seen on the x-ray. Which of the following types of renal stones is radiolucent (i.e., does not appear on a plain radiograph)?

    A. Calcium phosphate

    B. Struvite

    C. Calcium oxalate

    D. Uric acid

    E. Cystine

60-4. A 36-year-old woman who is 24-weeks pregnant presents to the ED with acute-onset left flank discomfort that radiates to the left lower quadrant. Urinalysis shows 2+ blood without evidence of infection. A fetal monitor shows a FHR of 146. You suspect a kidney stone. In order to minimize radiation exposure you consider an intravenous pyelogram (IVP) over CT scan. Which of the following is an absolute contraindication to IVP?

   A. Elevated creatinine
   B. Pregnancy
   C. Allergy to contrast material
   D. Diabetes mellitus
   E. Solitary kidney

 ANSWERS

60-1. C. Nephrolithiasis is the most likely cause of this patient's symptoms. A subsequent urinalysis showed 2+ blood without white cells, bacteria, or crystals. The patient most likely passed a small stone earlier when he experienced painful urination with hematuria. The least likely diagnosis is neoplasm, based on the patient's age. Neoplasm is important to consider in those with painless hematuria, especially in elderly patients with no other alternative explanation. In addition to renal calculi, urinary tract infection is a common cause of hematuria. Upper urinary tract etiologies of hematuria should also be considered, which include glomerulonephritis, pyelonephritis, and renal vein thrombosis.

60-2. C. Patients with nephrolithiasis who should be hospitalized include those with solitary kidney or other structural abnormalities, concomitant urinary tract infection, intractable vomiting, pain unrelieved by oral analgesics, and significant comorbidities. Patients with stones greater than 5 mm in size should have urology consultation from the ED. The patient in choice A has a structural abnormality, while the patient in choice B has significant comorbidities. The patient in choice D has intractable emesis and therefore will not be able to keep down his pain medications or enough fluids to stay hydrated while at home. The patient in choice E has a concomitant urinary tract infection as evidenced by her urinalysis.

60-3. D. Ninety percent of renal stones are radiopaque, with calcium phosphate and calcium oxalate stones being the most dense. Struvite (magnesium-ammonium-phosphate) stones and cystine stones are less dense but still radiopaque, while **uric acid and matrix**

stones are radiolucent. It is thus important to remember that even though a patient's plain abdominal film does not show a renal stone, the patient may still have one.

60-4. C. Two major contraindications to IVP are allergy to contrast material and renal failure. Patients older than 60 years and patients with renal disease, diabetes, or myeloma are also at risk for contrast-mediated nephrotoxicity. Dehydration, hypotension, hyperuricemia, hypertension, use of diuretics for cardiovascular disease, and recent (within 72 hours) administration of IV contrast dye are additional factors predisposing to radiocontrast-mediated nephrotoxicity. Although ultrasound is preferred over IVP for pregnant patients, a limited IVP can be performed if ultrasound is nondiagnostic.

SUGGESTED ADDITIONAL READINGS

Gillespie RS, Stapleton FB. Nephrolithiasis in children. Pediatr Rev 2004;25:131–139.

Safriel Y, Malhotra A, Sclafani SJ. Hematuria as an indicator for the presence or absence of urinary calculi. Am J Emerg Med 2003; 21:492–493.

Unwin RJ, Capasso G, Robertson WG, et al. A guide to renal stone disease. Practitioner 2005;249:18, 20, 24.

Webber R, Tolley D, Lingeman J. Kidney stones. Clin Evid 2005;(13): 1060–1069.

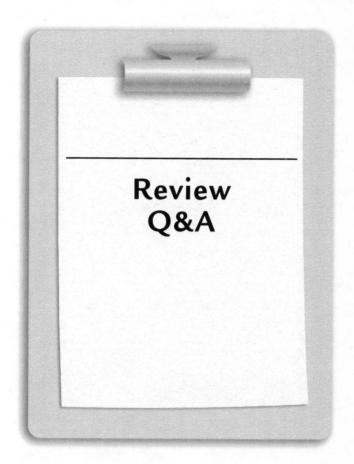

Review
Q&A

Questions

Directions: Each of the numbered items or incomplete statements in this section is followed by answers or by completions of the statement. Select the **one** lettered answer or completion that is best in each case.

1. A 19-year-old woman presents with 5 days of heavy vaginal bleeding and low abdominal cramps during which she is soaking up to 15 pads per day. Her last normal menstrual period was 6 weeks ago, but she has been having irregular periods with varying amounts of flow. She has never been pregnant and denies recent sexual activity. Her vital signs are normal. Her pelvic exam is unremarkable other than blood in the vault. Her hematocrit is 34% and a urine pregnancy test is negative. What is the most likely etiology of her vaginal bleeding?

  A. Normal period
  B. Uterine fibroids
  C. Ovarian cyst
  D. Anovulatory cycle
  E. Completed miscarriage

2. A 20-year-old helmeted hockey player gets knocked unconscious during a rough check into the side boards. His vital signs are HR 80, BP 110/74, RR 18, O$_2$ sat 99%. He is mildly confused but ambulatory. His friends bring him to the ED. Which of the following is appropriate management?

  A. Intubate, c-spine collar, primary and secondary survey, CT scan of head and c-spine.
  B. History and physical, then discharge with "head injury" instructions if patient can be accompanied for 24 hours by a competent adult.
  C. Immediate OR with neurosurgery for intracranial pressure monitor placement.
  D. C-spine collar, primary and secondary survey, head and c-spine CT.
  E. Primary and secondary survey, c-spine collar if any stepoffs palpated during exam, CT scan of head, CT scan of c-spine if stepoffs.

3. A 52-year-old woman presents to the ED with heavy vaginal bleeding that started today. She has soaked through 20 pads and now blood is coming out in a constant stream. She called 911 and arrives to the ED by ambulance. Her vital signs are HR 132, BP 88/46, RR 24, and oxygen saturation 98% on room air. She is placed on high-flow oxygen and two large-bore peripheral IVs are started, and then normal saline is hung. She looks pale but is alert and states that she has low abdominal cramping. Her last normal period was 4 months ago and she was told she is perimenopausal. You immediately begin to pack her vagina, from which blood is actively flowing. You ask the nurse to call for 4 units of type O-positive blood. What medicine should you administer now?

    A. Intravenous dopamine infusion
    B. Intravenous phenylephrine infusion
    C. Intravenous medroxyprogesterone infusion
    D. Intravenous estrogen infusion
    E. Oral medroxyprogesterone medication

4. A 38-year-old MVC patient with a small amount of extra-axial blood seen on initial head CT becomes markedly confused. After intubation, which of the following is appropriate in this patient's management?

    A. Rapid infusion of normal saline
    B. Mannitol 70 g IV
    C. Lasix 40 mg IV
    D. Trendelenberg position
    E. Hypoventilation to a goal pco_2 of 45 mm Hg

5. A 19-year-old woman with a history of ovarian cysts has acute-onset right lower quadrant abdominal pain. Her LMP 2 weeks ago was normal. She denies dysuria or vaginal discharge. She has vomited twice. She arrives in the ED one hour after the onset of pain. Her vital signs are normal. On exam, she has right lower quadrant abdominal tenderness below McBurney's point, with guarding and focal rebound. Pelvic exam reveals a right adnexal mass with tenderness; there is no cervical discharge. Her hCG is negative. What is the most important test to obtain for this patient?

    A. Hematocrit
    B. Urinalysis
    C. CT scan with IV and rectal contrast
    D. Transvaginal sonography with Doppler flow study
    E. Bedside ultrasound

6. A 26-year-old man is stabbed once in the chest. On arrival in the ED, his vital signs are HR 130, BP 80/palp, RR 35, O_2 sat 96%. His exam is notable for JVP of 15 cm, midline trachea, clear breath sounds bilaterally, distant heart sounds, soft nontender abdomen, and thready peripheral pulses. What has likely happened?

    A. Injury to the tracheobronchial tree

    B. Paralysis of the diaphragm

    C. Ruptured viscous

    D. Tension pneumothorax

    E. Cardiac tamponade

7. A 36-year-old G_3P_2 female with a positive home pregnancy test and an LMP 10 weeks ago presents with sudden onset of left lower quadrant abdominal pain. Her vital signs include HR 120, BP 86/46, RR 24, and oxygen saturation of 98% on room air. She is in moderate discomfort and appears pale. She is alert and has a palpable radial pulse. She has a mildly distended abdomen and is tender in the left lower quadrant with guarding. She is placed on oxygen; a 14-gauge antecubital IV is established, and a normal saline bolus is started. What should be the next action?

    A. Do a bedside ultrasound to look for free intraperitoneal fluid.

    B. Check a hematocrit and Rh factor.

    C. Obtain a pelvic ultrasound to look for evidence of an ectopic pregnancy.

    D. Obtain an upright CXR to look for free intraperitoneal air.

    E. Transport her immediately to the OR for exploratory laparotomy.

8. A 32-year-old man is stabbed in the upper chest just above the sternal notch. His vital signs are HR 90, BP 140/85, RR 28, O_2 sat 97% on room air. His exam is notable for a JVP of 6 cm, midline trachea, clear breath sounds bilaterally, subcutaneous crepitus near the skin wound, normal heart sounds, soft nontender abdomen, and 2+ peripheral pulses. Which of the following is this patient most likely to need?

    A. Exploratory laparotomy

    B. Left-sided tube thoracostomy

    C. Esophagoscopy

    D. Pericardiocentesis

    E. ED thoracotomy

9. A 26-year-old woman presents to the ED with right lower quadrant pain and vaginal spotting for one day. Her LMP was 6 weeks ago. Her vital signs are normal. Her exam is remarkable only for tenderness without guarding in the right pelvis. Labs show hematocrit 42%, serum hCG 1,600 mIU/mL, normal urinalysis, and Rh factor positive. A pelvic exam reveals a closed os, a small amount of blood in the vault, and right adnexal tenderness without an obvious mass. An ultrasound shows a normal uterus without an IUP and a 2-cm complex cystic mass in the right fallopian tube. There is no pelvic free fluid seen. What is the most appropriate management?

  A. Laparotomy for salpingectomy and removal of ectopic pregnancy
  B. Laparoscopy for salpingostomy and removal of ectopic pregnancy
  C. Culdocentesis to detect presence of free fluid in the pelvis
  D. Methotrexate therapy and outpatient follow-up
  E. Discharge and follow-up for 48-hour repeat hCG

10. A 33-year-old pregnant woman at 30 weeks gestation sustains a 10-cm leg laceration while on a camping trip. She received routine healthcare as a child growing up in Minnesota. She has no known drug allergies. Her last tetanus booster was 8 years ago. Which of the following is the best choice for her?

  A. No tetanus injections are needed; tetanus is up to date
  B. No tetanus injections should be given until after she delivers the baby
  C. Td
  D. DT
  E. Tetanus immune globulin

11. A 22-year-old G_2P_1 female with a history of therapeutic abortion presents to the ED with vaginal bleeding and low abdominal cramping. She soaked one pad, although did not notice clots or tissue. Her last menstrual period was 7 weeks ago, and she recently tested positive for pregnancy with a home pregnancy kit. Her vital signs are normal. On exam, her abdomen is soft and nontender. The pelvic exam reveals a small amount of dark blood in the vault, a closed cervical os, and a small, nontender uterus without adnexal masses. An ultrasound reveals an intrauterine yolk sac without a fetal pole. What is the diagnosis?

  A. Normal pregnancy
  B. Threatened abortion
  C. Inevitable abortion
  D. Incomplete abortion
  E. Complete abortion

12. A 19-year-old man sustains a 7-cm laceration to his left arm from a frat party brawl that occurred 2 hours earlier. He has a normal distal neurovascular exam. As you prepare to anesthetize the area before repair, he says that he had an allergic reaction to the anesthetic the last time this happened, one month prior. Which of the following is the best way to proceed?
  A. Do not use any anesthetic.
  B. Use local lidocaine.
  C. Use local diphenhydramine.
  D. Use local bupivicaine.
  E. Use general anesthesia in the OR.

13. A 68-year-old man saw his primary care doctor for a fever, difficulty urinating, and dysuria. A urinalysis showed 10 to 20 WBCs/hpf and was positive for nitrites and bacteria. He was sent home with trimethoprim/sulfamethoxazole (Bactrim) one tablet twice daily for 3 days. Five days later he presents to the ED with a fever to 40.1°C (104.2°F), rigors, continued dysuria, and low abdominal, perineal, and back pain. Which test is required to confirm the diagnosis?
  A. Urine culture
  B. Abdominal CT scan with IV and oral contrast
  C. Rectal exam
  D. Scrotal ultrasound
  E. Stool culture

14. A 54-year-old chronic alcoholic with no prior orthopedic injuries is brought in after a witnessed tonic-clonic seizure; there was no fall involved, as he had been lying on the ground prior to the seizure. He is no longer seizing but you notice a deformity on his exam. Which of the following does he likely have?
  A. Anterior shoulder dislocation
  B. Posterior shoulder dislocation
  C. Anterior hip dislocation
  D. Posterior hip dislocation
  E. Knee dislocation

15. A 24-year-old man with no prior medical history presents to the ED with sudden-onset severe right flank discomfort that radiates around to his right testicle. He is pacing and states that he can't find a comfortable position. His vital signs are normal. On exam, his abdomen is nontender, his testicles are nontender and without masses, and he has right flank tenderness. Which test is mandatory in this patient?
   A. CBC with differential
   B. Urinalysis
   C. Ultrasound of kidneys
   D. Testicular ultrasound
   E. KUB

16. A 16-year-old unrestrained male driver is involved in a high-speed head-on MVC during which there is no airbag deployment. EMS reports significant front-end damage to the car, as well as markedly dented dashboard in front of the driver's right knee. The patient complains of severe right hip pain and difficulty with moving the right leg. Which of the following is this patient most likely to also have injured?
   A. Femoral nerve
   B. Femoral artery
   C. Sciatic nerve
   D. Popliteal artery
   E. Iliac artery

17. The triage nurse informs you of a 3-week-old newborn who just arrived with a 6-hour history of vomiting. The baby's temperature at triage is 38.3°C (101°F), with a HR of 120 and BP of 65/38. The triage nurse relays that the baby is very fussy but otherwise appears relatively well. She vomited bilious fluid in triage and had a small stool that was hemoccult-positive. Which piece of information compels you to see this patient immediately?
   A. Rectal temperature of 38.3°C (101°F)
   B. Bilious emesis
   C. Hemoccult-positive stool
   D. Blood pressure of 65/38 mm Hg
   E. Heart rate of 120 bpm

18. A 60-year-old woman presents with weakness and dysuria. She denies chest pain or shortness of breath, and has no cardiac history. An EKG shows normal sinus rhythm at 68, normal axis, PR interval 180 ms, QRS duration 80 ms, QTc interval 500 ms, and no ST- or T-wave abnormalities. Urinalysis shows WBC 50 to 100/hpf, RBC 2 to 4/hpf, many bacteria, few squamous epithelial cells, and positive leukocyte esterase. She has no known drug allergies and she is neither nauseated nor vomiting. Which of the following antibiotics is the most likely to be problematic for her?

A. Levofloxacin
B. Trimethoprim-sulfamethoxazole (Bactrim)
C. Nitrofurantoin
D. Gentamicin
E. Ceftriaxone

19. The parents of a 10-month-old little girl bring her to the ED in the middle of the night because she had been having periods of irritability throughout the evening. She woke up an hour ago with a more severe episode, characterized by inconsolable crying and several bouts of nonbloody, nonbilious emesis. The entire episode lasted approximately 20 minutes and resolved on the way to the ED. She has had no diarrhea or bloody stools. Her vital signs are normal and exam unremarkable. There is a small amount of dark red blood on rectal exam. Which of the following is associated with this condition?

A. Female gender
B. Age 3 to 12 months
C. "Sausage-shaped" mass in right abdomen on exam
D. Ectopic gastric tissue in an embryonic outpouching of the ileum
E. "Olive-shaped" mass seen on ultrasound in the pylorus

20. A 71-year-old woman with history of TIAs presents with left-sided weakness and left facial droop. She was fine when she went to bed at 11 P.M. last night, but woke up with the symptoms 45 minutes ago at 7 A.M. Which of the following is the best treatment after a noncontrast head CT shows no bleeding?

A. Intravenous tPA
B. Intraarterial tPA
C. Intravenous heparin
D. Aspirin
E. Warfarin (Coumadin)

21. A 64-year-old woman with a history of atrial fibrillation on warfarin presents to the ED with a sudden onset of periumbilical abdominal pain 4 hours earlier. The pain is constant, boring, and does not radiate. She is anorexic but denies nausea or vomiting. She denies dysuria and has had normal bowel movements. She has no history of abdominal surgery. On exam, she is uncomfortable and she has diffuse abdominal tenderness with minimal guarding. Her stool is hemoccult-positive. Her lab results show a WBC count of 12 k/mm^3 with 82% PMNs, bicarbonate of 16 mEq/L, and INR of 1.2. A CT scan of the abdomen with IV contrast shows only very mild thickening of the ileum and ascending colon. What is the next best step in her management?

- A. Admission for broad-spectrum antibiotics and serial abdominal exams
- B. Immediate exploratory laparotomy
- C. Angiography to confirm vascular patency
- D. Colonoscopy for direct visualization of colonic mucosa
- E. Discharge home with antibiotic coverage for infectious colitis

22. A 59-year-old man with history of MI status post CABG 3 years ago, gout, viral meningitis diagnosed by lumbar puncture 1 month ago, prior ischemic stroke 2 months ago, and external hemorrhoids, presents with 1 hour of aphasia and right arm and leg flaccidity that began at the dinner table. Noncontrast head CT scan shows no blood. Which of the following is a contraindication to giving this man tPA?

- A. MI and CABG 3 years ago
- B. Gout
- C. Viral meningitis diagnosed by lumbar puncture 1 month ago
- D. Ischemic stroke 2 months ago
- E. External hemorrhoids

23. A 79-year-old woman presents to the ED complaining of 6 hours of diffuse abdominal pain with nausea and one episode of vomiting. She has had several loose bowel movements, the last one mixed with dark blood. She denies fevers or chills. Her vital signs are unremarkable. On exam, she appears uncomfortable but only has diffuse mild abdominal tenderness without guarding or rebound. Her labwork is remarkable for a WBC count of 18,000/mm³ with 86% PMNs, a bicarbonate of 18 mEq/L, and a lactate of 5.6 mmol/dL (normal <4 mmol/dL). What is the most common associated risk factor for this condition?

- A. Coronary atherosclerosis
- B. History of stroke
- C. History of cerebral aneurysm
- D. Prior deep venous thrombosis
- E. Atrial fibrillation

24. A 68-year-old man presents with crushing chest pain. He has a history of hypertension, CHF, BPH, and hyperlipidemia, and smokes 2 packs per day. His medications include atenolol, furosemide, tamsulosin (Flomax), and atorvastatin. He is allergic to sulfa, which causes a rash. He is afebrile with a heart rate of 98, blood pressure of 150/85, respiratory rate of 20, and oxygen saturation of 97% on room air. His EKG shows 2-mm ST elevations in leads II, III, and aVF. Which of the following do you want to be most careful about giving him?

- A. Oxygen
- B. Aspirin
- C. Nitroglycerin
- D. Metoprolol (Lopressor)
- E. Heparin

25. A 64-year-old man has several days of worsening right upper quadrant pain, fever to 38.9°C (102°F), chills, vomiting, and back pain. He is relatively healthy and has never had abdominal surgery. His vital signs are temperature 39.3°C (102.8°F), HR 110, BP 96/46, RR 26, and oxygen saturation 96% on room air. On exam, he is mildly jaundiced, and appears ill and dehydrated. His abdomen is tender in the right upper quadrant with guarding. There is no rebound. Labs are significant for a total bilirubin of 6.4 mg/dL, ALT of 900 units/L, alkaline phosphatase of 550 units/L, and lipase of 64 units/L (normal range 7–60 units/L). Abdominal ultrasound shows cholelithiasis without evidence of cholecystitis, and a common bile duct diameter of 8 mm. What is the most appropriate management of this patient?

A. Emergent endoscopic retrograde cholangiopancreatography (ERCP)

B. Emergent surgery for cholecystectomy and common bile duct exploration

C. Broad-coverage antibiotics and admission for observation

D. Hepatic iminodiacetic acid (HIDA) scan to confirm common bile duct obstruction

E. CT scan of the abdomen with oral and IV contrast to rule out an obstructing mass

26. A 71-year-old woman presents to the ED with shortness of breath and chest tightness that started 15 minutes ago. She has a past medical history significant for adult-onset diabetes, arthritis, and high cholesterol. Her EKG shows 1-mm ST elevations in leads V_1–V_4. Which of the following is a correct eligibility criterion for thrombolysis?

A. Age <75 years

B. New or presumed new RBBB

C. ST elevation of 1 mm or more in two or more contiguous precordial leads

D. Time from symptom onset <1 hour

E. Blood pressure <180/110 mm Hg after treatment

27. A 76-year-old woman presents to the ED with a 2-day history of right upper quadrant abdominal pain, nausea, occasional vomiting, and a fever to 39.3°C (101°F). She had knee surgery 2 months ago. Her temperature in the ED is 38.2°C (100.8°F), with HR 110, BP 112/78, RR 18, and oxygen saturation 100% on room air. On exam, she has right upper quadrant tenderness with guarding, especially upon deep inspiration. She has no peritoneal signs. Lab results reveal WBC 18,000/mm^3 with 90% PMNs, and normal LFTs, bilirubins, and lipase. An ultrasound shows a normal gallbladder that is tender when pressed with the ultrasound probe. What is the best course of action?

- A. Admit for antiobiotics and delayed laparoscopic cholecystectomy.
- B. Admit for antibiotics and delayed repeat ultrasound.
- C. Obtain CT scan of the abdomen with oral and IV contrast.
- D. Obtain hepatic iminodiacetic acid (HIDA) scan to confirm cystic duct obstruction.
- E. Discharge home with primary care follow-up the next day.

28. A 25-year-old man in good health goes on a climbing trip with his buddies to Mount Aconcagua, South America's highest peak at 22,840 feet. He has climbed a few smaller mountains in the past without problems. By the second night of the expedition, at 15,000 feet, he complains of shortness of breath on exertion that does not resolve with rest. He has also developed a cough, initially dry but now it has become productive of clear, watery sputum. What is the most important aspect of therapy for his condition?

- A. Furosemide (Lasix)
- B. Dexamethasone
- C. Bed rest
- D. Descent
- E. Nifedipine

29. A 78-year-old man is gardening with his wife when he complains of horrible abdominal and back pain, and then suddenly collapses. EMS detects a carotid pulse but is unable to obtain a blood pressure reading. A 14-gauge IV is established and normal saline run wide open. The patient is intubated. Upon arrival to the ED, he appears pale with a faint carotid pulse. The cardiac monitor shows a sinus tachycardia. A bedside ultrasound is performed, which shows a large fluid collection adjacent to the posterior wall of the aorta, measuring 5 cm in diameter. What is the most important action?

    A. Activate the OR for emergent laparotomy and aortic repair.
    B. Establish large single-lumen central venous access.
    C. Administer large-volume IV crystalloid.
    D. Fluid resuscitation and CT scan for operative planning.
    E. Obtain an upright chest x-ray.

30. A 55-year-old woman presents to the ED with complaint of nausea and vomiting for several days. She also reports loss of appetite, weakness, and constipation. She denies any chest pain or shortness of breath. On review of systems, she does feel like she is very thirsty and urinating more frequently, but denies dysuria or urgency. Her past medical history is significant for hypertension, high cholesterol, and breast cancer with bone metastases, for which she is currently undergoing chemotherapy. She is afebrile with HR 86, BP 150/80, RR 18, and O_2 sat 99% on room air. Neurologic exam shows hyporeflexia diffusely but no focal weakness. Urinalysis shows 0 to 2 WBCs/hpf. What is the most likely finding on her EKG?

    A. ST elevations in II, III, and F
    B. Long PR interval
    C. Short QT interval
    D. $S_1 Q_3 T_3$
    E. Delta wave

31. A 56-year-old man presents to the ED with a chief complaint of lower back pain that he thinks is musculoskeletal in nature. On abdominal exam, a pulsating mass is palpated above the umbilicus just to the left of the midline. An abdominal ultrasound is obtained, which shows a 6-cm infrarenal abdominal aortic aneurysm (AAA). Which of the following is true regarding this condition?

    A. Often associated with aortic dissection
    B. Not considered abnormal until it reaches at least 5 cm in diameter
    C. CT with IV contrast should be obtained to rule out rupture in this case
    D. Mortality is about 30% with elective operative repair
    E. Is usually palpated below the level of the umbilicus

32. A 78-year-old woman with a history only of hypertension and high cholesterol presents to the ED after witnessed tonic-clonic activity. She has no past seizure history, but her son says she had recently complained of several days of diarrhea. Her lab results are significant for a sodium value of 160 mEq/L. What is the major concern of correcting her sodium too quickly?

A. CHF
B. Central pontine myelinolysis
C. Overshoot hyponatremia
D. Cerebral edema
E. Hypocalcemia

33. A 9-month-old girl presents with several days of runny nose, cough, and fussiness. Mom states that she has very noisy breathing and does not want to eat. At home, she had a temperature of 37.6°C (99.6°F). She has had two episodes of wheezing in the past and Mom was told she may have asthma. In the ED, she is afebrile; her respiratory rate is 52 and her oxygen saturation is 92% on room air. On exam, she is mildly tachypneic but not ill-appearing. She has clear nasal discharge, normal oropharynx, and "junky" breath sounds bilaterally, with expiratory wheezing. Which of the following treatments is indicated acutely?

A. Nebulized epinephrine
B. Nebulized albuterol
C. Oral prednisolone 1 mg/kg
D. Endotracheal intubation
E. Humidified air

34. An 18-month-old boy presents with fever to 39.9°C (103.9°F) rectally. He was full term and has no significant past medical history; he is circumcised, and his immunizations are up to date. He appears happy and is playing with a toy car. His mother says that he is eating and drinking less than usual, but is having roughly the same number of wet diapers. Which of the following is the best approach after a thorough history and physical exam with no remarkable findings?

A. Discharge with pediatrician follow-up
B. CBC, blood culture, discharge with pediatrician follow-up
C. CBC, blood culture, U/A, urine culture, discharge with pediatrician follow-up
D. Empiric ceftriaxone 50 mg/kg IV with pediatrician follow-up
E. Admit for observation after CBC and blood culture

35. A 3-month-old infant is brought to the ED for noisy breathing. She began with sneezing, runny nose, and cough 2 days ago. Every time she feeds she appears to have difficulty breathing and gets irritable; her rectal temperature was 38.1°C (100.6°F) earlier today. On exam, the infant has increased work of breathing, with nasal flaring as well as intercostal and subcostal retractions. She appears congested, with audible noises during both inspiration and expiration. Rectal temperature is 37.6°C (99.6°F), HR is 170, BP is 80/60, RR is 66, and oxygen saturation is 91%. She has copious nasal secretions and on auscultation of her chest you hear bilateral diffuse inspiratory crackles and rhonchi as well as expiratory wheezes. What is the most likely cause of this child's respiratory distress?

A. Foreign body inhalation
B. Upper airway obstruction
C. Lower airway obstruction
D. Combined upper and lower airway obstruction
E. Epiglottitis

36. A healthy 34-year-old woman with no past medical history and no known allergies presents to the ED complaining of headache, dizziness, and abdominal cramping that started gradually when she was about to go to bed. She felt fine earlier today, and had a same-as-usual day except for going to dinner at a seafood restaurant, where she ordered mahi mahi. She has never had these symptoms before. The restaurant was very nice and seemed clean, she recalls, though her meal did seem a bit "peppery." On exam, she has facial flushing but otherwise unremarkable skin exam. What is the best management?

A. Epinephrine 0.3 mL of 1:1000 solution SC
B. Morphine 2-4 mg IV Q1 hr PRN
C. Acetaminophen 1000 mg PO and supportive care
D. Diphenhydramine 50 mg IV
E. Admit for IV fluids and observation, with endoscopy as needed

37. A 17-year-old boy presents with 3 days of sore throat, malaise, myalgias, rhinorrhea, and headache. He had a fever at home to 38.3°C (101°F) and felt chilled. He has increased pain with swallowing. In the ED, his temperature is 38.2°C (100.8°F), with otherwise normal vital signs. He does not appear toxic, and his oropharynx is erythematous with patchy white exudates. He has several small palpable cervical lymph nodes, and he can range his neck with minimal discomfort. His lungs are clear. He also has a fine maculopapular, erythematous rash over his torso and upper extremities. What is the most likely etiology of his condition?

    A. *Mycoplasma pneumoniae*
    B. Group A β-hemolytic streptococcus (GABHS)
    C. Viral
    D. Mononucleosis
    E. Diphtheria

38. A 24-year-old man presents to the local ED in a small town in the Bahamas, complaining of nausea, vomiting, diarrhea, and "burning feet." He has no past medical history and no known drug allergies, and was well up until a few hours after lunch. He is allergic to shrimp, but his allergy manifests as itching and hives all over his body. He further vehemently denies eating any shellfish, saying he clearly remembers having a delicious meal of broiled sea bass with lemon from a distinctive restaurant. He has had several episodes of profuse watery diarrhea over the last couple hours, and is especially perplexed by the fact that he thought a cold beer can felt hot to touch. He also says that his symptoms became much worse after he drank the beer. What is the best management?

    A. Metronidazole (Flagyl) 250 mg PO TID for 5 days
    B. Ciprofloxacin 500 mg PO BID for 5 days
    C. Transfer to the mainland for urgent brain MRI
    D. Diphenhydramine 50 mg IV
    E. Supportive care with IV fluids and analgesics as needed

39. A 13-year-old boy presents to the ED with a chief complaint of sore throat. He states that he has pain with swallowing and his voice seems high-pitched. He denies fevers, chills, cough, or earache, and does not feel particularly ill. The pain seemed to develop yesterday afternoon during football practice but he remembers no specific injury. His vital signs are normal. On exam, his oropharynx and tympanic membranes are normal. He has no posterior neck tenderness and his anterior neck is mildly taught with a "crackling" feeling. He has some discomfort with neck range of motion and his lungs are clear. What is the most likely diagnosis?

    A. Retropharyngeal abscess
    B. Epiglottitis
    C. Laryngeal fracture
    D. Cervical spine fracture
    E. Pneumomediastinum

40. A 39-year-old heavy-set man presents to the ED complaining of low back pain for several weeks, which he had just "put up with." Yesterday, however, his pain became severe and he also developed left leg shooting pains to below his knee. He works for a parcel delivery service and lifts heavy boxes all day long normally, but is unable to do anything today because of the pain. On exam, elevation of his right leg produces the shooting pain in his left leg. Which of the following is most likely?

    A. Spinal stenosis
    B. Cauda equina syndrome
    C. Spinal epidural hematoma
    D. Disc herniation
    E. Malingering

41. A 72-year-old man has a sudden onset of vision loss in his right eye. He describes it as a shade coming down over his eye. He has no pain or redness of the eye. On exam he has a 4-mm pupil that constricts with illumination of the opposite eye. His retina appears very pale with a small, bright red spot in the middle. He can only sense motion with his right eye. Which of the following is true?

    A. Digital orbital massage will exacerbate the problem.
    B. One aspect of treatment is to decrease Pco_2 to cause vasodilation.
    C. Associated carotid artery atherosclerotic disease is rare.
    D. Arterial thrombolytics are clearly helpful.
    E. One aspect of treatment is to decrease intraocular pressure.

42. A confused patient is brought to the ED by family and is found to have a blood sugar of 940 mg/dL with a high serum osmolarity. Which of the following is typical of this patient's diagnosis?
A. Hypertonic urine
B. Volume overload
C. Hypernatremia
D. Ketosis
E. History of type 1 diabetes

43. A 62-year-old woman presents to the ED with sudden-onset severe left eye and head pain. She has vomited twice and has abdominal pain as well. Her vitals include a HR of 86, BP of 164/94, RR of 18, and oxygen saturation of 98% on room air. On exam, she appears very uncomfortable; her left pupil is dilated, her cornea is cloudy, and her sclera is red and chemotic. The rest of her exam is unremarkable. Which is true regarding this condition?
A. Can be precipitated by walking into a dimly lit room
B. Has no effect on the optic nerve
C. Atropine eye drops are sometimes effective for treatment
D. Intravenous steroids are effective if started within 1 hour
E. First-line treatment is with pseudoephedrine

44. A 24-year-old woman with no past medical history returns to the ED after having been seen the prior day for nausea, vomiting, and diarrhea, thought due to viral gastroenteritis. She says that her vomiting and diarrhea have subsided, but that she awoke with her head turned sharply to the left and cannot move it from that position. Which of the following is likely to help her most?
A. Diazepam (Valium)
B. Ibuprofen (Motrin)
C. Oxycodone
D. Diphenhydramine (Benadryl)
E. Ranitidine (Zantac)

45. A 56-year-old man is receiving a blood transfusion for acute GI bleeding. Ten minutes into the transfusion, he develops hypotension and lightheadedness. Which is true regarding transfusion reactions?
A. Most common cause of ABO incompatibility is differences in non-ABO antigens.
B. ABO incompatibility is characterized by extravascular hemolysis.
C. Rh-related incompatibilities result in extravascular hemolysis.
D. The most common type of transfusion reaction is allergic, with rash or hives.
E. Febrile reactions are common and require repeat crossmatching.

46. A 29-year-old healthy woman comes to the ED with concern about rabies; one week ago, she woke up early when she heard a sound, and then saw a bat fly across her bedroom into the chimney of her bedroom fireplace. She did not come sooner because she was too anxious. She has not been vaccinated against rabies. Which of the following is appropriate?

- A. Human rabies immune globulin (HRIG) in and around the wound +IM
- B. Human diploid cell vaccine (HDCV) IM on days 0, 3, 7, 14, and 28
- C. HRIG IM and HDCV IM on days 0, 3, 7, 14, and 28
- D. No prophylaxis is warranted due to the one-week delay
- E. No prophylaxis is necessary because no bite occurred

47. A 42-year-old healthy woman is being treated in the ED with IV nafcillin for a cellulitis when she develops a rash. On exam, she is sitting upright in bed in moderate respiratory distress, audibly wheezing, with hives over her trunk and extremities. She has no obvious oropharyngeal swelling and no stridor. Her vital signs include heart rate 110, blood pressure 105/75, respiratory rate 32, and oxygen saturation 94% on room air. She is placed on high-flow oxygen. Which intervention is the most important at this point?

- A. Epinephrine 0.1 mL of 1:1000 solution subcutaneously
- B. Diphenhydramine (Benadryl) 50 mg IV
- C. Ranitidine (Zantac) 50 mg IV
- D. Nebulized albuterol 1 mg in 3 mL of saline
- E. Intubation and mechanical ventilation

48. A 62-year-old woman with a history of hypertension, bipolar disorder, PTSD, and polymyalgia rheumatica presents with complaint of sudden-onset nausea and vomiting. She also says she feels like either she or the floor is moving. On exam she has persistent rotatory nystagmus. When she stands with her feet placed together, arms to her sides, and closes her eyes, she sways widely and nearly falls over. She is also grossly ataxic when she tries to walk. What is the likely diagnosis?

- A. Carotid artery dissection
- B. Meniere's disease
- C. Labyrinthitis
- D. Cerebellar hemorrhage
- E. Conversion disorder

49. A 34-year-old man with AIDS is noncompliant with his anti-retroviral medications. He presents to the ED with several days of low-grade fever, cough, dyspnea, and malaise. His chest x-ray shows a diffuse perihilar infiltrate. Which of the following is true regarding this illness?

A. First-line treatment is pentamidine
B. Caused by a bacterium
C. Benefit of corticosteroids if oxygen saturation >90%
D. Associated with elevated LDH levels
E. Prophylactic treatment common if CD4 count <300 cells/mm^3

50. A 58-year-old chronic alcoholic presents to the ED with complaint of nausea, vomiting, and abdominal pain. He says he recently attended a party at which he had slightly more than his usual amount of daily beer and vodka, but hasn't had anything to drink for at least the last couple of days because of his vomiting. Urinalysis shows ketonuria without glucosuria. Which of the following is most useful in the treatment of his condition at this time?

A. Insulin 0.1 units/kg IV bolus followed by 0.1 units/kg/hr IV drip
B. D5NS IV
C. Bicarbonate IV
D. Glucagon IM
E. NS wide open

51. An 82-year-old man has had several days of fever to 38.9°C (102°F), chills, malaise, and a dry cough with left-sided pleuritic chest pain. He has also had abdominal cramps and watery, non-bloody diarrhea. In the ED, his temperature is 38.7°C (101.6°F), HR 110, BP 106/76, RR 24, and oxygen saturation 94% on room air. On exam he looks ill, has scattered rhonchi bilaterally, and has mild abdominal tenderness diffusely. He has bilateral patchy infiltrates on CXR. Which organism likely accounts for this presentation?

A. *Streptococcus pneumoniae*
B. *Staphylococcus aureus*
C. *Legionella*
D. *Listeria monocytogenes*
E. *Mycoplasma pneumoniae*

52. A 22-year-old woman with no past medical history and LMP 4 weeks ago presents to the ED with a complaint of left-sided pelvic pain that came on suddenly. Her vital signs are stable and cervical os closed. Serum hCG is negative. Transvaginal ultrasonography reveals normal Doppler flow to both ovaries, and a small amount of complex fluid near the left ovary. Of the following, which is the most likely explanation for her symptoms?

A. Ruptured ectopic pregnancy
B. Ovarian torsion
C. Mittelschmerz
D. Fibroid
E. Ruptured corpus luteum cyst

53. A 72-year-old woman with a history of CHF presents with sudden onset of shortness of breath that began 4 hours ago. In the ED her pulse is 140, blood pressure 88/46, respiratory rate 28, and oxygen saturation 90% on room air. She has elevated jugular venous pressure, an irregular heart rate without murmurs, and crackles at the bases of her lungs. Her EKG shows atrial fibrillation without obvious ischemia. Which would be a good agent to acutely control her heart rate?

A. Amiodarone
B. Metoprolol (Lopressor)
C. Verapamil
D. Digoxin
E. Adenosine

54. A 78-year-old man with a history of high cholesterol and smoking presents to the ED with substernal chest pressure and shortness of breath lasting "all night long" without any periods of relief. His EKG shows 2-mm ST depressions in leads V_1 and V_2 with large R waves in those same leads. Which of the following is likely?

A. Septal ischemia
B. Inferior ischemia
C. Posterior infarction
D. Anterolateral infarction
E. Lead placement error

55. An elderly woman with a history of CAD presents to the ED with sudden-onset of chest tightness and difficulty breathing. Her exam is remarkable for distended neck veins, an S_3 gallop with a loud systolic murmur best heard at the right upper sternal border with radiation into the right neck, crackles heard bilaterally halfway up, and trace peripheral edema. Her HR is 94, BP 96/46, RR 28, and oxygen saturation 92% on oxygen. Her EKG shows normal sinus rhythm with ST depressions in leads V_1-V_4. Which of the following would most likely cause precipitous hypotension in this scenario?

A. Continuous positive airway pressure (CPAP)
B. Metoprolol (Lopressor)
C. Heparin
D. Nitroglycerin
E. Furosemide (Lasix)

56. A 42-year-old woman presents to the ED with complaints of fever, palpitations, shortness of breath, and weakness. On review of systems, she has lost 35 lbs in the past month. She appears flushed, with wide-staring eyes. EKG shows sinus tachycardia in the 140s with PACs. Chest x-ray is consistent with CHF. Which of the following needs to be given at least one hour after initiating treatment?

A. Propylthiouracil (PTU)
B. Propranolol
C. Acetaminophen
D. Methimazole
E. Potassium iodide

57. A 64-year-old man with a history of MI, CHF, DM, and HTN, presents with sudden onset of palpitations, chest discomfort, and difficulty breathing. He appears pale and somewhat tachypneic. His vital signs are HR 158, BP 98/58, RR 26, and oxygen saturation 96% on room air. He is placed on a cardiac monitor. What is the most appropriate next step?

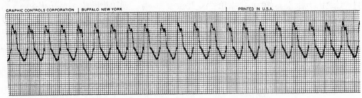

Rhythm strip showing ventricular rate of 158 bpm. (*Image reprinted with permission from Smeltzer SC, Bare BG. Textbook of Medical-Surgical Nursing, 9th Ed. Philadelphia: Lippincott Williams & Wilkins, 2000.*)

    A. Administer fentanyl 100 μg IV then electrical cardioversion at 100 J
    B. Lidocaine 100 mg IV bolus then continuous infusion
    C. Adenosine 6 mg IV
    D. Amiodarone 150 mg IV bolus followed by a continuous infusion
    E. Immediate electrical cardioversion at 200 J

58. A 29-year-old man with no significant past medical history is involved in a car accident during which the car explodes and he sustains 30% BSA second- and third-degree burns. His lab results are remarkable for an elevated BUN and creatinine. Which of the following would you expect to find?
    A. BUN/Cr ratio >10:1, UNa concentration >20 mEq/dL, FENa >= 1%
    B. BUN/Cr ratio <10:1, UNa concentration <20 mEq/dL, FENa >= 1%
    C. BUN/Cr ratio <10:1, UNa concentration >20 mEq/dL, FENa <1%
    D. BUN/Cr ratio >10:1, UNa concentration <20 mEq/dL, FENa <1%
    E. BUN/Cr ratio >10:1, UNa concentration <20 mEq/dL, FENa >= 1%

59. A 55-year-old woman presents to the ED with palpitations and difficulty breathing, especially with any exertion. The symptoms started one hour prior to arrival. She was previously healthy. Her vital signs include a pulse of 200, blood pressure 108/58, respiratory rate 20, and oxygen saturation 98% on room air. On exam she has mild pallor and rapid weak radial pulses. Her rhythm strip is shown below. What is the next best step in her management?
  A. Lidocaine 100 mg IV followed by a continuous infusion
  B. Electrical cardioversion at 50 J
  C. Amiodarone 150 mg bolus followed by a continuous infusion
  D. Verapamil 5 mg IV bolus
  E. Adenosine 6 mg IV bolus

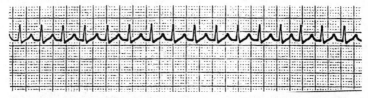

Rhythm strip showing ventricular rate of approximately 200 bpm. (*Figure reprinted with permission from Harwood-Nuss A, Wolfson AB, et al. The Clinical Practice of Emergency Medicine, 3rd Ed. Philadelphia: Lippincott Williams & Wilkins, 2001.*)

60. A 70-year-old man presents with shortness of breath, substernal chest tightness, nausea, and diaphoresis. He is found to be in complete heart block with a junctional escape rhythm at 45 beats per minute. Which of the following vessels is most likely involved?
  A. Left anterior descending artery
  B. Right coronary artery
  C. Posterior descending artery
  D. Left circumflex artery
  E. Obtuse marginal

61. A 68-year-old woman presents to the ED with severe midback pain and progressive right leg pain, numbness, and weakness. Her vital signs include a pulse of 88, blood pressure 198/92, respiratory rate 18, and oxygen saturation 98%. You notice she is unusually tall and thin, with long fingers. Her physical exam is remarkable for an absent right femoral pulse, a mottled leg, and diffusely decreased sensation in that leg. A portable chest x-ray shows a widened mediastinum. What is the most common risk factor for this disease process?

A. Hypertension
B. Atherosclerosis
C. Marfan's syndrome
D. Recent cardiac surgery
E. Ehlers-Danlos syndrome

62. A 19-year-old woman with history of eczema presents to the ED with a complaint of intermittent nonproductive cough for a couple months, ever since the weather turned cold. She grew up in Florida and just moved to Massachusetts to attend college, so has not previously had much exposure to cold weather. She says that her cough is especially bad if she is late for lecture and runs to class. She denies fever, chills, rhinorrhea, nasal congestion, sore throat, or any other symptoms. She also denies any sick contacts. On exam, lung sounds are clear. Chest x-ray is normal. Which of the following is likely to help her the most?

A. Home oxygen 2 L by nasal cannula
B. Azithromycin
C. Benzonatate (Tessalon Perles)
D. Albuterol
E. Guaifenesin (Robitussin) with codeine

63. A 42-year-old man presents to the ED with sudden-onset anterior chest pain with radiation to the upper back and difficulty breathing. His heart rate is 124, blood pressure 84/46, and oxygen saturation 98%. On physical exam, you notice jugular venous distension, distant heart sounds, and clear lungs. His abdomen and back are nontender. Large-bore IVs are established. What is the next appropriate step?

A. Take patient immediately to OR for repair of ruptured aortic aneurysm
B. Immediate CT scan to confirm diagnosis of aortic dissection
C. IV thombolysis for presumptive massive pulmonary embolus
D. Bedside ultrasound to confirm pericardial tamponade
E. Placement of right subclavian central venous catheter to measure right heart pressure

64. A 13-year-old boy is brought to the ED by his parents because they noticed he is limping. The boy says his left knee hurts. He has no significant past medical history other than always being a bit "chubby" for his age and height. In this past year, he has started to become more proportional as his growth spurt has begun. On exam, he is a stocky boy who sits with his left lower extremity out to the side, with no tenderness or swelling at the left knee, and full range of motion at the knee without discomfort. He clearly limps when asked to walk across the room, favoring the left side. What is the likely diagnosis?
  A. Transient synovitis of the left knee
  B. Septic left knee joint
  C. Occult bone metastasis
  D. Slipped capital femoral epiphysis
  E. Legg-Calvé-Perthes's disease

65. A 2-year-old boy presents to the ED with his mother for a persistent cough. The illness began with a runny nose 2 nights ago and the cough has progressed since then. This evening he continued to cough and was unable to sleep. His temperature is 37.1°C (98.8°F), his respiratory rate 28, and oxygen saturation 96% on room air. The toddler is mildly tachypeic with audible stridor and a very dry, hoarse, persistent cough; otherwise he looks well. He has clear nasal discharge. On lung exam you hear inspiratory stridor over the upper chest but no wheezes. Which treatment will have the greatest benefit over the next 15 minutes?
  A. Humidified oxygen
  B. Nebulized racemic epinephrine
  C. Dexamethasone 0.6 mg/kg by mouth
  D. Nebulized albuterol
  E. Encourage oral fluid intake

66. A 54-year-old woman with a history of two cesarean sections and appendectomy presents to your small community ED with complaint of abdominal pain, nausea, bloating, and constipation. She says the pain started yesterday morning and has not let up once, though sometimes it is worse than others. Her last bowel movement was 3 days ago and she doesn't remember when she last had flatus. On exam, her abdomen is diffusely distended and nonspecifically tender, with some voluntary guarding but no rebound. There is limited CT capability at your ED, and it is not currently available. What is the next best step for further management?
  A. Barium enema
  B. Manual disimpaction
  C. KUB and upright
  D. Ultrasound
  E. Colonoscopy

67. A 74-year-old man presents to the ED with a complaint of suicidal thoughts. He has no prior psychiatric illness and states he feels very depressed. His wife died 2 years ago and he has no family remaining; he also has no close friends. He has been drinking more than usual and needs at least three drinks to sleep at night. He owns a firearm and has been tempted to use it against himself. Which of the following is considered the most predictive of risk for future suicide?

- A. Ownership of a firearm and a plan to use it
- B. Male gender
- C. Age
- D. Lack of social support
- E. Excessive alcohol use

68. A 39-year-old woman complains of intermittent epigastric burning pain for several weeks, usually worse at bedtime and when she doesn't eat for a few hours. She gets partial relief with eating. She has a past medical history significant only for an ankle sprain for which she has been taking occasional ibuprofen when the ankle acts up. *H. pylori* testing comes back positive. What is the best treatment for her condition?

- A. PPI alone
- B. Bismuth alone
- C. PPI + amoxicillin + clarithromycin
- D. Bismuth + tetracycline + PPI
- E. Bismuth + tetracycline + H2-blocker

69. A chronic alcoholic is transported to the ED after being found unconscious in the street. He is minimally arousable in the ED but is breathing rapidly. His vital signs are a pulse of 126, blood pressure 88/46, respiratory rate 32, and oxygen saturation 98% on high-flow oxygen. His physical exam is unremarkable. Serum chemistry shows a sodium level of 136 mEq/L, chloride 96 mEq/L, potassium 5.2 mEq/L, bicarbonate 8 mEq/L, BUN 46 mg/dL, creatinine 1.6 mg/dL, and glucose 92 mg/dL. His urine is fluorescent green under a Wood's lamp (purple light) in the ED. Which of the following is true regarding his condition?

- A. Co-ingesting alcohol has a deleterious effect
- B. Associated with hypercalcemia
- C. Associated with blindness
- D. Associated with ingestion of isopropyl alcohol (rubbing alcohol)
- E. Amenable to hemodialysis

70. A 38-year-old man presents to the ED with complaint of sudden onset right-sided low abdominal pain earlier in the day. He has no past medical history and does not drink alcohol or smoke. On exam, he appears to be in mild discomfort but is non-toxic. Palpation of his abdomen in the right lower quadrant elicits moderate tenderness without guarding or rebound. Abdominal CT scan with contrast shows a normal-sized appendix with contrast filling the appendix to its tip and no peri-appendiceal fat stranding; there is a 2-cm oval-shaped mass in the paracolic area by the cecum, with thickened peritoneal lining and some fat stranding; the mass has Hounsfield units consistent with fat density. Which of the following is the best treatment for his condition?

A. Exploratory laparotomy
B. Laparoscopic appendectomy
C. Ibuprofen and oxycodone
D. Metronidazole and ciprofloxacin
E. Colon resection

71. A 26-year-old woman ingested 40 Extra Strength Tylenol tablets (500 mg each of acetaminophen) 4 hours ago as a suicide attempt. She presents to the ED entirely asymptomatic with a normal physical exam. Her vital signs are normal. Which of the following is true regarding acetaminophen toxicity?

A. A toxic ingestion is considered at least 200 mg/kg.
B. A toxic level is considered at least 140 μg/mL at 4 hours after ingestion.
C. Symptoms of toxicity usually develop only after 24 hours.
D. The oral preparation of *N*-acetylcysteine (NAC) should not be given IV.
E. NAC is significantly less effective if started after 4 hours of ingestion.

72. A 56-year-old woman with history of poorly controlled diabetes type I, diabetic retinopathy with hemorrhage 4 weeks ago,
poorly controlled high blood pressure, lung cancer with a known
metastasis to the brain, and status post appendectomy one year
earlier is brought in by ambulance with CPR underway after being
found unresponsive and hypotensive. Family members say that she
had recently taken a cross-country road trip to visit some friends,
returning just a few days ago. This morning the patient was visiting
her sister, complaining of new left leg swelling, when she suddenly
clutched her chest and said she couldn't breathe, then soon after collapsed. Which of the following is an *absolute* (rather than *relative*)
contraindication to thrombolysis for her condition?
  A. Diabetic retinopathy with hemorrhage 2 months ago
  B. Long-standing diastolic hypertension over 110 mm Hg
  C. Lung cancer with brain lesion resected 4 weeks ago
  D. CPR for 10 minutes
  E. Appendectomy 12 months ago

73. A 45-year-old man is rescued from a house fire, sustaining
second-degree burns estimated at 20% BSA. He is intubated in the
field due to confusion, respiratory distress, and hypoxia. In the ED,
the nurse points out a very bright appearance to the venous blood. A
venous blood gas is sent which reveals a pH of 7.14, P_vO_2 340 mm Hg,
P_vco_2 60 mm Hg, and HCO_3 of 14. His oxygen saturation is 100% on a
F_iO_2 of 1.0. What is the most likely etiology for these findings?
  A. Cyanide poisoning
  B. Carbon monoxide poisoning
  C. Hydrocarbon gas inhalation
  D. Inhalation pneumonitis
  E. Ammonia poisoning

74. A 29-year-old man with a history of severe asthma and two
prior intubations presents to the ED with a complaint of severe chest
tightness and shortness of breath that started after he attended a
picnic. On exam, he is in moderate distress with audible expiratory
wheezes throughout and a severely prolonged expiratory phase.
What is the first medication you want to give him?
  A. Methylprednisolone IV
  B. Ipratropium bromide via nebulizer
  C. Albuterol via nebulizer
  D. Theophylline IV
  E. Magnesium IV

75. An immigrant farm laborer presents to the ED after a day of heavy pesticide spraying with lethargy, vomiting, diaphoresis, difficulty breathing with wheezing, and incontinence. His exam is significant for miosis and bradycardia. This syndrome is mediated by which mechanism?

   A. Adrenergic stimulation
   B. Adrenergic inhibition
   C. Inhibition of acetylcholine degradation
   D. Inhibition of acetylcholine release
   E. Heat stroke resulting in decreased parasympathetic tone

76. A 3-year-old girl is brought to the ED by her father who says she placed a coffee bean in her nose an hour earlier. She is in no apparent distress, but on exam with a nasal speculum clearly has a brown foreign body in the left posterior naris. Which of the following is a good choice for initial management?

   A. Papoose
   B. Nebulized racemic epinephrine
   C. Magill forceps
   D. Blind probing with suction catheter
   E. Right-angle probe

77. A 34-year-old ice fisherman falls through thin ice and is submerged for 20 minutes before rescuers are able to bring him to the surface. He is unresponsive, apneic, and pulseless. After he is intubated and CPR is started, he is transported to the ED by EMS. By the time he reaches the ED, he has regained a carotid pulse but is still unresponsive. His pulse is 120, blood pressure unobtainable, and oxygen saturation 86% on F_iO_2 of 1.0. His lungs are rhonchorous bilaterally. His pupils are dilated and he is areflexic. A rectal probe temperature is 28°C (82°F). What is the most important intervention for this patient?

   A. Bilateral chest tubes and warm fluid lavage
   B. Administer vasopressors to increase cardiac output and tissue perfusion
   C. Gastric lavage with warmed fluid
   D. Cardiopulmonary bypass
   E. Deep tracheal suctioning

78. A 19-year-old college freshman presents to the ED with complaint of severe bilateral eye pain. He started a new welding class at school today, and says he had not realized the welding goggles had to be "turned on" to be UV protective. He was initially fine, but as the evening went on, developed worsening and severe bilateral eye pain. On slit lamp exam, you see diffuse uptake of fluorescein dye in both eyes. Which of the following outpatient treatment recommendations is likely to lead to a corneal ulcer?

A. Cyclopentolate
B. Ibuprofen
C. Oxycodone and acetaminophen
D. Proparacaine
E. Erythromycin eye ointment

79. A 46-year-old man is winter-camping in the Rocky Mountains when he is caught in a blizzard and gets lost. He is rescued the next day, found wandering in subzero temperatures. He is brought to the ED where he complains of foot numbness. The toes on both feet are dry and appear pale and waxy with mild swelling. He has sensation over the dorsum of both feet but not at the toes. What is true regarding this condition?

A. Does not require actual tissue freezing to occur.
B. Most common presenting symptom is pain.
C. Tetanus booster is not required.
D. Requires rapid rewarming by immersion in warm water.
E. Presence of hemorrhagic blebs would be reassuring.

80. A 40-year-old woman who is one-month postpartum presents to the ED with complaint of right leg pain and swelling of 2 days. She denies any chest pain or shortness of breath. On examination, her vital signs are stable, her lungs are clear, and her right leg is remarkable for tenderness and mild erythema at the distal thigh. You suspect superficial thrombophlebitis, but decide to get an ultrasound to be cautious. The ultrasound report comes back with a reading of "clot present in the superficial femoral vein." What is the best management?

A. Anticoagulation with low-molecular weight heparin until warfarin is therapeutic
B. Admit for IV heparin
C. Rest, elevation, local heat, and NSAIDs
D. Thrombolysis
E. Compression stockings

81. A 17-year-old boy presents to the ED with a fever. He is triaged to an open area, where he shortly begins to look very ill. An LP is performed because he has a headache and neck stiffness. He is diagnosed with bacterial meningitis, placed in an isolation room, and given broad-spectrum antibiotics. The Gram's stain later shows gram-negative diplococci. How should the care providers be treated for the exposure?

A. Oral rifampin single dose
B. Oral penicillin 4-day course
C. Oral ciprofloxacin single dose
D. Intravenous ceftriaxone single dose
E. Oral azithromycin 5-day course

82. A 42-year-old man presents to the ED after awakening and seeing his left eye was very red. He has no past medical history, does not recall trauma to the eye, and has never had anything like this before. He denies any pain in the left eye or visual changes. He denies any other symptoms. On exam, he has normal visual acuity on both sides and intact extraocular movements. His left eye is remarkable for an area on the lateral part of the bulbar conjunctivitis that is flat, bright red, smooth, and sharply demarcated at the limbus. What is the best management?

A. Erythromycin eye ointment
B. Emergent ophthalmology consult
C. Cold compresses for 24 hours
D. Topical timolol and IV acetazolamide
E. Prednisone

83. A 70-year-old woman presents with one day of high fever, headache and neck stiffness, and confusion. She is seen promptly in the ED, where she receives ceftriaxone 2 g IV for suspected bacterial meningitis. An LP shows 1,200 WBCs/hpf with 80% neutrophils, glucose 30 mg/dL (normal 50–80 mg/dL), protein 60 mg/dL (normal 15–45 mg/dL), and a Gram's stain showing gram-positive rods. What is the most important antibiotic to administer for this particular organism in addition to ceftriaxone?

A. Vancomycin
B. Nafcillin
C. Acyclovir
D. Ampicillin
E. Ciprofloxacin

84. A 5-year-old girl is brought in to the ED by parents who are panicked that she is choking after eating a hot dog. The girl initially appeared to be in distress, coughing violently, but just as they pulled up to the hospital, she became unresponsive. What should you do first?

   A. Finger sweep
   B. Back blows and abdominal thrusts
   C. Bag-mask ventilation
   D. Needle cricothyrotomy
   E. Chest compressions

85. A 24-year-old woman presents with 2 days of left knee swelling, pain, and difficulty with range of motion. She also has scattered papules on her trunk and extremities; these have pustular centers. On further questioning she had abnormal vaginal discharge several weeks ago that resolved. What is the most sensitive test to diagnose septic gonoccocal arthritis in this patient?

   A. Culture of joint fluid
   B. Cervical swab culture
   C. Gram's stain of joint fluid
   D. Fluid count > 50,000 WBCs/hpf
   E. Blood culture

86. A 14-year-old boy is brought to the ED by his mother, who says her son has been complaining of right lower abdominal pain and nausea for the past week. He has also had a low-grade fever and some diarrhea. On exam, he is very tender to palpation of the right lower quadrant, but not specifically at McBurney's point. There is no guarding or rebound, and he is guaiac-negative. His labs are significant for a WBC count of 18,000/mm³. CT scan shows a normal-filling appendix, multiple enlarged mesenteric lymph nodes, and some ileal wall thickening. What is the most likely etiology of his condition?

   A. Appendicolith
   B. Chronic constipation
   C. Viral
   D. *Yersinia enterocolitica*
   E. *Campylobacter jejuni*

87. A 56-year-old man with a history of gout presents to the ED with a 1-day history of right knee swelling and mild malaise. He is afebrile. His right knee is swollen and warm with a palpable effusion. He denies trauma to the knee. An arthrocentesis is performed and 10 mL of straw-colored fluid is obtained. The cell count shows 30,000 WBCs/hpf with 80% PMNs. It is 10 P.M. and the lab cannot analyze the fluid to look for negatively birefringent crystals. The patient feels much better after the procedure and wants to go home. Which test result is essential before he can be safely discharged?

A. Fluid culture result
B. Erythrocyte sedimentation rate
C. Fluid protein-to-glucose ratio
D. Crystal analysis
E. Gram's stain

88. A 45-year-old man presents to the ED with complaint of bright red blood on the toilet paper when he wipes, especially after a bowel movement. He feels something at his anus at times, which he pushes back inward; it is not painful. He is healthy overall, but is a very busy executive who does a lot of traveling; he says he doesn't have time to exercise or eat right, and is often constipated. On exam of the anal area, he has an internal hemorrhoid prolapsed at the anus, which is easily reducible. Which of the following do you recommend as the next step?

A. Linear incision and drainage
B. Emergent surgical referral for hemorrhoidectomy
C. Sitz baths, oral analgesics, stool softeners, high-fiber diet
D. Ellipitical incision and clot evacuation
E. Total excision

89. A 23-year-old man fractures his left midshaft fibula playing football. He is seen by an orthopedist and placed in a leg cast, immobilizing the knee and ankle, and sent home with crutches. He presents to the ED the next day with increased pain, numbness along the lateral aspect of his leg and dorsum of his foot, and difficulty dorsiflexing his toes. He has a strong dorsalis pedis pulse and his foot appears well perfused. Which structure is being compressed?

A. Anterior compartment of the leg
B. Saphenous nerve
C. Peroneal nerve
D. Anterior tibial artery
E. Tibial nerve

90. A construction worker presents to the ED after getting hot tar spilled on his right arm. The foreman on the scene immersed his arm in a pail of cold water. The tar is currently solidified and cool. Which of the following do you want to use to remove the tar?

- A. Naphthalene (aromatic hydrocarbon)
- B. Normal saline
- C. Viscous lidocaine
- D. Neosporin ointment
- E. None, to prevent further injury

91. A 46-year-old pedestrian is struck by a car at about 35 mph. Upon primary and secondary survey in the ED, his only injury appears to be to his left lower extremity, where he has tenderness over the lateral aspect of the mid-tibia. On exam he has extreme leg pain with passive ROM of the ankle. He has decreased sensation over the lateral dorsum of his foot. His distal strength is intact and he has a palpable dorsalis pedis pulse. An x-ray shows a minimally displaced midshaft tibial fracture. What is the appropriate management for this patient?

- A. Open reduction of fracture and fasciotomy to release compartment pressure
- B. MRI of the lumbar spine to look for occult spine contusion
- C. Ankle and foot x-rays
- D. Splinting, elevation, ice, and follow-up with orthopedics in one week
- E. Check compartment pressure with Stryker, fasciotomy if greater than 30 mm Hg

92. A 52-year-old man with history of hypertension and diabetes presents to the ED with complaint of left knee pain that has been excruciating since onset. He denies trauma to the knee. X-ray shows some soft-tissue swelling at the left knee. Joint fluid is obtained and is remarkable for negatively birefringent crystals with a negative Gram's stain. Which of the listed options is likely to help the most?

- A. Allopurinol
- B. Colchicine
- C. Ceftriaxone
- D. Oxycodone
- E. Probenecid

93. A 24-year-old woman is working in a restaurant when a pot of boiling grease spills onto her right arm. She has erythema over the dorsum of her arm extending from her elbow to her wrist. There are several blisters forming. Her arm is extremely painful and the burn is tender to touch. The wound is cleansed and debrided. What is the most important aspect to burn healing?

    A. Oral antibiotics that cover staphylococcus and streptococcus

    B. Sodium-chloride-soaked sterile fine-mesh gauze

    C. Twice daily wet-to-dry dressings

    D. Daily application of bacitracin

    E. Dry dressing with fluff gauze

94. A 40-year-old woman presents with pain and trouble with swallowing, pain with opening her mouth, and fevers. She also says her voice sounds hoarse. On exam, she has an erythematous oropharynx, purulent tonsillar exudates, inferomedial displacement of the right tonsil, and deviation of the uvula to the left. Which of the following does she likely have?

    A. Peritonsillar abscess

    B. Ludwig's angina

    C. Retropharyngeal abscess

    D. Pharyngitis

    E. Parapharyngeal abscess

95. A 22-year-old man is involved in a high-speed motor vehicle accident in which he is ejected from the car. On arrival to the ED he does not answer questions and he is intubated after placement of two large-bore IVs. He has clear breath sounds and thready femoral pulses. His pulse is 136, blood pressure 78/36, and oxygen saturation 96% intubated with F_iO_2 100%. A FAST exam shows no pericardial effusion but there is a peri-renal fluid stripe. A portable chest x-ray shows no pneumothorax and a normal mediastinum. A portable pelvis x-ray shows bilateral displaced pubic symphysis fractures. Uncrossmatched blood is administered, and his blood pressure is 80/42 after 20 minutes with continued thready pulses. What is the most appropriate next step in this patient's management?

    A. CT scan of head, c-spine, chest, and abdomen

    B. Rapid infusion of normal saline

    C. Bilateral chest tubes

    D. Transfer to OR for exploratory laparotomy and placement of intracranial bolt

    E. Diagnostic peritoneal lavage (DPL)

96. A 45-year-old man complains of acute onset of severe back pain in the setting of heavy lifting, followed by numbness and weakness in his legs. You find that he has a markedly decreased reflex at the right knee. For which spinal cord level is that concerning?

A. S1
B. L2
C. L3
D. L4
E. L5

97. A 62-year-old woman was smoking in bed when she fell asleep and her bed caught fire. She was rescued when her neighbors noticed the smoke. En route to the hospital she was intubated for altered mental status and soot in her throat. Upon arrival to the ED she is trying to pull at the tube. Her vital signs are a pulse of 120, blood pressure 150/94, and oxygen saturation 96%. She has first- and second-degree burns to her face, right chest, abdomen, and arm. What is the best management strategy regarding fluid administration?

A. Give 2 L normal saline over one hour followed by 4 mL/kg/hr for 24 hours.
B. Administer normal saline and titrate to a urine output of 0.5 mL/kg/hr.
C. Administer lactated ringers 4 mL/kg per % burn surface area over 12 hours.
D. Administer normal saline 4 mL/kg per % burn surface area over 12 hours.
E. Administer colloid solution for burn surface area greater than 20%.

98. A 79-year-old man with history of osteoarthritis presents to the ED following a motor vehicle collision in which he was rear-ended with significant force. He complains of neck pain and weakness in both of his arms. He has no trouble moving his legs. Which of the following is most likely?

A. Anterior cord syndrome
B. Central cord syndrome
C. Cauda equina syndrome
D. Brown-Séquard syndrome
E. Sciatica

99. The victim of a high-speed motor vehicle accident arrives to the emergency department by EMS awake but groggy. On primary survey his airway is intact but his breathing is shallow and labored. He has audible breath sounds bilaterally and palpable crepitus over the right chest. He is intubated using etomidate and succinylcholine, followed by tube confirmation by CO_2 capnometry. After intubation his pulse is 120, blood pressure 82/40, and oxygen saturation 84%. What is the most appropriate next step?

    A. Obtain a STAT portable chest x-ray to confirm tube placement.

    B. Administer 2 units of PRBCs rapidly to reverse circulatory shock.

    C. Perform a FAST exam to rule out intraperitoneal bleeding.

    D. Place a right-sided chest tube to relieve a presumed pneumothorax.

    E. Reconfirm tube placement with laryngoscopy.

100. A 38-year-old man with very poor dentition presents to the ED after a recent tooth extraction with a complaint of difficulty swallowing, neck swelling, and neck pain. On examination, there is bilateral submandibular swelling and the patient's tongue appears to be protruding out. Which of the following is the likely culprit of his problem?

    A. Polymicrobial

    B. Streptococci

    C. Staphylococci

    D. *Klebsiella* species

    E. *Bacteroides* species

Answers and Explanations

1. D	26. E	51. C	76. B
2. D	27. D	52. E	77. E
3. D	28. D	53. A	78. D
4. B	29. A	54. C	79. D
5. D	30. C	55. D	80. A
6. E	31. C	56. E	81. C
7. A	32. D	57. A	82. C
8. C	33. B	58. D	83. D
9. D	34. B	59. E	84. B
10. C	35. D	60. B	85. B
11. B	36. D	61. A	86. C
12. C	37. C	62. D	87. E
13. C	38. E	63. D	88. C
14. B	39. E	64. D	89. C
15. B	40. D	65. B	90. D
16. C	41. E	66. C	91. A
17. B	42. C	67. A	92. B
18. A	43. A	68. C	93. B
19. C	44. D	69. E	94. A
20. D	45. C	70. C	95. D
21. B	46. C	71. B	96. D
22. D	47. A	72. C	97. B
23. E	48. D	73. A	98. B
24. C	49. D	74. C	99. D
25. A	50. B	75. C	100. A

1. D. This woman has menometrorrhagia, defined as excessive bleeding at irregular intervals. **The most common cause of dysfunctional uterine bleeding during reproductive years is anovulation. During an anovulatory cycle, a corpus luteum fails to form in the latter part of the cycle, and thus progesterone is not secreted. This results in unopposed synthesis of estradiol and overproliferation of the endometrial wall. The normal period will be missed, but eventually the endometrial wall outgrows its blood supply and sloughs, resulting in heavier than normal vaginal bleeding.** The treatment in the short term is to initiate hormone therapy with an estrogen-progesterone combination regimen to restore regularity. An outpatient transvaginal sonogram (TVS) should be done to rule out fibroids or other structural abnormalities, as well as to rule out polycystic ovarian disease. Women who are older than 35 years of age should also have a uterine biopsy done to rule out the possibility of uterine cancer.

2. D. Given the patient's mechanism and confusion, c-spine collar should be applied immediately. The patient should not be discharged without a CT scan of the head because of his confusion. Clinical clearance of the c-spine can be done if the patient has a GCS of 15, is sober, has a normal neurologic exam, and has no major distracting injuries. There is no current indication for intubation in this patient; even if there were (e.g., vomiting, combativeness, marked mental status change, poor oxygenation), c-spine collar should be placed first and intubation would then be performed with inline c-spine stabilization.

3. D. This woman has signs of hemorrhagic shock. In addressing the ABCs, she is placed on high-flow oxygen, large-bore IV access is established, crystalloid infusion is initiated, and preparation for blood transfusion is undertaken. The next step is to stop the bleeding by placing vaginal packing. A technique is also described in which a Foley catheter is placed through the cervix into the uterus, the balloon is inflated, and then the tube is clamped. Vaginal packing, however, is usually effective. **In someone with this degree of hemorrhage, hormonal therapy should be started. For severe bleeding, estrogen (Premarin) can be given 25 mg IV over 10 to 15 minutes. This acutely causes uterine arterial vasoconstriction.** Heavy vaginal bleeding may require dilatation and curettage (D&C), or in extreme cases an emergent hysterectomy. Oral estrogen and progesterone agents can be started for moderate dysfunctional uterine bleeding. Of note, vasopressors are of little use in hemorrhagic shock.

4. B. The patient's deterioration is likely due to increased ICP from worsening EDH or SDH that was only seen initially as a small collection of extra-axial blood. **Raising the head of the bed by 30 degrees, hyperventilation to a goal pco$_2$ of about 35 mm Hg, and infusion of IV mannitol are conservative measures for decreasing ICP.**

5. D. This young woman has a presentation concerning for acute ovarian torsion, which is more common in women with a history of ovarian cysts. **Ovarian torsion is a gynecologic emergency and must be diagnosed promptly in order to prevent ovarian ischemia and death. Diagnosis is made by TVS with Doppler flow study to assess for adequate flow in the ovarian artery.** If ovarian torsion is found or suspected, the patient must be taken to the OR for laparoscopy and detorsion. Other diagnostic considerations include ruptured ovarian cyst, tubo-ovarian abscess, and appendicitis.

6. E. This patient likely has cardiac tamponade, as evidenced by Beck's triad of hypotension, muffled or distant heart sounds, and jugular venous distention; his penetrating stab wound to the chest furthermore provides a likely cause for acute tamponade. He may benefit from urgent pericardiocentesis in an attempt to rapidly improve his hemodynamics at risk of causing damage, for example, to the coronary arteries or lungs. Definitive management is by thoracotomy to repair the laceration to the heart from which blood is filling the pericardial sac. Whether the thoracotomy occurs in the ED or the OR depends on the stability of the patient. Injury to the tracheobronchial tree, paralysis of the diaphragm, and ruptured viscous would not be expected to cause JVD, hypotension, and distant heart sounds with normal lung and abdominal exam. Tension pneumothorax could similarly present with tachypnea, tachycardia, hypotension, and JVD; however, breath sounds would be absent on the affected side.

7. A. This woman, who is in her first-trimester of pregnancy, presents with signs of early hypovolemic shock, which is concerning for a ruptured ectopic pregnancy. As with any unstable patient, the ABCs are addressed. In this case, she does not require intubation, and she has large-bore IV access. Normal saline should be administered wide open and another large-bore IV established. Bloodwork should be sent, including a hematocrit and blood type and screen. **The first action, however, should be to obtain a bedside ultrasound if available to look for free intraperitoneal fluid, suggesting either a ruptured ectopic pregnancy or ruptured luteal cyst. Free fluid in the presence of persistent hypovolemic**

shock would be an indication for emergent laparotomy. This patient is too unstable to go for a formal transvaginal ultrasound at this time.

8. C. The location of the stab wound combined with the finding of subcutaneous emphysema point to a disruption of either the tracheobronchial tree or the esophagus, thus necessitating both bronchoscopy and esophagoscopy. However, tracheal injury is most likely given its anterior position. A stab at or below the level of the nipples should be considered potentially intra-abdominal, which would require exploratory laparotomy if the patient had peritoniteal signs or were unstable. A left-sided chest tube would be indicated in the setting of decreased breath sounds, tachypnea, or hypoxia. Pericardial tamponade should always be considered with anterior chest penetrating wounds. A pericardiocentesis would be performed if there were pericardial fluid present on the FAST exam, combined with hypotension, elevated JVP, and distant heart sounds (Beck's triad). ED thoracotomy would be indicated if the patient were to lose vital signs in the ED.

9. D. Patients with first-trimester vaginal bleeding must be ruled out for ectopic pregnancy. This is usually done based on a combination of physical exam, quantitative hCG levels, and transvaginal sonography. TVS should demonstrate an IUP at hCG levels greater than 1,500 mIU/dL. Signs of an IUP include a "double" gestational sac, fetal pole, or yolk sac. Signs concerning for ectopic pregnancy include an adnexal mass or free pelvic fluid in the absence of an IUP. For hCG <1,500 mIU/dL, benign physical exam, and ultrasound without IUP or adnexal masses, patients can be discharged for follow-up in 48 hours for a repeat hCG and ultrasound to confirm a normal increase in hCG. Patients who have significant tenderness with an indeterminate ultrasound should be admitted for observation or diagnostic laparoscopy. Patients with an hCG >1,500 mIU/dL and no IUP are presumed to have an ectopic pregnancy. If an ectopic pregnancy is confirmed, the treatment is based on patient stability and ectopic size. **Methotrexate can be used for stable mothers provided the ectopic pregnancy is less than 4 cm in diameter and that there is no evidence of rupture.** Large ectopic mass or mother instability are indications for laparotomy.

10. C. The patient would have received a full series of tetanus immunization as a child with routine healthcare in most parts of the United States. Her wound sustained while camping is presumed to be dirty, and thus she should have a tetanus toxoid booster (Td) if her last booster was more than 5 years ago. For clean wounds, Td should be given if the last booster was more than 10 years ago. Pediatric DT (diphtheria, tetanus) is for children in their primary immunization series and contains 8 times as much diphtheria toxoid as is in Td. There is no contraindication to tetanus toxoid during pregnancy. If the patient had said she was allergic to tetanus toxoid, which had previously caused her an immediate hypersensitivity reaction (e.g., hives, bronchospasm, shock), she could then be given tetanus immune globulin instead.

11. B. Miscarriages are common, with an estimate of about 30% to 50% embryonic or fetal loss after implantation of the zygote; however, most of these go undetected as simply a "missed" menstrual period. Approximately 20% of pregnant women will experience some degree of vaginal bleeding during the first trimester. The management of first-trimester vaginal bleeding depends on the pelvic exam and the ultrasound results. **A *threatened miscarriage* is defined as bleeding with a closed cervical os and evidence of an intrauterine pregnancy (IUP) on ultrasound. About 25% to 50% of these pregnancies will go on to miscarriage, depending on the degree of bleeding.** *Inevitable miscarriage* is defined as an open os with an ultrasound showing an IUP. *Incomplete miscarriage* is defined as products of conception (POC) present in the cervical os. *Complete miscarriage* is defined as passage of POCs with closing of the cervical os and contraction of the uterus.

12. C. The correct answer of the choices given is to use local diphenhydramine (Benadryl), diluted to 1%, which serves as an effective anesthetic. Not using any anesthetic or using general anesthesia in the OR are not reasonable options. Other possibilities for local anesthesia in someone allergic to lidocaine, of the amide class of anesthetics, are the ester anesthetics, including procaine, cocaine, tetracaine, benzocaine, and chloroprocaine. Other anesthetics in the amide class of anesthetics are bupivicaine, etidocaine, and mepivicaine; these should be avoided if a patient truly is allergic to lidocaine. More often, patients are actually allergic to the preservative (methylparaben) in multidose lidocaine; in these cases, single-dose lidocaine ("cardiac lidocaine"), which does not contain the preservative, can be used.

13. C. This patient has symptoms consist with bacterial prostatitis, characterized by fever, chills, urinary symptoms (frequency, urgency, dysuria, obstruction), and low back and perineal pain. It is sometime associated with complete urinary obstruction. The diagnosis is made entirely based on the history and the prostate exam. The prostate will be tender, swollen, warm, and

often boggy. Urethral discharge is sometimes present, and urinalysis is usually positive for WBCs and bacteria. Treatment consists of a 30-day course of trimethoprim/sulfamethoxasole (Bactrim) or a quinolone such as ciprofloxacin or levofloxacin. Patients who appear ill or toxic should be admitted for IV antibiotics, typically ampicillin plus gentamicin. Of note, an uncomplicated UTI in men should be treated with 7 days of oral antibiotics, as opposed to the 3-day course indicated for women with uncomplicated UTIs.

14. B. Posterior shoulder dislocations are classically associated with seizures and electrocution (or electroconvulsive therapy), occurring due to a strength imbalance between the internal and external rotators of the shoulder. Anterior shoulder dislocations are far more common than posterior dislocations overall, however.

15. B. This man presents with symptoms classic for an acute renal calculus that is migrating down the ureter. The pain is typically severe and colicky, and radiates to the groin or testicle. **The quickest and easiest way to secure the diagnosis is to check a urinalysis, which is also essential to check for concurrent urinary tract infection. These symptoms in the setting of microscopic hematuria, present in about 90% of cases, can be used as presumptive evidence of the diagnosis in someone with a history of renal stones.** Patients with first-time renal colic should undergo imaging to confirm the diagnosis, and to exclude other etiologies. CT scan of the kidneys and ureters is the most effective modality, as it can visualize a renal stone as small as 1 mm, detect hydronephrosis, and rule out other etiologies of pain and hematuria (e.g., renal mass, renal infarct).

16. C. The patient described has suffered a classic mechanism for posterior hip dislocation—posteriorly directed force against a flexed knee and flexed hip, as occurs with head-on motor vehicle collisions. **Injury to the sciatic nerve is associated with approximately 10% to 14% of posterior hip dislocations; this manifests as pain or decreased sensation in the distribution of the sciatic nerve (posterolateral aspect of calf and foot), and/or decreased ability to dorsiflex or plantarflex the foot.** Injury to the femoral nerve and femoral artery can occur with anterior hip dislocations. Injury to the popliteal artery can occur with knee dislocations.

17. B. Bilious emesis in an infant should be considered an emergency, and malrotation with an associated midgut volvulus is the most concerning diagnosis. These patients must be evaluated immediately as rapid decompensation will occur due to bowel ischemia. Intestinal malrotation is defined as the incomplete rotation and abnormal fixation of the gut during embryologic development. Because the intestine is not properly fixated, it is at risk for twisting on its own blood supply, a condition known as midgut volvulus. The diagnosis is made by an upper GI series, an x-ray with contrast administered via an NG tube. A positive test will reveal a "corkscrew" appearance of the contrast abutting the twisted bowel. Treatment is immediate surgical decompression. A blood pressure of 65/38 mm Hg is within normal limits for an infant of this age, and therefore should not be cause for alarm. Hypotension for term infants is defined as an SBP less than 60 mm Hg.

18. A. This woman needs an antibiotic for her urinary tract infection. Her EKG is significant for QT prolongation, so care should be given to avoid starting her on any medication that can prolong the QT interval further. QT prolongation can be congenital or drug induced; in either case, QT prolongation may lead to increased risk of ventricular tachyarrhythmias, which can cause syncope, cardiac arrest, or sudden death. **Levofloxacin is one such medication that can cause QT prolongation and thus should be avoided in this patient, whose QTc is 500 msec.**

19. C. This patient has intussusception, which is a telescoping of a proximal segment of bowel (*intussusceptum*) into a distal segment (*intussuscipiens*), most commonly the distal ileum into the ascending colon. It presents classically as intermittent colicky abdominal pain that resolves suddenly, as the intussusception often reduces spontaneously, only to recur again later. It can sometimes be palpated as a "sausage-shaped" mass in the right abdomen; however, this is not a sensitive sign. Prolonged intussusception can result in bowel wall ischemia, sloughing, and bloody stools, described as "currant jelly stools." The most common age of presentation is from 6 months to 2 years, and it can happen in either gender, although it occurs in males at least twice as often as females. Ectopic gastric tissue in an embryonic outpouching of ileum describes Meckel's diverticulum. An "olive-shaped" mass on ultrasound is found in infants with pyloric stenosis.

20. D. This patient's time of onset of stroke symptoms is 11 P.M. the previous night, or 8 hours and 45 minutes ago, and therefore she does not meet criteria for thrombolysis (onset of neurologic deficits within 3 hours). With a negative noncontrast head CT scan, she likely has an ischemic stroke of either thrombotic or embolic origin. In certain stroke centers, intraarterial tPA is being used if patients present within 6 hours of neurologic deficits, but this patient is again outside the required time window. Intravenous heparin is often started by neurologists if the patient has atrial fibrillation, known carotid atherosclerosis, or waxing and waning symptoms. Despite this practice, IV heparin has never been shown in large randomized-controlled trials to affect outcomes in acute stroke. **Aspirin, on the other hand, has been shown to decrease the incidence of stroke recurrence by 1% to 2% within one month after an acute stroke.** Oral Coumadin would take several days before effecting a therapeutic level of anticoagulation.

21. B. This woman presents with symptoms and signs classic for acute mesenteric artery occlusion, which occurs predominantly in the superior mesenteric artery (SMA) and mostly in women. The SMA supplies the distal duodenum, jejunum, ileum, ascending colon, and transverse colon to the splenic flexure. The most common risk factor is atrial fibrillation, and the classic presentation is abdominal pain "out of proportion to exam," meaning that the abdominal exam may not be very impressive. Intestinal mucosal ischemia will result in sloughing and hemoccult-positive stools. **CT scan is notoriously insensitive for mesenteric ischemia, especially early in its course.** The first signs to appear are bowel wall thickening in a single arterial distribution. Late cases are characterized by pneumatosis, or air seen within the bowel wall. This is an ominous sign. **The key to treatment is early surgical intervention.** It can be argued that this woman should be taken to the OR based on history and physical findings alone, even if the CT were normal.

22. D. Contraindications to tPA for ischemic stroke include the following: **stroke or head trauma within 3 months**; any prior history of intracranial hemorrhage; major surgery within 14 days; GI or GU bleeding within 21 days; MI within 3 months; arterial puncture at a noncompressible site or lumbar puncture within 7 days; rapidly improving symptoms; only minor or isolated neurologic signs; seizure at stroke onset; symptoms suggestive of SAH, mandating lumbar puncture; clinical presentation consistent with acute MI or post-MI pericarditis; refractory hypertension (BP >185/110, despite treatment); pregnancy or lactation; active bleeding or acute trauma; platelets <100,000/mm^3; serum glucose <50 mg/dL or >400 mg/dL; INR >1.7 if on warfarin; elevated PTT if on heparin; evidence of hemorrhage on head CT; and evidence of major early infarct signs, such as diffuse swelling of the affected hemisphere.

23. E. This woman has a presentation consistent with mesenteric ischemia, which is occlusion of either the superior mesenteric artery (SMA) or inferior mesenteric artery (IMA), resulting in intestinal mucosal ischemia. **Embolism is the most common etiology of**

mesenteric ischemia in about 50% of cases, with the embolic source being a cardiac mural thrombus in most cases. Risk factors include coronary artery disease, valvular disease, and atrial fibrillation, the last being the most common. The second most common etiology of mesenteric ischemia is in situ arterial thrombosis, most often occurring at the origin of the SMA where atherosclerotic plaque tends to form. Patients with mesenteric vessel atherosclerosis tend to have plaque formation elsewhere also, as in the coronary or carotid arteries. Patients with mesenteric venous thrombosis usually have a history of peripheral deep venous thrombosis. Mesenteric venous thrombosis tends to occur in younger patients and is more indolent clinically than arterial occlusion.

24. C. This patient has ischemic EKG changes in the inferior leads (II, III, and aVF). **Approximately 25% to 40% of patients with inferior MIs will also have right ventricular MIs, typically due to acute occlusion in the RCA occurring proximal to the right ventricular branch.** Patients with RV infarctions are extremely dependent on right-ventricular filling pressure in order to maintain cardiac output. **Nitroglycerin (e.g., sublingual nitroglycerin 0.4 mg tablets) in the setting of RV infarction causes vasodilation, decreased right-ventricular filling pressure, and potential hypotension.** If this occurs, aggressive fluid resuscitation should be undertaken. Nitroglycerin can still be given in RV infarction, but typically patients should receive an initial fluid bolus and then titratable IV nitroglycerin as the blood pressure tolerates. Oxygen, aspirin, β-blockers, and heparin are also useful in the setting of acute STEMI in conjunction with cardiac catheterization or thrombolysis.

25. A. This patient has evidence of ascending cholangitis that is described by Charcot's triad of right upper quadrant pain, fever, and jaundice. These patients can become rapidly septic and thereby develop hypotension and altered mental status, making Reynold's pentad. The etiology is typically obstruction, often from a gallstone but sometimes due to a mass or underlying sclerosis. The most prominent organism is *E. coli*, but other enteric organisms are often present, such as *Enterococcus*, *Klebsiella*, and *Bacteroides*. **Early broad-spectrum antibiotics are crucial in ascending cholangitis and should include ampicillin, gentamicin, and metronidazole or clindamycin. The key to treatment is decompression of the biliary tract. This can be accomplished either endoscopically by ERCP or by open laparotomy with common bile duct exploration.** This patient will need to have a cholecystectomy anyway, but it would ideally be done in a delayed fashion to allow for resolution of the infection. Given the likely distal position of a common bile duct (CBD) stone (i.e., CBD >6 mm and evidence of pancreatic duct obstruction by lipase), an ERCP would likely be more effective in extracting the obstructing stone.

26. E. Eligibility criteria for thrombolysis in ST elevation MI include the following: ST elevation of 1 mm or more in two or more contiguous limb leads, ST elevation of 2 mm or more in two or more contiguous precordial leads, new or presumed new LBBB, time from symptom onset <12 hours, blood pressure <180/100 mm Hg after treatment, and no other contraindications to thrombolysis. Age is not a definitive contraindication to thrombolysis, though patients over age 75 years have a higher incidence of hemorrhagic stroke as a result of therapy.

27. D. This patient has a classic history and physical exam for acute cholecystitis. Ultrasound will typically show gallstones, gallbladder wall thickening, pericholecystic fluid, and **a positive sonographic Murphy's sign (the presence of maximal tenderness elicited over a sonographically localized gallbladder); the last is thought to be the most specific indicator for acute cholecystitis.** In the absence of confirmatory findings on ultrasound, the diagnosis of acalculous cholecystitis must be entertained, as it is present in about 10% of cases. It tends to occur in older patients and in those who have had recent surgery. Its mortality is higher, probably because it often goes undiagnosed. **The most sensitive test for cholecystitis is hepatic iminodiacetic acid (HIDA) scan**, which involves IV administration of IDA. IDA is absorbed through the liver and secreted into bile ducts. Delayed nuclear scintigraphy illuminates the biliary tree. Illumination of the common bile duct without the gallbladder is highly suggestive of cystic duct obstruction, and thus acute cholecystitis.

28. D. This patient has high-altitude pulmonary edema (HAPE), which typically occurs with rapid ascent (i.e., greater than 14,000 feet in 1 to 2 days). HAPE is characterized by dyspnea that is not relieved by rest, cough that is initially dry but which becomes productive of copious amounts of clear, watery sputum and sometimes even blood, rales, cyanosis, hypoxemia, tachycardia, and tachypnea. **The most important aspect of treatment for HAPE is descent, in addition to oxygen and bed rest.** Lasix 80 mg twice a day may also be useful to promote diuresis. Nifedipine 10 mg sublingually every 4 to 6 hours can be useful to promote pulmonary vasodilatation. Dexamethasone is used in the treatment of high-altitude cerebral edema (HACE).

29. A. The priority when evaluating unstable patients is ABCs. "A" and "B" have already been addressed by intubation and mechanical ventilation. The problem with this patient is "C," or namely, massive internal exsanguination from a ruptured AAA. **Establishing large-bore central venous access and aggressive blood transfusion are critical in the case of a ruptured AAA if the patient is to survive. However, this is temporizing until the patient can get to the OR for definitive repair.** Therefore, activating the OR is of utmost importance. This patient requires multiple units of uncrossmatched type O blood immediately.

30. C. This woman has a classic history for hypercalcemia, though patients without cancer and without bone metastases can also develop hypercalcemia. Common signs and symptoms of hypercalcemia in malignancy include itching, fatigue, muscle weakness, hyporeflexia, lethargy, apathy, perceptual and behavioral disturbances, stupor, coma, polyuria, polydipsia, renal insufficiency, anorexia, nausea, vomiting, constipation, abdominal pain, hypertension, dysrhythmias, and sensitivity to digitalis. **In hypercalcemia, the QT interval on EKG is shortened. ED management for hypercalcemia, after ABCs, consists primarily of fluid hydration (IV or PO, depending on the patient's status) and furosemide (Lasix) to promote calcium diuresis.** After the acute period in the ED, management also involves addressing the underlying cause of hypercalcemia, further promoting calcium excretion (e.g., calcitonin), decreasing calcium removal from bone (e.g., calcitonin and bisphosphonates), and reducing calcium intake.

31. C. Abdominal aortic aneurysms (AAAs) occur mostly in aging men and are associated with atherosclerotic disease elsewhere. The pathophysiology involves degradation of elastin and collagen, the structural components of arterial walls. AAA has no association with aortic dissections; the latter involves dissection of blood into the medial wall of the aorta, usually originating just distal to the take-off of the left subclavian artery in the chest. AAA is defined as an aortic diameter greater than 3 cm. The risk of rupture increases dramatically after it reaches 5 cm in diameter. Elective surgery should be undertaken to repair an AAA, as mortality for elective repair is about 5%. **When performing an abdominal exam, it is important to know that the aorta bifurcates at the level of the umbilicus, and an aneurysm if present is palpated in the epigastrium. Given that this patient has back pain, a CT scan with IV contrast should be obtained to rule-out rupture.** In any case, this patient should be admitted for an elective repair given the size of his AAA.

32. D. This patient's hypernatremia is likely due to dehydration from her diarrhea and has led to a reactive seizure. The more common electrolyte abnormality causing seizures is actually hyponatremia.

Hypoglycemia and hypocalcemia are also associated with seizure activity. **Correcting hypernatremia too quickly can lead to cerebral edema, while correcting hyponatremia too quickly can lead to central pontine myelinolysis**.

33. B. This infant has bronchiolitis. Administration of supplemental oxygen is the first priority. This will help improve oxygenation, and the addition of humidified saline may help clear respiratory secretions. Use of a bulb syringe to clear nasal secretions may also be indicated in this situation. Although the patient has signs of respiratory distress, she is still alert and is perfusing well. Therefore, endotracheal intubation is not indicated at this point. **Nebulized albuterol is often helpful in patients with bronchiolitis to reverse bronchospasm, especially if the child has a prior history of reactive airway disease.** Similar to asthma, bronchiolitis results in lower airway obstruction as a result of airway inflammation and bronchoconstriction. Nebulized epinephrine is indicated in children with croup, but is not used in bronchiolitis. Oral steroids, such as prednisolone, have not been proven effective for children with bronchiolitis.

34. B. Well-appearing patients between ages 3 and 36 months with no medical history that would make them prone to infection should undergo a thorough history and physical exam. Children 3 months to 3 years with a fever greater than 39.0°C (102.2°F) should have a CBC and blood culture sent. Children 6 months of age or less, and children under 36 months who have not been completely immunized, should further have CBC, blood culture, urinalysis, and urine culture; if WBC >15,000/mm^3, patients should receive 50 mg/kg of parenteral ceftriaxone. Chest x-ray should be done if patients have symptoms suggestive of pneumonia or WBC >20,000/mm^3. For girls under age 24 months and uncircumcised boys 6 to 12 months old, urinalysis and urine culture should be sent as well. Well-appearing children can then be discharged home with pediatrician follow-up within 24 to 48 hours (24 hours if ceftriaxone was given). Ill-appearing patients should undergo a full laboratory workup, including lumbar puncture when indicated, and intravenous antibiotics.

35. D. This patient has symptoms classic for bronchiolitis. **Bronchiolitis refers specifically to a lower respiratory tract infection with bronchiolar inflammation that leads to increased edema and mucus plugging, causing airway narrowing. However, upper airway congestion is also usually present.** Clinically, patients usually begin with rhinorrhea and cough, progressing to tachypnea, increased work of breathing, and wheezing. Patients may have a low-grade fever, but are usually not ill appearing. Bronchiolitis affects young children with small airways, with children under 2 years of age most commonly affected. Bronchiolitis is caused by a viral infection, most commonly respiratory syncytial virus (RSV). In this child, inspiratory rhonchi reflect transmitted upper airway sounds and show some degree of upper airway obstruction. Expiratory wheezing reflects inflammation of the lower airways and obstruction of the bronchioles. Although foreign body ingestion is a common cause of respiratory distress in young children, infants typically have sudden onset of symptoms and are not otherwise ill.

36. D. This woman has scombroid fish poisoning, as evidenced by her history of ingesting mahi mahi and her characteristic complaints of flushing, headache, dizziness, and abdominal cramps that started roughly 20 to 30 minutes to a few hours afterwards. Scombroid is caused by bacterial heat-stable toxins (histamine and histamine-like substances) in dark-fleshed fish (e.g., tuna, mahi mahi, mackerel, bluefish) due to improper refrigeration and handling. **Treatment is with parenteral antihistamines, such as diphenhydramine (Benadryl) or cimetidine (Zantac).** Scombroid is not an allergic reaction, and thus patients need not avoid fish in the future.

37. C. This patient has classic symptoms of a viral pharyngitis, which is far more common than bacterial pharyngitis. It is difficult to differentiate the two, especially in the setting of pharyngeal exudates that can be present in both; however, bacterial pharyngitis tends to be associated with higher fevers and a greater degree of adenopathy. A throat culture should be sent if there is suspicion for a bacterial source. Group A β-hemolytic streptococcus (GABHS) is a common bacterial source, especially in children. A rapid strep test is about 70% sensitive, and should be followed by a culture if negative. GABHS can cause a diffuse, erythematous, sandpaper rash known as scarlet fever; however, viral illnesses are also often associated with similar-appearing exanthems. Complications of untreated GABHS include rheumatic fever and post-streptococcal glomerulonephritis. Mononucleosis should be suspected in young adults with prolonged symptoms, impressive pharyngeal exudates, and lymphadenopathy. Diphtheria should always be in the differential for pharyngitis; it is characterized by gray and white spots in the back of the throat that coalesce into a pseudomembrane. The diphtheria toxin can cause multisystem organ failure.

38. E. This patient has ciguatera fish poisoning, with the classic "hot-cold reversal" of temperature perception. Ciguatera poisoning occurs due to a lipid-soluble, heat- and acid-stable toxin that accumulates in larger predatory coral-reef fish, such as sea bass, grouper, barracuda, and red snapper. Symptoms general appear 2 to 6 hours after ingestion, with worsening after alcohol consumption.

Symptoms are gastrointestinal (e.g., nausea, vomiting, profuse watery diarrhea, crampy abdominal pain, diaphoresis) and neurologic (e.g., sensory reversal dysesthesia, paresthesias, ataxia, weakness, vertigo, confusion). **Treatment is mainly supportive, with IV fluid hydration and analgesics as needed.**

39. E. There are several important entities to consider in patients who present with a sore throat with a normal-appearing pharynx. Constitutional symptoms should alert infection, such as retropharyngeal abscess (RPA), epiglottitis, or bacterial tracheitis. The hallmark of RPA is neck pain with range of motion. It is common in small children, who will often be unwilling to move their heads. Epiglottitis will present with sore throat and a muffled, "hot potato" voice. Patients with bacterial tracheitis will often appear ill, have throat pain, and have a productive cough. Given his symptoms since football practice, trauma should be considered. He has no midline posterior neck tenderness, making a cervical fracture less likely; laryngeal fracture should be associated with a specific, recalled blow to the anterior neck. **Anterior neck fullness with crepitus, along with voice change and sore throat, should raise suspicion for pneumomediastinum. This can occur spontaneously, or often in association with some type of exertional or contact activity, in which increased intrathoracic pressure causes a small disruption in the bronchoalveolar tree.** The result is air tracking into the mediastinum and up into the soft-tissue planes of the neck. Diagnosis can be made by plain x-ray of the neck and chest.

40. D. Lumbar disc herniation classically causes back pain with radiculopathy (sharp, shooting, or burning usually) to below the level of the knee. Elevation of the ipsilateral leg ("straight leg raise" test) usually worsens or reproduces the radicular pain in that leg. Elevation of the contralateral leg ("crossover straight leg raise" test) reproducing radicular symptoms is thought to be pathognomonic for nerve root irritation from a herniated disc. Spinal stenosis usually involves diffuse back pain in older patients, with or without radiation down one or both legs, and is due to compression of the spinal cord from narrowing of the canal. Cauda equina syndrome is a neurosurgical emergency, involving central disc herniation large enough to compromise the spinal cord, with symptoms of saddle anesthesia, bowel and bladder retention or incontinence, and bilateral leg pain. A spinal epidural hematoma causes sudden, severe, and constant back pain, and eventually (over hours to days) neurologic deficits. Which deficits occur depends on the location and extent of bleeding. Malingering refers to pretense of illness for secondary gain, usually narcotics.

41. E. This patient has suffered central retinal artery occlusion, usually resulting from an embolic clot in the retinal artery. This disease is commonly associated with carotid artery atherosclerosis and many have transient events known as amaurosis fugax, or TIAs involving the retinal artery. **Treatment consists of three aspects: 1) dislodge the thrombus, 2) dilate the artery, and 3) decrease intraocular pressure.** The first is attempted through digital orbital massage, applying pressure for 10 to 15 seconds and suddenly releasing. The second is achieved through increasing Pco_2 levels, which can be done by breathing into a paper bag. The third is accomplished through agents that decrease IOP such as timolol. Anterior chamber paracentesis will also acutely decrease IOP and facilitate forward blood flow. Intravenous acetazolamide has the effect of both decreasing intraocular pressure and dilating the retinal artery.

42. C. This patient has hyperglycemic hyperosmolar nonketotic coma (HHNC), as evidenced by the very high blood sugar (usually above 600 mg/dL) and the elevated serum osmolarity (greater than 350 mOsm/L), as well as the typical symptom of confusion. **In HHNC, the patient is severely dehydrated, with hypernatremia, hyperosmolarity, hyperglycemia, and altered mental status.** HHNC is more common in patients with type 2 diabetes, chronic renal insufficiency, GI bleeding, and gram-negative pneumonia or sepsis. Patients with HHNC do not generally have ketosis and usually have hypotonic urine.

43. A. This patient presents with primary angle-closure glaucoma, a condition that occurs in people with narrow anterior chambers. These patients have a natural obstruction of aqueous humor flow from the posterior to anterior chamber, causing an outward bowing of the iris. **Sudden dilatation of the iris can result in total obstruction of the trabecular meshwork, resulting in outflow obstruction and increased intraocular pressure. The major complication is optic nerve ischemia and subsequent blindness. Simply walking into a dimly lit room can precipitate this.** Medications with anticholinergic (e.g., atropine, Benadryl) or sympathomimetic (e.g., pseudoephedrine) effects can also precipitate glaucoma. First-line treatment is timolol and pilocarpine drops, a β-blocker and anti-cholinesterase, respectively. Prednisolone drops are also useful. Intravenous acetazolamide can be administered for severe cases. These agents are temporizing until an ophthalmologist can surgically correct the problem.

44. D. This patient has a dystonic reaction, likely from prochlor-perazine (Compazine) or promethazine (Phenergan) given to treat her nausea on her previous ED visit one day earlier. Acute dystonia is thought to arise because of an imbalance in the dopaminergic–cholinergic system in the basal ganglia. **Treatment for dystonia is with diphenhydramine or benztropine IV in the ED, followed by oral therapy for 48 to 72 hours.**

45. C. ABO incompatibility is rare (1 in 40,000) and is usually a result of a clerical error or administration of the wrong blood. ABO incompatibility is due to a direct attack of anti-AB antibodies on the red cell, resulting in intravascular hemolysis, which rapidly leads to renal failure, DIC, and cardiovascular collapse. The key is to recognize it and stop the transfusion while making efforts to maintain urine output with aggressive IV crystalloid and furosemide. **Rh and non-ABO incompatibilities result in extravascular hemolysis, in which red cells are consumed within the spleen.** These reactions tend to be less severe. Fever is the most common reaction to a blood transfusion. It is usually the result of antibodies to white cells or platelets in the donor blood. This only requires temporary cessation or slowing of the transfusion, antipyretics, and diphenhydramine.

46. C. Rabies is almost universally fatal, except in a very few rare cases in which the patient had been given either pre-exposure or post-exposure prophylaxis. Therefore, prophylaxis is extremely important to consider for any patient in the ED with a possible rabies exposure. Generally speaking, "exposure" is considered to be a bite, or contamination of saliva to an open wound or mucous membrane, in animals that are thought to carry rabies. Examples of such animals include raccoons, skunks, foxes, coyotes, dogs, groundhogs (woodchucks), and bats. In the case of bats, exposures further include any direct contact between a human and a bat, including being in the same room as a bat while sleeping, because of reports of rabies transmission from such contacts. **For a patient who has not previously been vaccinated, prophylaxis consists of both human rabies immune globulin (HRIG) 20 IU/kg given in and around the wound, with any remainder given IM; plus human diploid cell vaccine (HDCV) 1 mL IM on days 0, 3, 7, 14, and 28.** Patients who have previously been vaccinated should receive only HDCV 1 mL IM on days 0 and 3. All patients with bites or other exposure sites should have thorough wound scrubbing with soap, water, and a virucidal agent (e.g., povidone-iodine) because rabies is killed by soap, sunlight, and drying.

47. A. Intubation is a reasonable thought, given that this patient is likely having an anaphylactic reaction to nafcillin. Even though her airway is patent now, it may begin to swell, making intubation impossible if delayed. Intubation should be performed at the first sign of upper airway swelling. All of the listed medications are indicated in the treatment of a severe allergic reaction or anaphylaxis. **Although not yet hypotensive, this woman has signs of a severe systemic allergic reaction that requires aggressive management. Subcutaneous epinephrine 0.1 mL of a 1:1000 solution (contained in small vial) should be administered.** Simultaneously, nebulized albuterol can be given in order to stimulate bronchial β_2 receptors and dilate constricted airways. Solumedrol, Benadryl, and Zantac should also be administered intravenously.

48. D. This patient's signs and symptoms are classic for posterior circulation disease, with sudden onset of nausea, vomiting, vertigo (sense of self or world spinning or moving), and positive Romberg test. Hypertension is furthermore a risk factor for intracranial hemorrhage, as is age greater than 40 years. The patient should undergo emergent CT scan of the head to look for acute blood. Vertebral artery dissection (not carotid artery dissection) could also present with signs of vertebrobasilar insufficiency. Carotid artery dissection would lead to ischemic symptoms in the anterior cerebral artery (ACA) territory, middle cerebral artery (MCA) territory, or both. Ménière's disease and labyrinthitis would also present with vertigo, nausea, and vomiting, but cerebellar signs such as positive Romberg and gait ataxia should not be present. Conversion disorder refers to a psychiatric condition in which a patient usually presents with sudden onset of a dramatic finding, though the symptoms are not under the patient's voluntary control. It would only be considered as a diagnosis of exclusion.

49. D. This patient has an illness consistent with *Pneumocystis carinii* pneumonia (PCP). This organism is a parasite that is common in AIDS patients with CD4 counts less than 200 cells/mm³, a level below which prophylactic treatment with trimethoprim/sulfamethaxazole (Bactrim) is indicated. Bactrim is also first-line treatment for acute illness, with pentamidine an alternative for those with sulfa allergy. There is evidence that corticosteroids (e.g., prednisone) improve outcome in patients with a P_aO_2 <70 mm Hg or an A-a gradient >35 mm Hg. In practice, instead of obtaining a blood gas, patients with an O_2sat <90% are started on prednisone. **PCP is associated with an elevated serum LDH level.**

50. B. The patient described has alcoholic ketoacidosis (AKA), an anion-gap metabolic acidosis thought due to starvation in the setting of chronically low glycogen stores, dehydration, an imbalance of counterregulatory hormones, and the metabolism of alcohol. This leads to lipolysis, ketogenesis, and ketosis. Patients typically present with nausea, vomiting, and abdominal pain a few days following a binge of alcohol consumption and decreased food intake. **Treatment for AKA is primarily with D5NS rehydration, as well as repletion of potassium and thiamine.** Insulin has no role in the treatment of AKA, and bicarbonate is not routinely used either. Glucagon is a counterregulatory hormone; it is not part of AKA treatment.

51. C. *Legionella* is a source of atypical pneumonia that is usually mild and self-limited in young, healthy people. In the elderly or immunocompromised, it can present as a more severe illness with high fever, toxic appearance, altered mental status, dry cough, and pulmonary infiltrates. **The distinguishing characteristic of *Legionella* is that it is often associated with GI symptoms such as abdominal cramping and diarrhea.** Mycoplasma also causes an atypical pneumonia with scattered infiltrates, but patients are not often ill appearing. *S. pneumoniae* and *S. aureus* both present as lobar pneumonias.

52. E. The most likely explanation for this patient's pain and findings is a ruptured corpus luteum cyst on the left. The corpus luteum forms after release of an egg from a follicular cyst and produces hormones that support a pregnancy should the egg become fertilized. Corpus luteum cysts are caused by excessive accumulation of blood, which appears as complex free pelvic fluid by ultrasound after cyst rupture. Corpus luteum cysts usually rupture during the latter 2 weeks of the menstrual cycle. This patient's hCG is negative, which effectively rules out ectopic pregnancy. Ovarian torsion symptoms usually start suddenly as well, but normal Doppler flow to both ovaries rules out the diagnosis. Mittelschmerz refers to abdominal pain experienced mid-menstrual cycle due to ovulation. Fibroids are benign smooth muscle tumors in the uterus and do not generally cause acute-onset pain, although this is possible if a fibroid degenerates. Fibroids would be visible on ultrasound.

53. A. This woman has evidence of acute CHF, likely a result of new-onset atrial fibrillation (AF) with rapid ventricular response (RVR). **The key to treating her heart failure will be controlling her heart rate. If she were frankly unstable, electrical cardiover-**

sion would be indicated. In this scenario, amiodarone would be an ideal agent as it does not significantly affect blood pressure. Both metoprolol (Lopressor) and verapamil are negative inotropes, so should not be used in the setting of hypotension. A reasonable approach would be first to administer normal saline 500 mL IV bolus along with furosemide, and then reassess blood pressure before administering nodal-blocking agents. Digoxin would be a good choice for long-term heart rate control for AF in the setting of a low ejection fraction, as it results in positive inotropy, but would not be useful to acutely control her rate.

54. C. This patient has EKG findings consistent with acute posterior-wall MI, characterized by ST depressions in leads V_1–V_2, which would be ST elevations in posterior leads if checked, and prominent R waves in V_1–V_2, which would correspond to Q waves in posterior leads. In approximately 90% of individuals, the RCA or its posterior descending branch supplies the posterior wall of the left ventricle. The left circumflex artery supplies that area in the remaining 10% of individuals. Posterior wall MIs in isolation are actually not common; they more often occur in association with inferior or lateral MIs.

55. D. This woman has evidence of acute CHF with resulting myocardial ischemia. The treatment for this is aspirin, β-blocker, heparin, furosemide, nitroglycerin, and CPAP. However, she also has a murmur consistent with aortic stenosis. **Patients with significant aortic stenosis must chronically produce a higher cardiac output to overcome the fixed obstruction. These patients are very sensitive to agents that reduce preload, such as nitroglycerin.** Nitroglycerin may still be used; however, it should be started as an intravenous drip at a very low rate and should be stopped if any signs of decreased cardiac output develop. Metoprolol (Lopressor), a β-blocker, must also be used with care in this scenario, as it will have a negative inotropic effect.

56. E. Thyroid storm is at the end of the spectrum of hyperthyroidism and thyrotoxicosis; untreated, it can result in death. Treatment begins with propylthiouracil (PTU) or methimazole to inhibit further synthesis of thyroid hormone. **Iodine, in the form of potassium iodide, Lugol's iodine solution, or sodium iodide, is given to block release of hormone stored in the thyroid colloid. Iodine should not be given for at least one hour after PTU or methimazole; otherwise the iodine can be used to synthesize new thyroid hormone and worsen symptoms.** Propranolol is a β-blocker that is used to reduce symptoms such as palpitations, restlessness, dysrhythmias, and tremor. PTU, propranolol, or dexamethasone can be used to block the peripheral conversion of T_4 to T_3.

57. A. **This is a wide-complex tachycardia (WCT) that is highly suspicious for ventricular tachycardia (VT), given his history of a previous MI. It may also represent SVT with aberrancy (e.g., LBBB). Regardless, given the symptoms and low blood pressure, he can be considered unstable. This is an indication for electrical cardioversion starting with 100 J.** It is very reasonable to give fentanyl, as it has little effect on blood pressure, for mild sedation and pain control prior to administering the shock. Lidocaine is an agent used in stable VT, as is amiodarone. As a note, administering β-blockers or calcium-channel blockers to VT can result in hypotension and degeneration of the rhythm into ventricular fibrillation.

58. D. This patient's elevated BUN and creatinine are most likely due to prerenal azotemia from volume loss due to his trauma and burns. **In prerenal azotemia, the typical findings are BUN/Cr ratio greater than 10:1, urine sodium concentration less than 20 mEq/dL, fractional excretion of sodium (FENa) less than 1%, and urine specific gravity increased.** In normal individuals, the BUN/Cr ratio is roughly 10:1. This increases in hypovolemic states because the rate of tubular reabsorption of urea in the kidneys is increased (urea is passively reabsorbed in the proximal tubules, linked to the reabsorption of sodium and water), whereas creatinine clearance remains at a relatively constant steady state (creatinine is produced by skeletal muscle and is not reabsorbed at the renal tubules). The BUN/Cr ratio can often exceed 20:1. The FENa reflects sodium handling by the kidneys, and is estimated as (UNa $\times$ PCr) / (PNa $\times$ UCr) $\times$100%, in which UNa is urine sodium, PNa is plasma sodium, UCr is urine creatinine, and PCr is plasma creatinine.

59. E. This is a narrow-complex tachycardia (NCT), too fast to tell if it is regular or irregular. Given the rate, however, it is likely that this is AV nodal re-entrant tachycardia (AVNRT), a result of rapid circulation of an electrical impulse at the AV node. AVNRT is one of several types of supraventricular tachycardia (SVT), with rapid atrial fibrillation and flutter included. After recognizing the rhythm, the next step is to determine whether the patient is stable or not. This woman does have symptoms, but she cannot be considered unstable (e.g., chest pressure, respiratory distress, hypotension, etc). Unstable patients with NCT require immediate cardioversion. **Adenosine acts transiently at the AV node to stop any conduction through it, which in effect resets it. AVNRT will often convert to normal sinus rhythm with adenosine.** Verapamil is a calcium-channel blocker that can be effective in slowing NCT; however, it has a potent negative inotropic effect and can cause hypotension. Amiodarone has little negative inotropic effect and is useful in patients with a known impaired ejection fraction.

60. B. The right coronary artery gives rise to the AV nodal artery in 90% of individuals, while the left circumflex does so in the other 10%. Ischemia of the AV node can lead to heart block, so patients with an acute inferior MI should be monitored carefully for this potential complication.

61. A. This is a case of aortic dissection that is characterized by tearing chest or back pain, depending on the location of the dissection in the aorta. **Aortic dissection is a result of aortic wall weakening over time, resulting in a tear in the intima of the aorta with blood tracking into the media. Hypertension is the most common risk factor associated with aortic dissection.** Longstanding hypertension results in repeated stress on the aortic wall with each heartbeat, with the most stress occurring at the point where the aorta dives into the posterior mediastinum, at the origin of the descending aorta. The patient in this case has the physical traits of Marfan's syndrome. About 40% of patients with Marfan's syndrome eventually develop aortic dissection, due to inherent connective tissue weakness in the aortic wall; however, only 5% of patients with aortic dissection have Marfan's syndrome. Of note, atherosclerosis is a risk factor for aortic aneurysm, not dissection. Ehlers-Danlos syndrome and recent cardiac surgery are also risk factors for aortic dissection.

62. D. Cough-variant asthma is commonly associated with wheezing and shortness of breath, but can present as an isolated symptom. This patient's history of eczema and her lack of any URI symptoms or chest x-ray findings, in addition to the fact that her symptoms come on with cold air or exertion, point toward the diagnosis. Peak expiratory flow rate (PEFR) may show a decrease as in classic asthma, but it is often normal in the absence of symptoms. **The diagnosis of cough-variant asthma is confirmed if one week of inhaled β-agonist therapy, such as albuterol, leads to improvement of cough symptoms.**

63. D. The patient presents with symptoms classic for thoracic aortic dissection, a disease that involves dissection of blood into the media layer of the aorta, usually at the level of the distal aortic arch at the branch of the left subclavian artery. A dissection usually propagates distally to involve the descending aorta, although it can also propagate proximally to involve the arch and ascending portion of the aorta. **A dissection that propagates to the aortic root can result in aortic regurgitation, coronary artery occlusion, and pericardial tamponade. The last is characterized by hypotension, distant heart sounds, and elevated jugular venous pressure (Beck's triad).** This patient is unstable and therefore unfit to go to CT scan. Although it is possible for a pulmonary embolus to present with acute chest or back pain and shortness of breath, administration of thrombolytics would be lethal in the setting of aortic dissection. **The best action is to do a bedside ultrasound to confirm pericardial tamponade such that an emergent pericardiocentesis can be done to stabilize the patient.** If the patient remains unstable, the patient should be intubated, undergo transesophageal echocardiogram (TEE) to make the diagnosis of aortic dissection, and go to the OR for repair. If stable, the patient can go to CT scan to make the diagnosis.

64. D. Hip pain will often be referred to the knee, necessitating a thorough evaluation of the hips in any patient who complains of knee pain or limp. **Slipped capital femoral epiphysis (SCFE) classically occurs in boys more often than girls, around the time of their growth spurt at approximately age 13, and especially in those who are overweight. SCFE is thought to be due to weakness in the physeal cartilage, exacerbated by rapid growth and overweight body. Although the symptoms usually come on gradually, patients usually present once the parents notice their child limping.** Exam will reveal tenderness over the hip, pain with range of motion of the hip along with decreased range of motion, and an abducted, externally rotated thigh. Given the benign examination of this patient's left knee, the diagnosis of pathology at that joint is much less likely. Transient synovitis refers to a common nonbacterial inflammation with unclear etiology that usually affects the hip or knee; septic arthritis must first be ruled out by arthrocentesis before transient synovitis can be given as a diagnosis. Legg-Calvé-Perthes's disease refers to avascular necrosis of the femoral head; this usually afflicts boys more than girls, between the ages of 2 and 10 years.

65. B. **This child has a persistent cough worse at night and inspiratory stridor on exam, findings consistent with croup.** Classically, the cough is described as a "barking seal." Patients with croup benefit from humidified oxygen, as it helps clear respiratory secretions and makes them feel comfortable. **Nebulized racemic epinephrine is indicated for evidence of respiratory difficulty, as it causes arteriole vasoconstriction and a reduction in subglottic edema, which reduces upper airway obstruction and improves breathing.** Steroids are proven to decrease inflammation and edema that contribute to respiratory distress. The steroid will take effect after 4 to 6 hours, and it will minimize rebound swelling that can occur with epinephrine. Albuterol, a β-agonist, may have a small effect but it acts primarily as a bronchodilator in asthma.

66. C. This patient clinically has a bowel obstruction, likely large-bowel (LBO) given the degree of her abdominal distention. **Barium enema is more sensitive for making the diagnosis of LBO than plain radiography. In this case, however, a KUB and upright should first be obtained to rule out perforation. Additionally, most cases of volvulus will be seen by plain radiography.** Her obstruction is likely due to cecal or sigmoid volvulus, in which case a cause for the volvulus (e.g., cancer) must be sought. Treatment for volvulus is initially rectal tube placement or rigid sigmoidoscopy. If this fails to reduce the volvulus, then surgery is indicated.

67. A. Elderly white men are at by far the highest risk for completing suicide, accounting for approximately 80% of suicide deaths. All the answers listed are risk factors for suicide based on the SAD PERSONS criteria listed in Case 24: 1) **S**ex (male); 2) **A**ge (<19 or >45); 3) **D**epression or hopelessness; 4) **P**revious suicide attempts or psychiatric admissions; 5) **E**xcessive alcohol or drug use; 6) **R**ational thinking loss (psychotic features that are affecting ability to think rationally); 7) **S**eparated, divorced, or widowed; 8) **O**rganized or serious attempt; 9) **N**o social supports; 10) **S**tated future intent. Of these, numbers 3, 6, 8, and 10 are considered higher-risk attributes. Therefore, **the fact that this man has a firearm and a plan to use it is the most ominous sign for future completed suicide.**

68. C. The classic symptoms of duodenal ulcer are pain in the epigastrium described as burning, indigestion-type symptoms such as belching or bloating, and reflux-type symptoms; symptoms typically come on 2 to 5 hours after eating or with an empty stomach. NSAIDs such as ibuprofen are known to predispose patients to ulcer formation. **Patients with *Helicobacter pylori* (*H. pylori*) confirmed by serology testing should be given treatment to eradicate the *H. pylori* given its association with peptic ulcer disease.** Four possible treatment regimens include: (1) **PPI + amoxicillin 1000 mg + clarithromycin 500 mg (each BID × 2 weeks)**; (2) PPI + metronidazole 500 mg + clarithromycin 500 mg (each BID × 2 weeks); (3) Bismuth subsalicylate 525 mg QID + metronidazole 500 mg QID + tetracycline 500 mg QID + PPI BID (each × 2 weeks); (4) Bismuth subsalicylate 525 mg QID + metronidazole 500 mg QID + tetracycline 500 mg QID + H2-blocker (each × 2 weeks + 2 additional weeks of H2-blocker).

69. E. This patient presents with toxic alcohol poisoning, characterized by profound mental status depression, hypotension, and anion-gap acidosis. His tachypnea is secondary to acidosis and a physiologic response in attempt to eliminate serum carbonic acid in the form of CO_2. The two most dangerous toxic alcohols are methanol and ethylene glycol. Both cause CNS depression, profound anion-gap acidosis, renal failure, and death. Methanol is typically associated with blindness. Ethylene glycol toxicity is usually the result of drinking radiator fluid, hence the fluorescent urine under a Wood's lamp. **Toxic metabolites of methanol and ethylene glycol, formic acid and oxalic acid, respectively, are produced by the enzyme alcohol dehydrogenase. This reaction can be inhibited by co-ingesting alcohol, which itself is metabolized by alcohol dehydrogenase. Fomepizole (4-methylpyrazole, or 4-MP) is a medication given intravenously that inhibits the enzyme as well. The goal is to prevent metabolism of methanol or ethylene glycol until hemodialysis can be done to remove the substances.** Of note, oxalic acid binds calcium and results in both serum hypocalcemia and urine calcium oxalate crystals.

70. C. Epiploic appendagitis (EA) refers to a condition in which one of the epiploic appendages, located on the external surface of the colon, torses or twists at the appendage pedicle, leading to inflammation and usually acute-onset pain. Symptoms can mimic that of appendicitis or diverticulitis, but it is easily distinguishable by CT scan, which will classically show a 2- to 3-cm, fat-density, oval-shaped, paracolic mass with thickened peritoneal lining and peri-appendageal fat stranding. **Treatment for EA is conservative, as the natural course of epiploic appendagitis is benign and self-limited. Ibuprofen plus narcotic pain medications as needed is the regimen usually recommended.** Exploratory laparotomy would be indicated for a patient who is hemodynamically unstable due to an intraabdominal process. Laparoscopic appendectomy is not indicated because the CT scan reveals a normal, contrast-filling appendix. Metronidazole and ciprofloxacin are the treatment regimen for diverticulitis.

71. B. Acetaminophen overdose is very serious because it can result in liver failure and death, despite initial symptoms in the first few days after ingestion that may be relatively mild. **Toxic ingestions are those greater than about 140 mg/kg body weight, or about 7 to 8 grams, 14 to 16 extra-strength tablets in an adult. A toxic level is considered a serum concentration of 140 µg/mL at 4 hours after ingestion, based on the Rumack-Matthew nomogram.** Symptoms within the first 24 hours include nausea, vomiting, malaise, and abdominal discomfort. These symptoms typically resolve, which can be falsely reassuring. At 24 to 48 hours, liver injury ensues, heralded by the recurrence of abdominal pain and constitutional symptoms, as well as elevations in ALT and AST. Maximal liver injury occurs at 3 to 4 days after ingestion. Fulminant hepatic failure can result. *N*-acetylcysteine (NAC), if administered within 8 hours of ingestion, can entirely prevent liver toxicity. If the oral preparation is not tolerated, it can be given in a diluted form intravenously. The dose is 140 mg/kg initially, followed by 70 mg/kg every 4 hours for 17 doses.

72. C. This woman has a presumptive massive pulmonary embolus leading to hemodynamic instability. **Absolute contraindications to thrombolysis for PE include active major external bleeding, active internal bleeding (even if minor), recent neurosurgery in the past 8 weeks, recent hepatic or renal biopsy, recent ocular surgery in the past 8 weeks, and diabetic retinopathy with recent hemorrhage.** Relative contraindications include major trauma, recent surgery including organ biopsy, recent major vessel puncture unless the cannula is still in place, immediately postpartum, recent past history of GI bleeding, hypertension uncontrolled at the time of thrombolysis, long-standing diastolic hypertension over 110 mm Hg, recent prolonged CPR, current pregnancy, bacterial endocarditis, and CNS cancer.

73. A. Inhalation injury is the leading cause of mortality in closed-space fires, due primarily to resulting upper airway edema and airway obstruction. Inhalation pneumonitis can also result from the transit of noxious substances into the bronchoalveolar system. This would cause alveolar exudates, impaired alveolar membrane diffusion, and low blood oxygen tension. Carbon monoxide (CO) poisoning should also be a consideration in closed-space fires. CO binds hemoglobin with 240 times the affinity of oxygen, thereby drastically reducing the oxygen-carrying capacity of blood. Oxygen saturation, the measurement of dissolved oxygen in serum, will remain unaffected. Symptoms of severe toxicity include altered mental status, seizures, hypotension, and metabolic acidosis. **Cyanide poisoning should additionally be considered in closed-space fires, especially in the setting of a profound metabolic acidosis. Cyanide inhibits oxidative phosphorylation, thus halting aerobic metabolism. Oxygen is therefore not absorbed by peripheral tissues, resulting in an unusually high oxygen tension in venous blood, giving it a bright, arterial appearance.**

74. C. Acute exacerbations of asthma can be quite severe, sometimes termed "status asthmaticus," and require immediate intervention.

After rapidly assessing ABCs, pharmacologic treatment should start with inhaled β-agonists, the quickest way of reversing bronchoconstriction and therefore improving airflow obstruction. β-agonists furthermore help by reducing bronchial mucosal edema. Albuterol, a selective β_2-agonist, is the mainstay of treatment for initial bronchodilator therapy. Inhaled ipratropium bromide, an anticholinergic agent, may also add to bronchodilation by a different mechanism. Intravenous methylprednisolone, as well as other corticosteroids, is thought to potentiate the β-responsiveness of airway smooth muscle, reduce mucosal edema and inflammatory cell infiltration, and decrease mucus secretion. The beneficial effects of corticosteroids may take up to several hours to begin. Theophylline, a systemic β-agonist, has not been shown in trials to improve outcome. Magnesium sulfate has been shown to improve outcome in moderate to severe asthma attacks.

75. C. This farm worker presents with symptoms of organophosphate poisoning, which acts by inhibition of acetylcholinesterase and prevents the degradation of acetylcholine. As a result, a cholinergic syndrome ensues, characterized by a hypersecretory state (e.g., salivation, lacrimation, bronchial secretions, vomiting, diarrhea, abdominal cramps, and incontinence). Also characteristic are lethargy, miosis, and bradycardia. The initial concern is for airway obstruction secondary to tracheobronchial secretions. A secondary concern is respiratory muscle weakness due to nicotinic receptor stimulation in the neuromuscular junction of skeletal muscles, including the diaphragm. Initial fasciculations are followed by muscle paralysis, similar to the result of administering succinylcholine for intubation. The treatment is high-dose atropine, the classic anticholinergic agent, 2 to 5 mg IV every 5 minutes until respiratory secretions dry up. Patients need to be on a cardiac monitor with a defibrillator in place because atropine can precipitate ventricular fibrillation in hypoxic patients.

76. B. Whichever the method used for foreign body removal from the nose, nebulized racemic epinephrine pretreatment will cause vasoconstriction of the nasal mucosa and thus facilitate removal. Pretreatment with a topical anesthetic, such as benzocaine spray, can also help by allowing the patient (often a child) to cooperate better. Magill forceps can be critical in removal of certain foreign bodies, especially in the airway, but would not fit in a useful way in the naris to grasp a coffee bean. Blind probing with any instrument is dangerous, as a nasal foreign body can become dislodged or driven posteriorly into the nasopharynx, with subsequent risk of aspiration. A right-angle probe may be useful for getting

behind certain foreign bodies to facilitate removal, but is less useful for the case of a coffee bean that does not have free space surrounding it. A papoose or other type of physical restraint is often necessary to safely permit examination and removal attempts in very young children. **Another method of removal after pretreatment with a vasoconstrictive agent is by use of positive pressure given through the patient's mouth while the unobstructed naris is gently occluded with a finger.** This can be accomplished either with a manual ventilation bag, or with a "kiss" from the parent.

77. E. This patient has suffered severe hypothermia, defined as a core body temperature of 28°C or less. Despite his initial prolonged water immersion and cardiac arrest, victims of prolonged immersion in cold water should be resuscitated aggressively due to numerous reports of favorable outcome. **As with any patient, the ABCs are of primary importance. This patient requires immediate deep tracheal suctioning to remove water that may have been aspirated.** The next priority would be arranging for emergent cardiopulmonary bypass, the most effective means of rewarming. Thoracic and gastric lavage are also means of active rewarming that can be utilized. More simple means of active rewarming include heat lamps and warmed IV fluid. Vasopressors will be of little use in hypothermia-induced circulatory shock.

78. D. UV keratitis, or Welder's keratitis, occurs from exposure of the eyes to natural or artificial sources of UV radiation, such as a welder's arc, the sun, suntanning lights, and lightning, resulting in diffuse irritation of the superficial corneal epithelium. On fluorescein staining, there is diffuse uptake due to superficial punctate epithelial surface irregularities. This condition is also known as superficial punctate keratitis. Treatment consists mainly of ibuprofen and narcotic analgesia for the inflammation and pain, which should improve significantly within 24 to 48 hours. A short-acting cycloplegic drop, such as cyclopentolate, can be used to help relieve pain from reflex ciliary spasm. Topical antibiotic ointment, such as erythromycin, can also be applied. **Patients should never be discharged home with a topical anesthetic due to delayed epithelial healing and possible corneal ulcer formation, as well as predisposition to further injury due to lack of corneal sensation.**

79. D. This man has suffered frostbite to his toes. **Frostbite occurs when tissues are exposed to subfreezing temperatures and ice crystals form, resulting in cellular damage and microvascular thrombosis.** This can initially look relatively benign, presenting primarily with numbness and a "dead weight" feeling of hands or feet. Initial appearance may be of pale, waxy-appearance, and immobile subdermal tissue. Clear vesicles can form early and are akin to second-degree burns involving the dermis. Hemorrhagic blebs develop late and indicate subdermal vascular injury, akin to third-degree burns and associated with poorer outcome. **The treatment is rapid rewarming with warm-water immersion, which will result in hyperemia, edema, and pain. After rewarming, frostbite is treated like a burn with elevation and sterile dressings.** Clear vesicles can be debrided to prevent thromboxane-mediated tissue injury. Hemorrhagic blisters should be left intact to reduce risk of infection. Tetanus booster should be given if not up to date.

80. A. **The "superficial femoral vein" is actually a deep vein, and thus this patient has a DVT rather than superficial thrombophlebitis. The treatment for DVT is anticoagulation with either IV heparin or SC low-molecular weight heparin as a bridge until the patient's warfarin (Coumadin) level is therapeutic.** Because this patient is hemodynamically stable and otherwise well, she can be treated at home. Rest, elevation, local heat, and NSAIDs are used for superficial thrombophlebitis. Compression stockings are additionally often used for superficial or deep clots in the lower extremities. Thrombolysis is usually done for catheter-associated clots; the catheter should be removed in such instances.

81. C. The rate of transmission to household contacts of meningococcus is about 5%; therefore, it is recommended that contacts, including care providers, receive antibiotic prophylaxis. **Rifampin is considered the first-line agent at a dose of 600 mg by mouth twice daily for 4 days. Single-dose alternatives are ciprofloxacin 500 mg by mouth, azithromycin 500 mg by mouth, or ceftriaxone 250 mg IM.**

82. C. **This patient has a subconjunctival hemorrhage, which results from rupture of small subconjunctival blood vessels. Patients may or may not recall any preceding traumatic incident. It can also be precipitated by transient increases in intraocular pressure such as in sneezing, coughing, or bearing down. Treatment is cold compresses for 24 hours to the affected eye; these resolve on their own after 2 to 3 weeks.** It is important to tell patients that the appearance of the eye may look worse before improving on its own. Erythromycin eye ointment would be indicated for conjunctivitis as well as several other conditions. Emergent ophthalmology consult is not indicated for subconjunctival hemorrhage, and outpatient follow-up with ophthalmology is also generally not necessary. Topical timolol and IV acetazolamide are part of the treatment regimen for acute angle-closure glaucoma,

which presents with a painful eye. Prednisone is needed in certain eye conditions, such as vision loss due to temporal arteritis.

83. D. It is important to rapidly administer ceftriaxone 2 g IV when meningitis is suspected, given the rapid increase in mortality with delayed treatment in bacterial meningitis. This will not alter the findings on LP other than decrease the sensitivity of CSF cultures after 6 hours. **When bacterial meningitis is confirmed by cell count, protein, and glucose, antibiotic coverage should be expanded to include vancomycin to cover resistant streptococcus and staphylococcus, ampicillin to cover *Listeria*, and acyclovir to cover herpes meningoencephalitis.** Coverage can be narrowed based on culture results and sensitivities the next day. *Listeria* **(a gram-positive rod), is more prevalent in the elderly, accounting for 25% of cases in patients ages 60 and older.** Overall, *Streptococcus pneumoniae* (gram-positive cocci in pairs) is the most common organism, followed by *Neisseria meningitidis* (gram-negative diplococci). The latter is the most common organism in young adults.

84. B. Back blows and abdominal thrusts are attempted first to try to dislodge an airway foreign body either entirely out or to a position where it can be removed under direct visualization. Blind finger sweeping should not be attempted, as this can push a foreign body from the oropharynx further back, possibly converting a partially obstructed airway to a fully obstructed airway. If back blows and abdominal thrusts are unsuccessful, direct laryngoscopy may allow direct visualization of the foreign body and then Magill forceps can be used to attempt removal of the foreign body. If still unsuccessful or if the foreign body is not visualized on direct laryngoscopy, the endotracheal tube can be advanced past the carina, in an attempt to push a foreign body into one bronchus. The endotracheal tube can then be pulled back to above the carina; this should allow temporary oxygenation and ventilation of the unobstructed lung while awaiting definitive intervention in the OR.

85. B. Disseminated gonococcal infection can occur in up to 3% of patients with untreated mucosal infections, more commonly occurring in women. A diffuse pustular rash can develop in days to weeks after the primary infection, usually in the extremities but also on the trunk. Thereafter, the infection can result in a septic arthritis, usually monoarticular. Despite the purulent nature of the arthritis, the fluid count is usually less then 50,000 WBCs/hpf. Both joint fluid and blood cultures have a sensitivity of less than 50%. The Gram's stain is more sensitive, at 60% to 70%. **The most sensitive test, however, is a culture of the primary mucosal site, yielding a sensitivity of 80%.** Another important distinction from non-gonorrheal septic arthritis is that joint washout is not usually indicated; the treatment is IV ceftriaxone.

86. C. Mesenteric adenitis is characterized by inflamed mesenteric lymph nodes, usually in the right lower quadrant, and can be confused with acute appendicitis. **Mesenteric adenitis, however, is a benign and self-limited disease, most often caused by viruses.** Other pathogens include *Yersinia enterocolitica*, *Helicobacter jejuni*, *Campylobacter jejuni*, *Salmonella* species, and *Shigella* species. A bacterial etiology with ileal thickening would more likely result in bloody diarrhea, or heme-positive stools. An appendicolith is often the cause of acute obstruction of the appendix, leading to acute appendicitis. Chronic constipation is associated with problems such as diverticulosis and diverticulitis.

87. E. Septic arthritis must always be considered when assessing a warm, red, painful knee. The problem sometimes lies in the fact that other more common inflammatory processes of the knee, namely gout and pseudogout, can present in exactly the same way. To complicate matters even more, sometimes there is not a large effusion and fluid aspiration can be challenging. If there is very little fluid obtained, the most important test is a fluid culture, followed by a Gram's stain and cell count with differential. **A cell count of greater than 50,000 WBCs/hpf is very concerning for septic arthritis and should prompt admission for IV antibiotics and a knee washout if the Gram's stain or culture is positive. A cell count between 5,000 and 50,000 WBCs/hpf is less specific and management is based on the Gram's stain and the crystal analysis. If the patient insists on going home, at least make sure that the Gram's stain is negative. Keep in mind, however, that this is only 50% to 70% sensitive for septic arthritis.**

88. C. External hemorrhoids are those that arise from below the dentate line, while internal hemorrhoids arise from above the dentate line. Thrombosed external hemorrhoids (deep purple and hard) are the only type that can be evacuated in the ED for relief of pain and to prevent skin tag formation; an *elliptical incision* is made after appropriate local anesthetic, and the clot is removed. *Linear incision* is used for drainage of an abscess, but should not be used for evacuating clot in a thrombosed external hemorrhoid due to likely early closure of the incision and reaccumulation of blood. *Total excision* of hemorrhoids is not indicated in the ED due to potential infectious and bleeding complications. This is an outpatient surgical procedure. Thrombosed internal hemorrhoids are not reducible and can become gangrenous; these require emergent surgical hemorrhoidectomy. **Patients with any other types of internal**

or external hemorrhoids can be discharged on the "WASH" regimen (warm water, analgesic agents, stool softeners, and high-fiber diet) with elective surgical follow-up.

89. C. When placing a leg cast or splint, it is important to provide padding at the proximal head of the fibula in order to prevent compression of the peroneal nerve, which courses inferiorly around the head of the fibula from posterior to anterior just before it breaks off into the deep and superficial peroneal nerves. The deep peroneal nerve enters the anterior compartment, along with the anterior tibial artery, and innervates the extensor muscles that allow dorsiflexion of the foot. It also provides sensation to the first web space. The superficial peroneal nerve provides sensation to the lateral aspect of the leg and dorsum of the foot. The saphenous nerve provides sensation to the medial aspect of the lower leg. The tibial nerve runs in the deep posterior compartment and innervates the flexor muscles responsible for foot plantarflexion.

90. D. Hot tar burns should be managed by first using cold water until the tar is hardened and cool. The tar should then be removed to prevent bacterial growth at the site of injured skin; this requires breaking the bond of the tar with the hair on the skin. Organic solvents can theoretically be useful for this purpose, but can be systemically absorbed and cause their own ill effects. **Neosporin ointment does not cause systemic or local toxicity but allows for tar removal due to its petrolatum ointment component, while also providing antibacterial effects.** Other options, especially when very large surface areas are involved, include sunflower oil, butter, or baby oil.

91. A. This patient has clinical evidence of compartment syndrome. The most sensitive signs are tenderness over the compartment and pain with passive ROM of the muscle contained within the compartment. Other signs include paresthesias and motor weakness, resulting from nerve compression. Arterial insufficiency (with absent distal pulses or pallor) is the latest sign. If the diagnosis is in doubt, compartment pressures can be measured with a Stryker device. Pressures greater than 30 mm Hg are suggestive of the diagnosis. **This patient has clinical evidence of compartment syndrome in addition to a fracture that requires operative repair.**

92. B. Colchicine is used in acute gout attacks, diagnosed by joint fluid having a negative culture but presence of negatively birefringent crystals under a polarizing microscope. Colchicine inhibits microtubule formation and the inflammatory response to crystals in the joint. NSAIDs, classically indomethacin, are useful in combination with colchicine in an acute attack. Ceftriaxone is not indicated in gout; ceftriaxone is indicated in patients with septic arthritis due to gonorrhea. Allopurinol and probenecid are used for long-term therapy to try to prevent further gout attacks, via decreasing uric acid production and increasing uric acid excretion, respectively; they are not useful in an acute attack. Oxycodone may be helpful for pain, but does not address the inflammatory nature of the disease.

93. B. Minor first- and second-degree burns are very common in the emergency department and can be managed as an outpatient. Admission criterion for a partial-thickness burn is 10% to 20% BSA involvement. It is important to cleanse the burn surface, ideally with a sponge and water. Large blisters should be debrided. Application of bacitracin and daily dressing changes with reapplication of bacitracin is a reasonable approach. The problem is that patients often do not fully cleanse the old bacitracin before reapplying the new due to pain, which can result in increased risk of infection. **A recommended approach is the application of sterile fine-mesh gauze soaked with 0.9% sodium chloride, then a layer of fluff gauze, and all covered by a roller-gauze.** The patient should have follow-up in 2 days, at which time the outer layer is removed. If the fine-mesh gauze is covering dry, pink wound, then it can be left in place for the next 7 days. If there is evidence of infection, the gauze is removed, the wound cleaned, and silver sulfadiazine cream applied twice daily after cleansing the wound thoroughly. Oral antibiotics have no role in preventing infection.

94. A. Peritonsillar abscess (PTA, or "quinsy") usually occurs following acute tonsillitis that then spreads to the peritonsillar tissues. PTA is the most common of the deep space infections of the head and neck in the adult. It is characterized by pain and difficulty swallowing, trismus, "hot potato" voice, fever, malaise, dehydration, and rancid breath. Exam is usually significant for erythematous oropharyngeal mucosa, purulent tonsillar exudates, and inferomedial displacement of the tonsil on the involved side with contralateral deviation of the uvula. Ludwig's angina refers to infection involving the connective tissues of the floor of the mouth and neck. Ludwig's angina has potential to cause acute airway obstruction due to extensive edema and soft-tissue swelling in the sublingual and submaxillary spaces. Retropharyngeal abscess (RPA) occurs in the retropharyngeal space or prevertebral space, and is characterized by sore throat, dysphagia, odynophagia, drooling, muffled voice, neck stiffness, neck pain, and fever. Pharyngitis is limited to the pharynx and/or tonsils. Parapharyngeal abscess (PPA) arises from dental, tonsillar, and pharyngeal infections, or contiguous spread from other deep neck space infections. PPA is characterized by pain and swelling of the neck, odynophagia, medial tonsillar displacement, posterolateral pharyngeal wall bulge, fever, and trismus.

95. D. This patient has sustained blunt traumatic injury with potential intracranial injury and hypotension. Given his mental status, the first priority is intubation. The next priority is a search for the cause of hypotension. Sources to consider include pericardial tamponade, hemothorax, aortic rupture, intraperitoneal bleeding, and pelvic or retroperitoneal bleeding. This patient has evidence of intraperitoneal bleeding and the potential for pelvic bleeding as well. The patient is too unstable to go to CT scan. Rapid administration of normal saline is reasonable; however, uncross-matched type O blood should be administered as soon and as rapidly as possible. If responsive to fluid and blood resuscitation, then CT scans can be performed. However, **if there is no response to initial resuscitation, immediate exploratory laparotomy is indicated to control intraperitoneal bleeding.** Pelvic angiography may be necessary if hypotension persists in order to embolize bleeding pelvic vessels. Neurosurgery should meanwhile place an intracranial bolt in the OR until the patient is stable enough to go for CT scan of the head.

96. D. A lesion at L4 would result in loss of the patellar reflex as well as difficulty with abducting at the hip. A lesion at S1 would result in loss of the Achilles reflex and trouble with plantar flexion of the foot. The other options listed do not have specific reflexes associated, but L2 can be tested with hip flexion, L3 can be tested with hip adduction, and L5 can be tested with dorsiflexion of the foot.

97. B. Fluid resuscitation is recommended in burns greater than 20% BSA due to gastrointestinal ileus and significant insensible losses. Traditionally the Parkland formula was used, which calculates the 24-hour crystalloid requirement at 4 mL/kg per % BSA of second- and third-degree burns. So for a 20% burn in a 70-kg person, the fluid required over 24 hours would be $4 \times 70 \times 20$, or 5,600 mL. Half this total amount is given over the first 8 hours, the rest over the next 16 hours. This formula often results in overhydration, with adult respiratory distress syndrome (ARDS) as a consequence. Therefore, **current recommendations are to titrate crystalloid (normal saline or lactated ringers) to urine output of about 0.5 mL/kg/hr, or about 30 to 40 mL/hr in a normal adult.** In theory colloid solution might benefit burn patients, increasing intravascular osmotic pressure and decreasing third-spacing (i.e., soft-tissue edema, ARDS). However, there are no data that show this practice improves outcome.

98. B. Central cord syndrome is due to trauma or spinal cord pathology (e.g., syrinx) that affects the central part of the spinal

cord, leading to loss of motor function in the arms bilaterally more than the legs, with variable sensory disturbances. In the setting of trauma, it is thought to be due to hyperextension injury with buckling of the ligamentum flavum leading to central cord injury. Anterior cord syndrome refers to bilateral loss of motor function and sensation to pain and temperature below the level of the spinal cord injury; this is usually due to hyperflexion or axial load injury to the neck. Cauda equina syndrome involves disc herniation in the distal spinal cord, which leads to saddle anesthesia, urinary retention, decreased rectal tone, severe low back pain with shooting pains down the leg(s), and lower extremity weakness. The Brown-Séquard syndrome refers to hemisection of the spinal cord, usually from penetrating trauma, leading to ipsilateral loss of motor function, proprioception, and sense of vibration, with contralateral loss of pain and temperature sensation. Sciatica refers to pain in the distribution of the sciatic nerve due, for example, to lumbar disc herniation.

99. D. The primary survey in trauma resuscitation consists of assessing the ABCs in conjunction with establishing "IV-O_2-monitor." During the primary survey, intubation is performed if airway patency is in jeopardy (e.g., decreased mental status, blood in the airway), breathing is inadequate, or circulatory shock exists. The need for rapid chest tube placement should also be considered in a patient with respiratory difficulty. **The two things to consider with circulatory shock and hypoxia after intubation are improper tube placement and tension pneumothorax.** CO_2 capnometry is the most effective means to confirm tube placement; it is more reliable than visual confirmation, auscultation, or chest x-ray. **This patient has a right-sided pneumothorax as is evident by chest wall crepitus. Optimally in this case a right-sided chest tube would be placed in conjunction with intubation.**

100. A. **The patient described has Ludwig's angina, which is usually a polymicrobial disease of the normal mouth flora.** The other options listed, including streptococci, staphylococci, *Klebsiella* species, and *Bacteroides* species, are possible organisms within this mix.

Index

Page numbers followed by *f* or *t* refer to figures or tables, respectively.

Abdominal aortic aneurysm (AAA)
  clinical presentation, 297–298
  diagnostic evaluation, 300–301, 412, 449
  immediate actions, 298, 412, 449
  management, 299
  pathophysiology, 449
  risk factors, 300
  rupture rate, 301
  rupture risk, 301, 449
Abdominal pain. *See also* Pelvic pain
  diffuse, with nausea and vomiting, 321
  with hypotension, 297–299
  in infants, 334–335, 336*t*, 339–340
  left lower quadrant, 314–317
  lower, in young woman, 302–304, 373–376, 375*t*, 403
  right upper quadrant, 308–310
  with vaginal odor, 380–381
Abdominal trauma
  blunt
    clinical presentation, 11–13, 13*f*
    diagnostic evaluation, 12
    immediate actions, 12, 435, 471
    with chest trauma, 23
    hematuria in, 16
    laparotomy indications, 15–16
ABO incompatibility, 417, 454
Abortion
  classification, 362
  spontaneous, 362–363, 404, 443
Acetaminophen overdose/poisoning, 129*t*, 427, 462–463
Acid-base disorders, 200, 419, 456
Acquired immunodeficiency syndrome (AIDS). *See* Human immunodeficiency virus (HIV) infection
Activated charcoal, 128, 131–132
Acute chest syndrome, 83
Acute mesenteric ischemia, 408–409, 446–447
Acute rheumatic fever, 253

Adenosine, 458
Airborne precautions, 270–271
Albuterol
  for asthma exacerbation, 220
  for bronchiolitis, 289, 450
Alcohol abuse
  adverse effects, 124*t*, 125, 312
  withdrawal syndrome
    clinical presentation, 121
    immediate actions, 121
    management, 122–124
    pathophysiology, 121–124
    seizures in, 146
Alcohol metabolism, 124
Alcohol poisoning, 129*t*, 426, 462
Alcoholic ketoacidosis, 419, 456
Aldosterone, 201
Altered mental status
  diagnostic evaluation, 88, 95
  etiologies, 89*t*
  with fever, 94–96
  with fever and seizure, 120–121
  with headache, 87–89, 90*f*, 92
  with hyperthermia, 107–109
  with toxic ingestion. *See* Toxic ingestion
Amaurosis fugax, 453
Amiodarone, 194
Anaphylaxis
  clinical presentation, 226, 229
  differential diagnosis, 229
  etiology, 228–229
  immediate actions, 226, 229
  management, 227, 418, 455
  pathophysiology, 226–227
  prevention of relapse, 229
  respiratory compromise in, 229
Aneurysm
  abdominal aortic. *See* Abdominal aortic aneurysm
  berry, 89, 90*f*
Angiography, CT, 37
Angulation, fracture, 60, 60*t*
Ankle dislocation, 68–69
Anterior cord syndrome, 472
Anthrax, 136, 138
Antiarrhythmics, 194

Antibiotics
  for aerobic organisms, 319
  for anaerobic organisms, 319
  for anthrax, 138–139
  for ascending cholangitis, 447
  for bacterial tracheitis, 288
  for chlamydial cervicitis, 384
  for colonic pathogens, 319
  for epididymitis, 360
  for epiglottitis, 288
  for impetigo contagiosa, 267
  for Lyme disease, 274
  for meningitis, 95–96
  for necrotizing fasciitis, 264–265
  for pelvic inflammatory disease, 382
  for perirectal abscesses, 349
  for peritonsillar cellulitis, 288
  for pharyngitis, 288
  for plague, 140
  for pneumonia, 217
  prophylactic
    for meningococcal meningitis, 96,
      431, 466
    for wounds, 55, 57
  for *S. aureus*, 75
  for sepsis, 105
  for STI prophylaxis, 371
Anticholinergics
  for asthma exacerbation, 220
  overdose/poisoning, 128t, 129t, 131
Anticoagulation
  for deep venous thrombosis, 430, 466
  for pulmonary embolism, 209–210, 212
  in stroke, 446
Antidotes, 129t
Antivirals
  for herpes zoster, 271
  for HIV prophylaxis, 371
Aortic aneurysm. *See* Abdominal aortic
  aneurysm
Aortic dissection
  classification, 180
  clinical presentation, 424, 459–460
  complications, 179–180
  diagnostic evaluation, 177, 178f, 180
  immediate actions, 177
  management, 177–178, 180
  risk factors, 424, 459
Aortic stenosis, 186–187, 457
Aortic thrombus, 261–262
Aortogram, 180
Aplastic crisis, in sickle-cell disease,
  79, 82
Appendicitis
  clinical presentation, 302, 307,
    336t, 375t
  diagnostic evaluation, 304, 304f, 375t

differential diagnosis, 303–304, 336t
  fever in, 307
  perforation in, 307
  in retrocecal appendix, 306
Arterial occlusion, 261–262
Arthritis, septic. *See* Septic arthritis
Ascending cholangitis, 312, 410, 447
Aspiration, foreign body, 290–294,
    432, 467
Asthma
  acute exacerbation
    chest radiograph in, 223
    clinical presentation, 219
    differential diagnosis, 223
    immediate actions, 220, 428, 463–464
    indications for hospital admission, 224
    management, 220–222, 224, 455–456
    pathophysiology, 223
  cough-variant, 424, 459
  preventive measures, 221
  risk factors for poor outcome, 221, 221t,
    223–224
Atrial fibrillation, 194–195
Atropine
  indications, 201
  mechanisms of action, 201
  for nerve gas exposure, 135–136
  for organophosphate poisoning, 464
AV nodal re-entrant tachycardia, 458.
    See also Tachycardia
Axillary temperature, 280

Bacillus anthracis, 138
Bacteremia. *See also* Sepsis
  in infants, 277–278, 278t, 281
Barium enema, in intussusception, 337f
Beck's triad, 403, 441
Benign positional vertigo, 156–157
Benzodiazepines
  for alcohol withdrawal syndrome, 122
  overdose/poisoning, 129t
  for seizures, 142
  for vertigo, 159
Berry aneurysm, 89, 90f
β-adrenergic agonists, 220
β-blockers
  in aortic dissection, 177
  in atrial fibrillation, 194–195
  overdose/poisoning, 129t
  topical, 234
β-human chorionic gonadotrophin
    (βhCG)
  in ectopic pregnancy, 363, 366, 442
  in pregnancy evaluation, 363, 363t, 365
Biliary disease. *See also* Cholecystitis
  ascending cholangitis, 312, 410, 447
  risk factors, 312

Biological weapons
  anthrax, 138
  mustard gas, 139
  nerve gas, 134–136
  plague, 139–140
  smallpox, 139
Bites, dog. *See* Dog bites
Blunt trauma
  abdominal. *See* Abdominal trauma, blunt
  with pelvic pain. *See* Pelvic fracture
Body surface area, 50, 51*f*
Boerhaave's syndrome, 345
Bowel obstruction
  clinical presentation, 321–322
  diagnostic evaluation, 315, 316*f*, 322–323, 324*f*, 425, 461
  etiology, 325–326
  functional vs. mechanical, 322
  incidence, 325
  management, 323
  mortality rate, 325
Bronchiolitis, 289, 413–414, 450–451
Brown-Séquard syndrome, 472
Brudzinski's sign, 99
Bubonic plague, 140
Bulimia, 345
Burn injuries
  body surface area estimate, 50, 51*f*
  chemical, 48
  classification, 47–48
  clinical presentation, 46–48
  criteria for burn unit admission, 50–51
  fluid resuscitation, 436, 471
  hot tar, 434, 469
  immediate actions, 47
  inhalation injury in, 47, 50, 428, 463
  minor, management, 435, 470
  prerenal azotemia in, 422, 458
Buttock pain, 347

Calcium channel blockers
  for atrial fibrillation, 195
  overdose/poisoning, 129*t*
Calcium oxalate stones, 397
Carbon monoxide poisoning, 47, 463
Cardiac bypass, for core rewarming, 118
Cardiac output, 206
Cardiac tamponade, 403, 441
Cardioversion, 194–195
Carotid artery dissection, 455
Casts, leg, 433, 469
Cauda equina syndrome
  clinical presentation, 257–259, 261, 452, 472
  management, 259
Cellulitis, in puncture wounds, 56

Central cord syndrome, 436, 471–472
Central retinal artery occlusion, 234, 237*f*, 239, 416, 453
Central retinal vein occlusion, 237*f*, 239
Cephalosporins, 371
Cerebellar hemorrhage, 418, 455
Cerebrospinal fluid analysis
  in herpes encephalitis, 98
  in meningitis, 97*t*, 99
Cervicitis, chlamydial, 384
Charcot's triad, 312, 447
Chemical burns
  eye, 245
  skin, 48
Chest
  pain. *See* Chest pain
  penetrating trauma
    abdominal injuries in, 23
    cardiac tamponade in, 403, 441
    clinical presentation, 17, 19, 19*f*
    diagnostic evaluation, 18–19
    immediate actions, 18
    management, 18–19, 403, 441
    wound inspection in, 22–23
  radiograph. *See* Chest radiograph
Chest pain. *See also* Aortic dissection; Myocardial infarction
  crushing, 169–170
  differential diagnosis, 171, 177, 180–181
  with dyspnea, 208–209
  exercise stress test after, 174
  with fever, 213–215, 215*f*
  immediate actions, 170, 170*f*, 174, 177, 180
  radiating to back, 176–177
  with syncope, 186
Chest radiograph
  in asthma exacerbation, 223
  in congestive heart failure, 223
  in croup, 285*f*
  in epiglottitis, 286*f*
  in penetrating chest trauma, 19, 19*f*
  in pneumonia, 215*f*
  in pulmonary edema, 204*f*
  in pulmonary embolism, 211–212
  in suspected hemothorax, 26
  in trauma evaluation, 26
Chest tube. *See* Tube thoracostomy
CHF. *See* Congestive heart failure
Chlamydia, 384
Choking, in child, 290–294
Cholangitis, ascending, 312, 410, 447
Cholecystitis
  clinical presentation, 308, 411, 448
  differential diagnosis, 309–310, 310*f*, 411, 440
  immediate actions, 309

Cholecystitis (*cont.*)
  management, 310
  risk factors, 312
Cholinergics, overdose/poisoning, 128*t*
Ciguatera fish poisoning, 415, 451–452
Cisplatin, 360
"Clenched-fist" injury, 57
Clostridium, 268
Coccidioides immitis, 218
Colles' fracture, 63. *See also* Radius
        fracture, distal
Coma cocktail, 128
Compartment syndrome
  anatomy, 41*f*
  clinical presentation, 40, 42, 44
  complications, 44
  diagnosis, 42, 42*t*, 469
  management, 434, 469
Complete abortion, 362, 443
Computed tomography (CT)
  in abdominal aortic aneurysm,
        300–301
  angiography, 37
  in appendicitis, 304*f*
  in blunt abdominal trauma, 12
  in diverticulitis, 320
  in epidural hematoma, 6*f*
  in intracranial hemorrhage, 5–6*f*, 8
  in penetrating chest trauma, 18
  in stroke, 149, 150*f*
  in subarachnoid hemorrhage, 5*f*, 90*f*
  in subdural hematoma, 5*f*
  vs. ultrasound in woman with low
        abdominal pain, 375–376
  in ureteral stones, 394
Conduction, 111
Congestive heart failure (CHF)
  acute exacerbation
    clinical presentation, 202–203
    diagnostic evaluation, 204, 204*f*
    etiology, 203
    immediate actions, 203
    management, 203–204, 206–207,
        420–421, 456–457
    pathophysiology, 206
  chronic, 207
  differential diagnosis, 223
  right-sided, 206
Conjunctivitis
  clinical presentation, 242
  differential diagnosis, 242–243
  management, 243
  neonatal, 245–246
Conscious sedation, 66
Contact lens wearers, conjunctivitis
        in, 243
Contact precautions, 270

Continuous positive airway pressure
        (CPAP), 207
Contraception, postcoital, 371
Contrast-mediated nephrotoxicity, 398
Convection, 111
Corneal abrasion, 242–243, 245
Coronary arteries, 172*t*
Coronary revascularization, 171
Corpus luteum cyst, ruptured, 375, 375*t*,
        378, 420, 456
Corticosteroids
  for asthma exacerbation, 220
  for croup, 283, 286
  stress-dose, in sepsis, 103, 105–106
Cosyntropin test, 106
Cough
  barking, in a child, 282–283. *See also*
        Croup
  intermittent nonproductive, 424, 459
Croup
  vs. aspirated foreign body, 294
  chest radiograph in, 285*f*
  clinical presentation, 282, 285, 289, 425
  vs. epiglottitis and bacterial tracheitis,
        284*t*
  management, 286–289, 425, 460
Crush injury, extremity
  anatomic considerations, 40, 41*f*
  clinical presentation, 39–40, 42–43
  compartment syndrome and, 40, 41*f*,
        42, 42*t*, 44
  complications, 40
  immediate actions, 39
  management, 42
Cryptococcus neoformans, 218
CT. *See* Computed tomography
Cullen's sign, 88
"Currant jelly stool," 334
Cyanide poisoning, 129*t*, 428, 463
Cystic teratoma, 378

DeBakey classification system, aortic
        dissection, 180
Deep venous thrombosis (DVT), 209,
        430, 466
Defibrillation, 198–200
Delirium tremens, 122
Depression, suicide risk in, 164
Dermoid cyst, 378
Dexamethasone
  for croup, 283, 286
  stress-dose, 103, 105–106
Diabetes
  hyperglycemia in. *See* Diabetic
        ketoacidosis
  hypoglycemic episode in,
        144, 146

Diabetic ketoacidosis
  clinical presentation, 327
  complications, 332
  diagnostic triad, 328–329
  immediate actions, 328
  management, 329–330, 332
  pathophysiology, 328, 331
  precipitants, 331–332
Diagnostic peritoneal lavage
  in blunt abdominal trauma, 12
  in hemoperitoneum, 16
  in penetrating chest trauma, 19, 23
Diarrhea, infectious, 319
Diazepam, for nerve gas exposure,
    135–136
Digoxin
  for atrial fibrillation, 195
  overdose/poisoning, 129t
Diphenhydramine
  for anaphylaxis, 226–227
  for dystonic reaction, 417, 454
  as local anesthetic, 405, 443
Diphtheria, 451
Disc herniation, 416, 452
Dislocation
  ankle, 68–69
  elbow, 68
  hip, 69
  knee, 69
  shoulder. *See* Shoulder dislocation
Displacement, fracture, 60, 60t
Diverticulitis
  clinical presentation, 314, 320
  complications, 316–317, 317f
  diagnostic evaluation, 315
  differential diagnosis, 315
  incidence, 320
  management, 316–318
  risk factors, 320
Diverticulosis, 320
Dix-Hallpike maneuver, 157
Dizziness. *See also* Vertigo
  clinical presentation, 155–156
  definition, 156
  diagnostic evaluation, 157
Dog bites
  clinical presentation, 53–55
  immediate actions, 54
  management, 54–55
Dopamine, 106
Droplet precautions, 270, 274
Duodenal ulcer, 426, 461
DVT (deep venous thrombosis), 209
Dysfunctional uterine bleeding,
    387–388, 401–402, 440
Dysmenorrhea, 382
Dyspnea

  with chest pain, 208–209
  in a child, 290
  with fatigue, 202–203
  with wheezing, 219–221
Dysrhythmias, syncope in, 187
Dystonic reaction, 417, 454

Early goal-directed therapy (EGDT), for
    sepsis, 102, 105
Ectopic pregnancy
  βhCG levels in, 303, 363
  clinical presentation, 375t,
    403–404, 441
  diagnostic evaluation, 404, 442
  management, 366, 441
  ruptured, 366
Eikenella, 57
Elbow
  dislocation, 68
  radial head subluxation, 69
Electrocardiogram (EKG)
  in hypercalcemia, 412, 449
  in hyperkalemia, 201
  in hypothermia, 116f, 118
  in myocardial infarction, 170f
  in pulmonary embolism, 211
Electrocautery, 249, 251
Encephalitis
  herpes simplex virus, 96, 98
  mosquito-borne, 271
Endocarditis
  bacteria causing, 261
  in intravenous drug abusers,
    258, 261
Endoscopy, in gastrointestinal bleeding,
    345
Epi-Pen, 229
Epididymitis
  clinical presentation, 355
  differential diagnosis, 356
  etiology, 359
  incidence, 359
  management, 357, 359–360
Epidural abscess, spinal, 258
Epidural hematoma, 6f, 9, 15
Epiglottitis
  antibiotics for, 288
  vs. aspirated foreign body, 294
  chest radiograph in, 286f
  clinical presentation, 284t, 452
  vs. croup and bacterial tracheitis, 284t
  etiology, 255–256
  management, 284t, 288
Epinephrine
  for anaphylaxis, 226–227, 229, 418, 455
  for croup, 283, 286, 460
  nebulized racemic, 429, 464

Epiploic appendagitis, 427, 462
Epistaxis. *See* Nosebleed
Epstein-Barr virus (EBV), 253
Erythema migrans, 273–274
Esophagus
  bleeding, 345
  foreign bodies in, 294
Estrogen, for dysfunctional uterine
    bleeding, 440
Ethylene glycol poisoning, 129*t*,
    426, 462
Evaporation, 111
Exercise stress test, after chest pain
    episode, 174
Extremity weakness, acute, 262
Eye injuries
  chemical burns, 245
  corneal abrasion, 242–243, 245
  foreign body, 245
  UV keratitis, 430, 465

Fall, on outstretched hand, 58–59.
    See also Fracture
FAST exam
  in blunt abdominal trauma, 12, 13*f*
  in suspected hemoperitoneum, 26
Fat emboli syndrome, 29–30
Febrile seizures, 147
Femoral neck, 62–63
Fever
  in infant, 276–278, 278*t*, 413, 450
  in intravenous drug user, 257
  measurement, 280
  with painful head and neck rash,
    269–270
  with sore throat, 252–253. *See also*
    Pharyngitis
Firearms, suicide risk and, 164
Fitz-Hugh-Curtis syndrome, 378, 384
Flank pain
  clinical presentation, 393
  differential diagnosis, 394–395
Flecainide, 194
Flexor tenosynovitis, 56–57
Fluid resuscitation, 436, 471
Fontanelles, in infant with meningitis,
    280
Food allergy, 228
Food-borne disease, 414–415, 451–452
Foreign body
  aspiration, 290–294, 432, 467
  in eye, 245
  in nose, 429, 464–465
  swallowed, 294
Fournier's gangrene, 267
Fracture

definition, 69
fat emboli syndrome and, 29–30
hip. *See* Hip, fracture
humerus, 45
pelvic. *See* Pelvic fracture
radius. *See* Radius fracture
Salter-Harris classification, 64
supracondylar. *See* Supracondylar
    fracture
terminology, 60*t*
Frank-Starling curve, 206
Frostbite, 118–119, 430, 465–466

GABHS. *See* Group A β-hemolytic
    Streptococcus
Gangrene
  Fournier's, 267
  gas, 268
Gas gangrene, 268
Gastrointestinal bleeding
  clinical presentation, 341, 345
  differential diagnosis, 342, 344
  immediate actions, 342
  management, 342–343, 345
Germ cell tumors, 378
Glaucoma
  acute angle-closure, 234, 239, 242,
    417, 453
  primary open-angle, 239
  risk factors, 242
Glucagon, in diabetic ketoacidosis, 329
Glyburide, 146
Gonorrhea, disseminated, 74,
    432, 467
Gout, 434, 469–470
Group A β-hemolytic *Streptococcus*
    (GABHS)
  in impetigo contagiosa, 267
  in necrotizing fasciitis, 265
  in pharyngitis, 253, 451
Group B *Streptococcus*, in meningitis, 96
Gunshot wound
  chest. *See* Chest, penetrating trauma
  neck, 38. *See also* Neck, penetrating
    trauma

Haemophilus influenzae B (HIB), 255
Hampton's hump, 212
HAPE (high-altitude pulmonary edema),
    411, 448
Head trauma
  clinical presentation, 3–4, 9
  diagnostic evaluation, 8–9
  immediate actions, 4, 401, 440
  increased intracranial
    pressure in, 6

intracranial hemorrhage in, 4, 5–6*f*
management, 6–7, 401, 440
Headache, with confusion, 87–90,
90*f*, 92
Hearing loss, sensorineural, 158–159
Heart block, 174, 423, 459
Heart failure. *See* Congestive heart
failure
Heat exhaustion, 108
Heat stroke, 108, 110–111
Helicobacter pylori, 426, 453
Hematemesis, 341–343
Hematoma
epidural, 6*f*, 8–9
intracerebral, 8
subdural, 5*f*, 8–9
Hematuria
in abdominal trauma, 16
painful, 397
painless, 397
Heme-positive stool, 344
Hemolytic crisis, in sickle-cell disease, 78
Hemoperitoneum, 16, 26
Hemorrhoids, 433, 468–469
Hemothorax, 26
Heparin, 209. *See also* Anticoagulation
Hepatic iminodiacetic acid (HIDA)
scan, 448
Hepatitis
alcoholic, 312
prophylaxis, 57, 372
Herpes simplex virus
corneal infections, 243
encephalitis, 96, 98
in neonatal conjunctivitis, 246
Herpes zoster
clinical presentation, 269–271
eye involvement, 243, 246, 272, 274
management, 271–272
HHNC (hyperglycemic hyperosmolar
nonketotic coma), 417, 453
High-altitude pulmonary edema
(HAPE), 411, 448
Hill-Sachs deformity, 69
Hip
dislocation, 69, 406, 444
fracture
clinical presentation, 62–63
femoral neck. *See* Femoral neck
fracture
intertrochanteric, 63
limp in a child, 425, 460
Histoplasma capsulatum, 218
Horner's syndrome, 152–153
Human immunodeficiency virus (HIV)
infection

C. neoformans in, 218
P. carinii pneumonia in, 217, 419, 455
prophylaxis after high-risk
exposure, 371
Hutchinson sign, 246, 274
Hymenoptera sting, 225, 228
Hyperaldosteronism, 201
Hypercalcemia, 412, 449
Hyperglycemia. *See* Diabetic
ketoacidosis
Hyperglycemic hyperosmolar nonketotic
coma (HHNC), 417, 453
Hyperkalemia
clinical presentation, 196
EKG findings, 201
etiology, 196, 201
management, 196–197
Hypernatremia, 413, 450
Hypersensitivity reactions. *See*
Anaphylaxis
Hypertension, 424, 459
Hyperthermia
clinical presentation, 107, 111
differential diagnosis, 108
immediate actions, 108
management, 109–111
risk factors, 111
Hyperthyroidism, 421, 457
Hypoglycemia
altered mental status in, 88
seizures in, 142, 144, 146
Hypokalemia
clinical presentation, 201
in diabetic ketoacidosis, 329, 332
Hyponatremia, 450
Hypotension
in blunt trauma, 26
categories, 114, 115*t*
in heat stroke, 111
in sepsis, 105–106
Hypothermia
clinical presentation, 113
immediate actions, 114, 429, 465
management, 115, 116*f*, 118, 465
stages, 114, 117–118
Hypoxia, 88

Ibutilide, 194
Impetigo contagiosa, 267
Incomplete abortion, 362, 443
Inevitable abortion, 362, 443
Inhalation injury, 428, 463
Insect-borne diseases, 271. *See also*
specific diseases
Insecticide poisoning.
See Organophosphate poisoning

Insulin, in diabetic ketoacidosis, 329, 332
Intersphincteric abscess, 349f, 351
Intertrochanteric fracture, 63
Intracerebral hematoma, 8
Intracranial pressure, increased, 6, 402, 441
Intravenous drug abusers
    endocarditis in, 261
    fever in, 257–258
Intravenous pyelogram, 397
Intussusception
    clinical presentation, 333, 336t, 407, 445
    diagnostic evaluation, 337, 337f
    differential diagnosis, 334–335, 336t
    lead point, 339
    management, 336t, 337
Iodine, 421, 457
Ipecac, 132
Iron overdose/poisoning, 129t
Ischiorectal abscess, 349f, 351–352
Isolation precautions, 270–271

Joint fluid analysis, in septic arthritis, 72

Keratitis, ultraviolet, 430, 465
Kerley B lines, 223
Kernig's sign, 99
Ketoacidosis
    alcoholic, 419, 448
    diabetic. See Diabetic ketoacidosis
Kiesselbach's plexus, 251
Knee
    dislocation, 69
    pain, in a child, 425, 460
    pain with fever, 71–73
Korsakoff's psychosis, 125

Labetalol, in aortic dissection, 177
Labyrinthitis, 158
Lacunar stroke, 153
Laparotomy, in abdominal trauma, 12, 15–16
Large bowel obstruction, 323, 326, 425, 461. See also Bowel obstruction
Lead poisoning, 129t
Legg-Calvé-Perthes disease, 460
Legionella, 217–218, 419, 456
Levofloxacin
    contraindications, 407, 445
    for sepsis, 105
Lidocaine, 194
Limp, in a child, 425, 460
Lisfranc injury, 69
Listeria monocytogenes, 96, 467

Lithium overdose/poisoning, 132
Local anesthetics, 405, 443
Low back pain
    diagnostic evaluation, 261, 452
    differential diagnosis, 452–453
    management, 261
Ludwig's angina, 437, 470, 472
Lumbar disc herniation, 416, 452
Lumbar puncture
    in meningitis, 97t
    in severe headache, 92
    in subarachnoid hemorrhage, 92
Lyme disease, 271, 273–274

Malingering, 453
Mallory-Weiss syndrome, 345
Marfan's syndrome, 424, 459
Matrix stones, 397
McBurney's point, 304, 306
Meckel's diverticulum, 339
Median nerve injury, 63
Meningitis
    aseptic, 274–275
    bacterial vs. viral, 97t
    cerebrospinal fluid analysis, 97t, 99, 275
    clinical examination, 99
    clinical presentation, 94–96
    complications, 98
    differential diagnosis, 95–96
    immediate actions, 95, 431, 467
    in infant, 280
    prophylaxis, 96, 431, 466
Menometrorrhagia, 387, 401, 440
Menopause, 391
Menorrhagia
    clinical presentation, 386–387
    diagnostic evaluation, 389, 389f
    management, 392
Menstrual cycle, 387–388, 388f
Mesenteric adenitis, 432, 468
Mesenteric ischemia, 408, 447
Metabolic acidosis
    in alcoholic ketoacidosis, 419, 456
    in diabetic ketoacidosis.
        See Diabetic ketoacidosis
    etiology, 200
Methanol poisoning, 129t, 426, 462
Methotrexate, for ectopic pregnancy, 366, 442
Methylprednisolone, for anaphylaxis, 226–227
Metoprolol, for atrial fibrillation, 195
Metronidazole, for sepsis, 105
Metrorrhagia, 387
Midgut volvulus, 336t, 339–340, 406, 444–445

Miscarriage. *See* Spontaneous abortion
Missed abortion, 362
Mittelschmerz, 456
Mononucleosis, 253, 451
Morison's pouch, 12, 13*f*
Mosquito-borne diseases, 271
Multiple sclerosis, optic neuritis in, 235
Murphy's sign, 306, 310
Muscarinic receptor blockade, 131
Mustard gas, 139
Mycoplasma pneumoniae, 83
Mydriasis, 131
Myocardial infarction
  altered mental status in, 88
  clinical presentation, 169–170
  complications, 174–175
  diagnostic evaluation, 174, 420, 449
  differential diagnosis, 171
  immediate actions, 170, 170*f*
  management, 171–174, 409, 447
  thrombolytic therapy in, 171, 409, 448
Myonecrosis, clostridial, 268

N-acetylcysteine, 463
Nasal pack
  complications, 250–251
  for nosebleed, 249, 251
Neck
  anatomical zones of, 34, 37–38
  penetrating trauma
    clinical presentation, 32–33, 35
    diagnostic evaluation, 37
    immediate actions, 33
    management, 33, 37–38
    signs of significant injury, 35*t*,
      37–38
Necrotizing enterocolitis, 336*t*, 340
Necrotizing fasciitis
  clinical presentation, 263
  differential diagnosis, 264–265
  immediate actions, 264
  management, 265
Needle-stick exposure, hepatitis risk
    after, 57
Neisseria gonorrhoeae
  disseminated infection, 74, 432, 467
  in neonatal conjunctivitis, 246
  in septic arthritis, 74–75
Neisseria meningitidis, 96
Nephrolithiasis, 397–398
Nephrotoxicity, contrast-mediated, 398
Nerve gas, 134–136
Nimodipine, in subarachnoid
    hemorrhage, 92
Nitroglycerin, 409, 421, 439, 447, 457
Nitroprusside, in aortic dissection, 177

Norepinephrine, for hypotension in
    sepsis, 106
Nosebleed
  clinical presentation, 247
  etiology, 248, 251
  immediate actions, 248
  management, 248–249
"Nursemaid's elbow," 69

Obturator sign, 306
Octreotide, for gastrointestinal
    bleeding, 343
Ogilvie's syndrome, 326
Opioids, overdose/poisoning, 128–129*t*
Optic neuritis
  clinical presentation, 233
  differential diagnosis, 234–235
  immediate actions, 234
  management, 235
Organophosphate poisoning
  antidotes, 129*t*
  clinical presentation, 133, 464
  immediate actions, 135
  management, 135–136, 464
  pathophysiology, 429, 464
Osborne J waves, 116*f*, 118
Osteomyelitis, puncture wounds and, 56
Otitis media, 281
Ovarian cysts, 381–382
Ovarian torsion
  clinical presentation, 303, 373, 375*t*
  diagnostic evaluation, 375–376, 376*f*,
    402, 441
  management, 378, 433

Pancreatitis, 312
Parainfluenza virus, 284*t*, 289. *See
    also* Croup
Paralysis, left-sided, 148–149
Parapharyngeal abscess, 470–471
Parkland formula, 471
Pasteurella, 57
Pelvic fracture
  associated injuries, 27, 31
  clinical presentation, 25–26, 28–29, 28*f*
  hemorrhage in, 26–27
  immediate actions, 26
  management, 27
  stabilization, 27, 31
  urologic injury in, 30–31
Pelvic inflammatory disease (PID)
  clinical presentation, 375*t*, 382
  diagnostic evaluation, 382
  management, 382
  risk factors, 385
  sequelae, 384

Pelvic pain
  acute vs. chronic, 381
  etiologies, 381–382
  with vaginal odor, 380–381
  with vaginal spotting in pregnancy,
    361–362
Penetrating trauma
  chest. *See* Chest, penetrating trauma
  neck. *See* Neck, penetrating trauma
Penicillin
  anaphylactic reaction to, 228
  in "clenched-fist" injury, 57
  cross-reactivity with cephalosporins,
    371
Perianal abscess, 348, 349*f*, 352
Peritonsillar abscess, 435, 470
Perirectal abscess, 348–349, 349*f*, 351–352
Peritonsillar cellulitis, 288
Peroneal nerve, 433, 469
Peyer's patches, 339
Pharyngitis
  in children, 255
  clinical presentation, 252
  complications, 253, 255
  differential diagnosis, 253, 415, 451
  etiology, 253
  immediate actions, 253
  management, 254
Phenobarbital, 142, 147
Phenytoin, 142, 147
Pilonidal cyst
  clinical presentation, 348
  differential diagnosis, 348
  immediate actions, 348
  management, 349–350, 352
Pneumocystis carinii pneumonia (PCP),
  217, 419, 447
Pneumomediastinum, 416, 452
Pneumonia
  atypical, 217, 419, 456
  clinical presentation, 213
  diagnostic evaluation, 215, 215*f*
  differential diagnosis, 214
  in elderly patients, 214, 218
  etiology, 217–218
  immediate actions, 214
  Legionella, 217–218, 419, 448
  management, 215, 217
  P. carinii, 217, 419, 455
  pneumococcal, 218
  risk factors, 217
Pneumonic plague, 139–140
Pneumothorax, 441
Poisoning. *See* Toxic ingestion
Polycystic kidney disease, subarachnoid
  hemorrhage and, 93
Popliteal artery injury, 69

Potassium, in diabetic ketoacidosis,
  329, 332
Potassium iodide, 421, 457
Pralidoxime chloride (2-PAM), 129*t*,
  135–136
Pregnancy
  first-trimester bleeding, 404, 442
  Lyme disease in, 274
  ultrasound findings, 363*t*, 365*f*
  vaginal spotting and pelvic pain in,
    361–362
Prerenal azotemia, 422, 458
Priapism, in sickle-cell disease, 82–83
Procainamide, 194
Propafenone, 194
Prostatitis, 405, 443–444
Pseudomonas, 57, 243
Psoas sign, 99, 306
Pulmonary arteriogram, 209
Pulmonary edema. *See also* Congestive
    heart failure
  acute, 202–203
  high-altitude, 411, 448
Pulmonary embolism
  clinical presentation, 208
  diagnostic evaluation, 209–210
  differential diagnosis, 209
  EKG findings, 211
  immediate actions, 209
  management, 209–210
  with right heart strain, 212
  risk factors, 214
Puncture wounds, 56
Pyloric stenosis, 336*t*, 339

QT prolongation, 407, 445
Quinsy, 435, 470

Rabies, 418, 454
Radial head subluxation, 69
Radial nerve injury, 45
Radius fracture, distal
  associated injuries, 63
  clinical presentation, 58–59, 59*f*
  management, 61
Ranitidine
  for anaphylaxis, 226–227
  for gastrointestinal bleeding, 343
Ranson's criteria, 312
Rapid sequence intubation (RSI), 92
Rash
  dermatomal distribution, 271
  in Lyme disease, 271, 273–274
  painful head and neck, with fever,
    269–270
  in Rocky Mountain spotted fever, 271
  in toxic shock syndrome, 268

Rectal bleeding
  in elderly patient, 344
  in infant, 333–334
Rectal temperature, 280
Red eye, 241
Red skin. *See also* Rash
  rapidly spreading, 263–264
  in toxic shock syndrome, 268
Reduction, 66–67
Respiratory acidosis, 20
Respiratory alkalosis, 224
Respiratory syncytial virus (RSV),
  289, 451
Retropharyngeal abscess, 452
Rewarming, 118–119
Reynold's pentad, 447
Rh incompatibility, 417, 454
Rhabdomyolysis, 44
RhoGAM, 364
Rinne test, 158
Rocky Mountain spotted fever, 271
Romberg test, 418, 455
Rovsing's sign, 99, 306
Rule of 9s, 50, 51*f*

SAD PERSONS mnemonic, 161–162, 461
"Saddle anesthesia," 259
Salicylates, overdose/poisoning, 129*t*
Salter-Harris classification, 64
Sarin gas, 134–136
Sciatica, 261, 472
Scombroid fish poisoning, 414, 443
Scrotal pain, 355
Seizures
  alcohol-related, 146
  differential diagnosis, 142–143, 143*t*
  in electrolyte abnormalities, 413, 449
  febrile, 147
  immediate actions, 142, 147
  management, 142, 144, 147
  in overdose/poisoning, 131
  shaking, 141–142
  shoulder dislocation in, 405, 444
Seminomas, 360
Sensorineural hearing loss, 158–159
Sepsis. *See also* Bacteremia
  clinical presentation, 100–101, 103–104
  early goal-directed therapy,
    102–103, 105
  immediate actions, 101, 105
  management, 102–103
  pathophysiology, 101–102
  stress-dose steroids for, 103, 105–106
  vasopressors for, 106
Septal perforation, 251
Septic arthritis
  clinical presentation, 71–73

  differential diagnosis, 72, 433, 468
  immediate actions, 72
  joint fluid analysis in, 72
  N. gonorrhoeae, 74–75, 467
  risk factors, 74–75
  treatment, 75
Sequestration crisis, in sickle-cell
  disease, 78–79
Sexual assault
  clinical presentation, 367–368
  immediate actions, 368
  management, 368–369
Sexually transmitted infections
  antibiotic prophylaxis, 371
  N. gonorrhoeae, 74–75
Shingles. *See* Herpes zoster
Shoulder dislocation
  clinical presentation, 65–66
  complications, 69
  diagnostic evaluation, 66, 67*f*
  management, 66–67
  mechanisms, 68
  recurrent, 69
  in seizure, 405, 444
Sickle-cell disease
  acute chest syndrome in, 83
  aplastic crisis, 79, 82
  hemolytic crisis, 78
  hip and sternum pain in, 77–80, 80*f*
  priapism in, 82–83
  sequelae, 79
  sequestration crisis, 78–79
  vaso-occlusive crisis, 78
Sickle-cell trait, 82
Silver nitrate
  eye drops, in neonate, 245
  for nosebleed, 249, 251
Sinus tachycardia, 190, 211
Sinusitis, after nasal packing, 251
Skin infections
  Fournier's gangrene, 267
  impetigo contagiosa, 267
  rapidly spreading, 263. *See also*
    Necrotizing fasciitis
Slipped capital femoral epiphysis,
  425, 460
Small bowel obstruction. *See* Bowel
  obstruction
Smallpox, 139
Smoke inhalation, 50
Sodium polystyrene sulfonate, 199
Soft-tissue infection
  Fournier's gangrene, 267
  rapidly spreading. *See* Necrotizing
    fasciitis
Sore throat. *See also* Epiglottitis;
  Pharyngitis

Sore throat (*cont.*)
  with fever, 252–253
  with normal-appearing pharynx,
    416, 452
Sotalol, 194
Spinal cord lesions, 436, 471
Spinal epidural abscess, 258
Spinal epidural hematoma, 452
Spinal stenosis, 452
Spontaneous abortion, 362–363,
    404, 443
Sprain, 69
Stanford classification system, aortic
    dissection, 180
Staphylococcus aureus
  antibiotic coverage, 75
  in endocarditis, 261
  in toxic shock syndrome, 268
Status epilepticus, 142, 147
"Steeple sign," 285*f*
Stool, heme-positive, 344
Strain, 69
Streptococcus pneumoniae
  in infants, 281
  in meningitis, 96, 467
Streptococcus viridans, 261
Stridor, in young child
  clinical presentation, 282
  etiology, 283, 284*t*
Stroke
  clinical presentation, 148–149
  diagnostic evaluation, 149, 150*f*
  etiologies, 153
  immediate actions, 149
  ischemic, 150, 153
  management, 151, 407, 445–446
  thrombolysis in, 150, 408, 446
  vertebrobasilar, 153
Struvite stones, 397
Subarachnoid hemorrhage
  clinical presentation, 87–89
  diagnostic evaluation, 5*f*, 8, 90*f*
  immediate actions, 88
  lumbar puncture in, 92
  nimodipine for, 91–92
  risk factors, 93
Subconjunctival hemorrhage, 431, 466
Subdural hematoma, 5*f*, 8–9
Subluxation, 69
Substance abuse. *See* Alcohol abuse;
    Intravenous drug abusers
Suicide attempt
  clinical presentation, 160–161
  risk factors, 161–162, 164, 426, 461
Superior mesenteric artery occlusion,
    408, 446–447
Supracondylar fracture

clinical presentation, 44
complications, 45
management, 45, 63–64
Supralevator abscess, 349*f*
Supraventricular tachycardia (SVT),
    190, 458. *See also* Tachycardia
Sympathomimetics,
    overdose/poisoning, 128*t*, 131
Syncope
  cardiac, 187
  with chest pain, 186
  clinical presentation, 182–183
  diagnostic evaluation, 183–184
  etiology, 183
  immediate actions, 183
  medication-related, 186
  vasovagal, 186–187, 229

Tachycardia
  classification, 190
  narrow-complex
    clinical presentation, 188, 189*f*,
      423, 423*f*
    etiology, 190
    immediate actions, 190
    management, 190–191, 192*f*,
      423, 458
  wide-complex
    clinical presentation, 196, 197*f*,
      422, 422*f*
    etiology, 198
    immediate actions, 198
    management, 422, 458
Tar removal, 434, 469
Temporal arteritis, 235, 238
Tension pneumothorax, 441
Terrorism. *See* Biological weapons
Testicular torsion, 356, 359
Testicular tumors, 360
Tetanus immunization, 55, 404,
    442–443
Thermometers, 280
Thiamine (vitamin B$_1$) deficiency, 125
Thoracotomy, 18, 22
Threatened abortion
  clinical presentation, 361
  definition, 362, 443
  management, 364, 365–366
Thrombolysis
  contraindications, 150, 173, 408, 428,
    446, 463
  in myocardial infarction, 171, 410, 448
  in pulmonary embolism with right
    heart strain, 212
  in stroke, 150, 445
Thyroid storm, 421, 457
Tick-borne diseases, 271

Toxic ingestion. *See also* Toxidromes
  acetaminophen, 427, 462–463
  antidotes to specific toxins, 129*t*
  clinical presentation, 126–127, 128*t*
  ethylene glycol, 462
  immediate actions, 127, 132
  management, 128–129, 129*t*, 132, 462
  methanol, 462
  seizures in, 143, 143*t*
Toxic inhalation
  anthrax, 138
  carbon monoxide, 63, 463
  mustard gas, 139
  nerve gas, 134–136
  organophosphates. *See*
    Organophosphate poisoning
Toxic shock syndrome, 250–251,
    268, 384
Toxidromes. *See also* Toxic ingestion
  Anticholinergic, 127, 128*t*
  Cholinergic, 127, 128*t*
  Opioid/sedative, 127, 128*t*
  Sympathomimetic, 127, 128*t*
Tracheitis, bacterial
  antibiotics for, 288
  vs. croup and epiglottitis, 284*f*
Transfusion reactions, 417, 454
Transient ischemic attacks (TIAs), 154
Transient synovitis, 460
Trauma
  abdominal. *See* Abdominal trauma
  chest. *See* Chest, penetrating trauma
  crush injury. *See* Crush injury,
    extremity
  head. *See* Head trauma
  initial management, 435, 437, 471, 472
Tricyclic antidepressants,
    overdose/poisoning, 129*t*, 131, 143
Troponins, in myocardial infarction, 174
Tube thoracostomy, 23
Tubo-ovarian abscess
  clinical presentation, 375*t*, 382
  diagnostic evaluation, 375*t*
  management, 378, 384
Tympanic membrane temperature, 280

Ulnar nerve compression, 45
Ultrasonography
  in abdominal aortic aneurysm, 300
  in blunt abdominal trauma, 12, 13*f*
  in cholecystitis, 310*f*
  vs. CT in woman with low abdominal
    pain, 375–376
  in hemoperitoneum, 16
  in ovarian cyst, 376*f*
  in pregnancy, 363*t*, 365*f*
  in uterine fibroids, 389*f*

Ultraviolet keratitis, 430, 465
Universal precautions, 270
Ureteral calculus
  clinical presentation, 393, 406
  diagnostic evaluation, 444
  differential diagnosis, 394–395
  management, 395
Uric acid stones, 397
Urinary tract infection, in infant, 277
Uterine fibroids
  clinical presentation, 387–388,
    389*f*, 456
  diagnostic evaluation, 389,
    389*f*, 456
  management, 389, 391–392

V/Q scan, in pulmonary embolism,
    209, 212
Vaginal discharge, 382
Vaginal odor, 380–381
Vaginal packing, 440
Valgus, 60
Vancomycin, for sepsis, 105
Variola virus, 139
Varus, 60
Vaso-occlusive crisis, in sickle-cell
    disease, 78
Vasopressors, for hypotension in
    sepsis, 106
Vasovagal syncope, 186–187, 229
Ventricular arrhythmias, 174, 200–201,
    422, 458. *See also* Tachycardia
Vertebral artery dissection, 455
Vertebrobasilar stroke, 153
Vertigo
  causes, 156, 158, 455
  characteristics, 156
  clinical presentation, 155
  diagnostic evaluation, 157
  drug-induced, 159
  management, 159
Vision loss, acute, 233–239
Vitamin B$_1$ (thiamine) deficiency, 125
Vomiting
  blood, 341–343
  with episodic irritability in an infant,
    333
  with weakness, 327
Von Willebrand's disease, 300

Warfarin, 209. *See also* Anticoagulation
Waterhouse-Friderichsen syndrome, 98
Weakness
  with fever, 104–105
  with malaise, 100–101
Weber test, 158

Welder's keratitis, 430, 465
Wernicke-Korsakoff syndrome, 125
Wernicke's encephalopathy, 125
West Nile virus, 271
Westermark's sign, 212

Xanthochromia, 92

Yersinia pestis, 139–140
Yuzpe method, emergency
    contraception, 371

Zoster. *See* Herpes zoster